T0374350

"A valuable contribution that enhances the regional understanding of maternal and child health issues. The book will contribute towards evidence-based policy-making to improve MCH indicators."

—K.S. James, *Director, International Institute for Social Sciences, Mumbai*

"Improving national averages disguise the unacceptable inequities in social and economic progress that continue to plague India. This book makes an important contribution to identifying some of the disparities in maternal and child health between and within the Empowered Action Group (EAG) states, as well as making practical policy recommendations to improve the health situation of those most disadvantaged. Its findings should be taken seriously."

—Alaka M. Basu, *Former Professor, Department of Global Development, Cornell University*

Health and Nutrition of Women and Children in Empowered Action Group States of India

This book tracks the progress of maternal and child health (MCH)—part of SDG3—in empowered action group states in India. It lays bare regional disparities and unfolds a range of issues relating to inequalities in access to MCH services, complex dynamics behind poor nutrition, health expenditure and impoverishment, structural bottlenecks of health system that hinder effective implementation of programmes; best practices adopted for improving MNCH indicators and appropriate strategies required for more informed policy.

The volume:

- Examines the changing features of health and nutrition of mothers, new-borns and children between pre and post National Rural Health Mission (NRHM)
- Studies reproductive health and well-being of mother and children
- Explores linkages between food, nutrition and health
- Examines the underlying factors determining poor health and nutrition
- Probes into health expenditure, their impoverishment and its bearing on access to maternal and child healthcare services
- Proposes strategic interventions to reduce maternal, neonatal and child mortality and improve nutritional status

The volume will be of great interest to scholars and researchers of public health, especially maternal and child health specialists, gender studies, development studies and public policy.

Sandhya R Mahapatro is Assistant Professor, Economics Division, at the A. N. Sinha Institute of Social Studies, Patna, India. She pursued her doctoral and postdoctoral research in migration studies. Her current research areas include issues related to health economics, migration, maternal and child health and gender.

Udaya S Mishra, a Statistician/Demographer, is Professor in the Department of Epidemiology and Bio-statistics at the International Institute for Population Sciences, Mumbai, India, with research contributions in the areas of aging, health and nutrition, in addition to population policy and programme evaluation. His current research interest includes measurement issues in health and equity focusing on the evaluation of outcomes.

Shubh Swain is an implementation scientist and a policy thought leader in the multi-sectoral areas of gender, nutrition, food systems and global health. He has worked in several regions, including South Asia and East Africa. He works as a Research Associate at the Tata Cornell Institute, Cornell University, USA. Shubh's current work focuses on developing strategies to involve men in achieving better nutritional status for women in low- and middle-income countries.

Health and Nutrition of Women and Children in Empowered Action Group States of India

Status and Progress

Edited by Sandhya R Mahapatro,
Udaya S Mishra and Shubh Swain

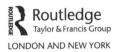

Routledge
Taylor & Francis Group

LONDON AND NEW YORK

First published 2024
by Routledge
4 Park Square, Milton Park, Abingdon, Oxon OX14 4RN

and by Routledge
605 Third Avenue, New York, NY 10158

Routledge is an imprint of the Taylor & Francis Group, an informa business

© 2024 selection and editorial matter, Sandhya R Mahapatro, Udaya S Mishra and Shubh Swain; individual chapters, the contributors

British Library Cataloguing-in-Publication Data
A catalogue record for this book is available from the British Library

ISBN: 978-1-032-37487-1 (hbk)
ISBN: 978-1-032-56235-3 (pbk)
ISBN: 978-1-003-43063-6 (ebk)

DOI: 10.4324/9781003430636

Typeset in Sabon
by Deanta Global Publishing Services, Chennai, India

Contents

List of Figures   *x*
List of Tables   *xii*
List of Contributors   *xvi*
Foreword by P.M. Kulkarni   *xviii*
Acknowledgements   *xxi*

Introduction: Perspectives on Maternal and Child Health and
Nutrition in Empowered Action Group States   1
SANDHYA R. MAHAPATRO, UDAYA S. MISHRA, AND SHUBH SWAIN

PART I
Regional Pattern, Causes and Implications   9

1   Maternal Mortality: Role of EAG States   11
     ANJALI RADKAR

2   Nutritional, Bio-Demographic and Socioeconomic
     Determinants of Neonatal Mortality in the EAG States of India   24
     PRAVAT BHANDARI AND SURYAKANT YADAV

3   Disparities in Health Outcome of Empowered Action Group
     States of India: A Panel Data Approach   37
     ADITYA KUMAR PATRA

PART II
Access and Utilisation: Gaps and Challenges   55

4   Differential Access to Maternal and Child Health Across Social
     Groups: Issues and Challenges of Discrimination   57
     SANGHMITRA S. ACHARYA

5   Continuum of Care for Maternal and Child Health in India
    and EAG States   78
    RINJU AND ABHISHEK SHARMA

6   Place of Hospitalization and Residence, and Their Effect on
    Caesarean Section Out-of-Pocket Expenditure in India   89
    PUSHPENDRA SINGH AND SANDHYA MAHAPATRO

7   Understanding Maternal Healthcare Deprivation in Bihar   104
    BRAJESH KUMAR

PART III
Nutrition and Well-being   119

8   Nutritional Status of Mothers and Children: Trends and
    Determinants   121
    NEHA YADAV AND KRISHNA KUMAR CHOUDHARY

9   Association between Parental Migration and Undernutrition
    Among the Children Left Behind in Rural Empowered Action
    Group (EAG) States, India   138
    MONALISHA CHAKRABORTY AND SUBRATA MUKHERJEE

10 Utilisation of Integrated Child Development Services (ICDS)
    and Nutritional Outcomes in Empowered Action Group (EAG)
    States of India: Evidence from Two National Surveys   156
    RUDRA NARAYAN MISHRA

11 Implication of Household Food Security on Child
    Health: Evidence from Rural Jharkhand   188
    NEHA SHRI

PART IV
Health Governance, Policies and Programmes   203

12 Factors Affecting Inequity in Institutional Delivery and
    Choice of Providers: The Role of Janani Suraksha Yojana and
    Community Health Workers in Bihar   205
    KAKOLI DAS AND SASWATA GHOSH

13 Men's Role in Unpaid Activities and Maternal Health Care in
    India: How Far Women Get Support from Men?   229
    ADITI B PRASAD AND APARAJITA CHATTOPADHYAY

14 Quality of Maternal Health Care in Public Hospitals of Uttar
    Pradesh: A Case Study of Lucknow District   251
    SONIA VERMA AND C S VERMA

15 Assessment of Health System Governance in Empowered
    Action Group States in India   261
    PRAVIN KUMAR

    Emerging Concerns and a Way Forward   286
    SANDHYA R. MAHAPATRO

Figures

1.1 Maternal Mortality Ratio, India, and States Subgroups,
1997–98 to 2018–20   15
1.2 Age Distribution of Maternal Deaths, India, 2001–03 and 2018–20   15
3.1 Infant Mortality Rate in Six Major States of India   39
3.2 Investment in Health System Resources and Other Health
Determinants   42
4.1 Social and Occupational Composition of Study Population   64
4.2 Plurality of Healthcare Services in Kusumpur Pahadi   65
4.3 Composite Score on Factors of Well-Being Across Social Groups   73
4.4 Composite Index of Well-Being: Across Domains and Social Groups 74
5.1 Percentage of CoC Maternal and Child Health in the EAG
States, NFHS-4 PR: Pregnancy Registration, MCH Card:
Maternal and Child Health Card, ANC: Antenatal Care,
ID: Institutional Delivery, M-PNC: Mother Postnatal Care,
C-PNC: Child Postnatal Care   81
5.2 Percentage of any MCH Services and Child Full Immunization
in the EAG states, NFHS-4   82
5.3 Percentage of Full CoC Services and Child Full Immunization
in the EAG States, NFHS-4   83
6.1 Percentage of Caesarean Delivery in EAG States   91
7.1 Comparison of ANC, Delivery Care, and PNC Among the
EAG States and India   106
8.1 Conceptual Framework of Undernutrition   123
8.2 Prevalence of Malnutrition (%), Across the State, NFHS-4
and NFHS-5   125
8.3 Declining Percentage Point Prevalence of Malnutrition Among
Children from NFHS-4 to NFHS-5   128
8.4 Prevalence of Lower Birthweight (>2.5kg) Babies, NFHS-5,
2019–21   129
8.5 Prevalence of Malnutrition (BMI > 18.5kg/m^2) Among
Women, NFHS-5   130
8.6 Prevalence of Nutrition-Specific Intervention Indicators,
NFHS-5, 2019–21   131
9.1 Undernutrition Among Children by Parent's Migration Status   146

10.1 Maternal and Child Nutrition Framework: UNICEF 161
10.2 Use of Any ICDS Among Pregnant Mothers: EAG States and All India – Urban 167
10.3 Use of Any ICDS Among Pregnant Mothers: EAG States and All India – Rural 168
10.4 Use of Any ICDS Among Breastfeeding Mothers: EAG States and All India – Urban 172
10.5 Use of Any ICDS Among Breastfeeding Mothers: EAG States and All India – Rural 172
10.6 Use of Any ICDS Among Children Below Six Years: EAG States and All India – Urban 176
10.7 Use of Any ICDS Among Children Below Six Years: EAG States and All India – Rural 177
10.8 Received Any Financial Assistance During Childbirth: EAG States and All India – Urban 180
10.9 Received Any Financial Assistance During Childbirth: EAG States and All India – Rural 181
11.1 Prevalence of Child Food Security by Ethnic Group 196
11.2 Prevalence of Adult Food Security by Ethnic Group 197
11.3 Prevalence of Household Food Security by Ethnic Group 197
12.1 Status of Continuum of MCH Care Services (in percent) in Bihar and Adjacent States between NFHS-3 (2005–06) and NFHS-5 (2019–21) 213
13.1 Conceptual Model for Gendered Division of Labour 234
13.2 Double Burden of Work on Women 237
13.3 Females Aged 6 Years and Above Participating in Different Activities in a Day at Different Levels of Education (%) 238
13.4a Men Who Were Present at Any Antenatal Check-Up (%), 2019–21 239
13.4b Men Ever Told What to Do If Child's Mother had Any Pregnancy Complication (%), 2019–21 241
15.1 Percentage Shortage in Health Infrastructure 272
15.2 Ranking of State Based on Patients and Health Human Resources Ratios 277

Tables

1.1	Maternal Mortality Ratio, India, 1957–20	14
1.2	Maternal Mortality Ratio, India and EAG States 1997–98 to 2017–19 and 2018–20	17
1.3	Maternal Mortality Ratio, India and Top Three States 1997–98 to 2018–20	18
1.4	Correlation Coefficients between MMR and Determinants of Maternal Mortality	19
1.5	Selected Determinants of Maternal Mortality, 1997–98 (NFHS-2) and 2019–21 (NFHS-5), India and EAG States	20
1.6	Share of Births and Maternal Deaths, 1997–98 to 2014–16, EAG States and Kerala	21
1.7	Causes of Maternal Deaths from 2001 to 2003 Special Survey of Death (in percentages)	21
2.1	Distribution of Selected Risk Factors for Neonatal Mortality in the EAG States of India, 2015–16 and 2019–21	28
2.2	Association between Neonatal Death and Several Risk Factors in the EAG States of India, 2019–21	30
3.1	Childhood Mortality Rate among the States of India	40
3.2	Population Served per Medical Facility	44
3.3	Non-Health Sector Parameters	45
3.4	Maternal Healthcare Indicators	47
3.5	FEM and REM Estimation of Stochastic Frontier Analysis	49
3.6	Relative Efficiency Score (in %) and Rank	49
3.7	Efficiency Dispersion Analysis	50
3.A	Appendix Table	53
4.1	Problems in Accessing Health Care Across Social Groups	61
4.2	Healthcare Providers and Access to Public Institutions for Child Delivery	61
4.3	Trends in Infant and Child Mortality Difference across Social Groups	63
4.4	House Type and Facilities and Amenities across Social Groups (in percentage)	64
4.5	Distribution of Services Ever Used in Last Five Years across Social Groups	66

4.6 Level of Satisfaction on RCH Services Availed 67
4.7 Domains and Indicators of Index of Maternal and Child
    Health and Well-Being 72
4.8 Standardized Scores for Domains of Well-Being Across Social
    Groups 72
5.1 Proportion of CoC Services Examine by Maternal and Child
    in the EAG States 82
5.2 Multinomial Regression Model Predicting the Relative Risk Ratio
    of a Women Continuum of Care of Maternal and Child Health 84
6.1 Percentage Distribution of Place of Hospitalization
    for Normal and Caesarean Section Birth and Delivery
    Expenditure by Level of Care in India, 2018–19 94
6.2 Adjusted Odds Ratio and 95% Confidence Interval (CI) of
    Caesarean Births Associated With Place of Hospitalization
    Among the Rural/Urban Area 97
6.3 Coefficient of Log-Linear Regression and 95% Confidence
    Interval (CI) of OOPE on Caesarean Delivery with Place of
    Hospitalization Among the Rural/Urban Area 98
7.1 Dimensions, Indicators, Weight, and Deprivation Cut-Off 108
7.2 Maternal Healthcare Deprivation for Different Cut-Offs 110
7.3 Dimension/Indicator-Wise Composition of MHC Deprivation 111
7.4 Subgroup Decomposition of MHC Deprivation 112
7.5 Dimensional Decomposition of MHC Deprivation as Evident
    from NFHS-4 114
8A1 Prevalence of Anaemia Among Women (15–49 Years) and
    Children (0–59 Months) Across States 135
8A2 Trends in Nutritional Status of Children NFHS-4 and
    NFHS-5 Across States 136
9.1 Inter-State Out-Migration Among Working Age Population
    (15–64 Years) from the EAG States to Five Major States
    and Delhi 140
9.2 Percentage of Population Below Poverty Line in the EAG
    States, 2011–12 (Tendulkar Methodology) 142
9.3 Select Summary Statistics 145
9.4 Logistic Regression Model Results for Undernutrition Among
    Children (0–14 Years) 147
10.1 Prevalence of Undernutrition Among Children Below Six
    Years of Age in Selected Anthropometric Indicators and Anaemia 163
10.2 Prevalence of Undernutrition (BMI and Anaemia) Among
    Women of Reproductive Age (15–49 Years) 165
10.3 Utilisation of Any ICDS for Pregnant Mothers by Social Groups 169
10.4 Utilisation of Any ICDS for Pregnant Mothers by Wealth Quintiles 171
10.5 Utilisation of Any ICDS for Breastfeeding Mothers by
    Social Groups 174

10.6 Utilisation of Any ICDS for Breastfeeding/Lactating
Mothers by Wealth Quintiles 175
10.7 Utilisation of Any ICDS for Children Below Age Six Years
by Social Groups 178
10.8 Utilisation of Any ICDS for Below Six Years by Wealth Quintiles 179
10.9 Received Any Financial Assistance During Childbirth by
Social Groups: EAG States and All India 182
10.10 Received Any Financial Assistance During Childbirth by
Wealth Quintiles: EAG States and All India 183
11.1 Overview of Surveyed Villages 191
11.2 Demographic Characteristics of Samples 192
11.3 Household Food Security by Background Characteristics 193
11.4 Food Consumption Score and Household Dietary Diversity
Among Sampled Households 195
11.5 Household Dietary Diversity by Different Forms of Malnutrition 195
12.1 Background Characteristics of Currently Married Women
(Aged 15–49), AHS 2012–13, Bihar, and EAG States 212
12.2 Distribution of Home Delivery, Institutional Delivery, and
Type of Providers According to Respondent's Selected
Background Characteristics, Bihar, AHS 2012–13 214
12.3 Adjusted Odds Ratios with 95% CI of Preference for
In-Facility Delivery and Choice of Specific Provider, Bihar,
AHS 2012–13 216
12.4 Understanding the Effects of *Janani Suraksha Yojana* on
Safe Delivery in Bihar – A Decomposition Analysis 219
13.1 Percentage Aged 15–59 Participating in Different Activities
in a Day 236
13.2 Average Time (in Minutes) Spent in a Day Per Participant
Aged 15–59 237
13.3 Male Involvement in Maternal Care by Background
Characteristics, India (NFHS 5, 2019–21) 240
13.4 Main Reason for not Receiving ANC Reported by
Husbands (NFHS-5, 2019–21) 241
14.1 Responses of the Care Seekers 255
15.1 Healthcare Regulations and Healthcare Protections Schemes 265
15.2A Public Health Expenditure 2014–2015 267
15.2B Public Health Expenditure 2018–2019 267
15.2C Increase/Decrease in Public Health Expenditure 268
15.3 Trend of Medical Expenditure on Inpatient and Outpatient
Care (₹) of Households at 2018 Prices in the EAG States of
India, 2004–18 269
15.4 Healthcare Human Resources among EAG States 271
15.5 Status of Health *Infrastructures (Hospitals)* 272
15.6A Health Indicators 1999–2022 in India 273

15.6B Health Indicators between 1999–2022 in India as well as
the EAG States   274
15.7A A Ranking of State Based on Public and Household
Expenditure   276
15.7B Ranking of State Based on Health Infrastructure   278
15.7C Ranking of States Based on the Reduction in Mortality Rates   278
15.8   Difference between SDGs Target and Achievement   279

Contributors

P. M. Kulkarni is Former Professor, Centre for the Study of Regional Development, Jawaharlal Nehru University, New Delhi, India.

Rinju is Research Scholar, Tata Institute of Social Studies, Mumbai.

Sanghmitrra S Acharya is Professor, Centre of Social Medicine and Community Health, School of Social Sciences, Jawaharlal Nehru University, New Delhi, India.

Pravat Bhandari is Research Scholar, International Institute for Population Sciences, Mumbai, India.

Monalisha Chakraborty is Research Scholar, Institute of Development Studies, Kolkata, India.

Aparajita Chattopadhyay is Professor, International Institute for Population Sciences, Mumbai, India.

Krishna Kumar Choudhary is PhD Scholar, Centre for Social Medicine and Community Health, Jawaharlal Nehru University (JNU), New Delhi, India.

Kakoli Das is Research Scholar IDSK & Assistant Professor, Vidyasagar University, India.

Saswata Ghosh is Associate Professor, Institute for Development Studies, Kolkata, India.

Brajesh Kumar is Assistant professor, B.B. Ambedkar University, Lucknow, India.

Pravin Kumar is PhD Scholar, Department of Public Policy and Public Administration Central University of Jammu, Jammu, India.

Subrata Mukherjee is Associate Professor, Institute of Development Studies, Kolkata, India.

Aditya Kumar Patra is Associate Professor, Maharaja Sriram Chandra Bhanja Deo University, Odisha.

Aditi B Prasad is Research Scholar, International Institute for Population Sciences, Mumbai, India.

Anjali Radkar is Professor, Gokhale Institute of Politics and Economics, Pune, India.

Abhishek Sharma is PhD fellow in Population studies in the Department of Public Health and Mortality, International Institute for Population Science, Mumbai, India, India.

Neha Shri is Research Scholar, International Institute for Population Sciences, Mumbai, India.

Pushpendra Singh is Assistant Professor, K. Soumiya Institute, Mumbai, India.

Neha Yadav is PhD Scholar, Centre of Social Medicine and Community Health, Jawaharlal Nehru University (JNU), New Delhi, India.

Rudra Naryan Mishra is Assistant Professor, Gujarat Institute of Development Research, Gujarat, India.

Suryakant Yadav is Assistant Professor, International Institute for Population Sciences, Mumbai, India.

Soniya Verma is Senior Research Associate, Giri Institute of Development Research, Lucknow.

C.S. Verma is Associate Professor, Giri Institute of Development Research, Lucknow.

Foreword

P.M. Kulkarni

Longevity of the human population experienced an unprecedented rise during the twentieth century. For India, longevity increased from about 23 years at the beginning of the last century to 63 years towards the end of the century, and recent estimates show that it has risen further to 70 years. A number of factors, such as advances in preventive and curative medicines, improvements in nutrition, sanitation and hygiene and enhanced access to health services, contributed to this development. Various programmes on health, nutrition and sanitation services have been introduced and implemented over the years in India. The health of women and children has received special attention in India's health policy. The health programmes have been refined, modified and expanded over the years through various policy initiatives. The network of primary health centres introduced during the early phase of India's planning process made basic health services accessible to rural populations. The Maternal and Child Health (MCH) component of the public health services facilitated pregnancy, delivery and post-natal care. The primary healthcare system was expanded and strengthened with the introduction of the tier of community health centres and increase in the density of the primary health centres. Two major initiatives of the National Rural Health Mission, namely, the Janani Suraksha Yojana and the Accredited Social Health Activists (ASHA), gave a huge boost to maternal and child healthcare. Making ambulance facilities available in remote areas facilitated emergency obstetric care. Immunization programmes have been in operation for a long time and have been strengthened over the years. Supplementary nutrition schemes for children and pregnant and lactating women are in place. Health schemes such as the Pradhan Mantri Ayushman Bharat/Jana Arogya Yojana and Pradhan Mantri Matru Vandana Yojana have been launched to meet the needs of the poor and vulnerable sections of society. Besides, there has been overall socio-economic development: a notable rise in literacy and the level of education and an increase in incomes. An impressive decline in fertility has occurred, lowering the reproductive burden on women and allowing greater attention to pregnancy and delivery care. The age at marriage has risen, thereby preventing many early pregnancies. We have seen a remarkable decline in infant and early childhood mortality and also in maternal mortality. By 2020, the infant mortality rate had fallen below 30 per thousand and the maternal mortality ratio had fallen below 100 per 100000 births.

Yet, there are issues of concern. The maternal and child health indicators vary substantially across states and regions. In spite of an overall improvement in maternal and child health conditions, it is seen that while some states have achieved fairly low infant and maternal mortality, the level is moderately high in some other states. In addition to the spatial variations, conspicuous differentials are seen by income and social background. The poor do not fare well and are burdened by high out-of-pocket expenditures on healthcare. Socially marginalised populations face difficulties in accessing public health services. Moreover, though mortality has declined rapidly, progress in improving the nutritional status of children has not been satisfactory.

Clearly, there is a need and scope for further improvement of the programmes. A number of questions arise. Why have some states done quite well and others not so? Is this attributable to differences in governance? In India, most of the health services are delivered by the state governments. Programmes by the central government are also administered by the state government institutions. Besides, many states have initiated their own health schemes which supplement and complement the central programmes. Moreover, health conditions are influenced by socioeconomic development, and it is known that the level of development varies across states. There are huge inter-state differences in the levels of education and income. While some convergence seems to be occurring in education, income gaps persist. Furthermore, transport and communication infrastructures play a crucial part in the delivery of services, and notable differences in such infrastructures are found across states. Besides, there is climatic diversity among regions. Naturally, the health situation is not expected to be uniform throughout the country. It is imperative, therefore, to identify specific factors that cause inter-state variations and try to find ways to improve conditions in states that have been lagging in progress. Spatial differences have also been found within states with some hotspots of poor health detected, and it is necessary to find out why these exist. New initiatives bring in additional inputs and strategies, but these need to function within the existing system of health services. The success of the new schemes depends on how seamlessly they work in conjunction with the existing health infrastructure and personnel and contribute to good health. Therefore, it is desirable to examine the functioning of specific interventions and initiatives in maternal healthcare and their impacts on health outcomes. Such analyses are valuable in detecting weak links in implementation and, in turn, in refining the programme. Nutrition is well recognised as an essential factor in the promotion of health, and schemes on supplementary nutrition to women and children have been functioning for long time in India and have been periodically reinforced to improve their effectiveness. Household food security also has an important role to play, and there are schemes towards enhancing food availability for the poor. How much impact have the various schemes on nutrition and food security made?

Health indicators show that the marginalized sections of the population fare poorly. Is this due to poor access to services on account of low incomes or isolation or is it attributable to social discrimination in the delivery of services? Traditionally, maternal and child healthcare has been considered a matter in the domain of women, with men playing only a marginal role. There is now greater recognition of the importance of male involvement in these vital matters. But to what extent is it occurring?

These questions call for systematic analyses of the health situation of women and children and of implementation of the programmes to identify strengths as well as deficiencies in inputs and strategies. This volume is a valuable effort in this direction. The focus of the volume is on the states in the empowered action group (EAG) which includes relatively backward states that show poor health indicators. The collection contains contributions from a number of scholars engaged in health research in India. The papers have been coordinated and edited by Dr. Sandhya Mahapatro of the A.N. Sinha Institute of Social Studies, Patna; Prof. U.S. Mishra, International Institute for Population Sciences, Mumbai, and Dr. Subh Swain, Tata-Cornell Institute, USA.

This volume makes a notable addition to our knowledge of the maternal and child health situation in India and particularly in the EAG states. The rigorous analyses by the contributors and the insights they bring in will certainly deepen our understanding of the health situation and functioning of the health programmes. The findings would provide directions for strengthening, modifying and refining the existing programmes and give clues for further initiatives. This volume is a rich source of information and ideas for policymakers and programme managers in the field of maternal and child health.

Acknowledgements

This volume is a collective effort of several authors who have presented their research work in an international seminar organized at A.N. Sinha Institute of Social Studies, Patna, in 2019. More than 80 papers were presented in the seminar; this volume contains only 15 selected papers. Each chapter in the book highlighted an important aspect of maternal and child health which is thought-provoking and important from a policy perspective. We are deeply indebted to the authors for their patience and co-operation in revising and updating the chapters as per the requirement of the book and making this volume readable.

We are thankful to UNICEF, Bihar, and Tata-Cornell Institute, USA, for providing financial support to organize the event at ANSISS without which this work would not have been possible. An immense sense of gratitude to Dr. Syed Hubbe Ali, former Health Specialist, UNICEF, Bihar for his constant support in this regard. The editors are grateful to Prof. K.S. James, International Institute for Population Sciences, Director; Prof S. Irudaya Rajan, Chair of International Institute for Migration and Development and former Professor, Centre for Development Studies, Mr. Asangba Chuba Ao, IAS, former Director, A.N. Sinha Institute of Social Studies and Education Secretary, Government of Bihar for their constant encouragement, suggestions and motivation. Thanks to Ms Dhanasree Ramdas, Senior Research Officer at ANSISS for helping us in formatting the chapters and other editorial support. We would also like to record our sincere appreciation to Routledge, India, for publishing this edited volume.

Introduction

Perspectives on Maternal and Child Health and Nutrition in Empowered Action Group States

Sandhya R. Mahapatro, Udaya S. Mishra, and Shubh Swain

Health and nutrition of women and children are fundamental to the state of health of any nation-state. Emphasis on this aspect of development is desirable given its impetus on human capital development, economic growth, and social development of the nation. Reduction in mortality levels, specifically infant and child mortality, is the precondition for fertility transition and is well recognized in demographic transition theory. The emphasis on maternal and child health and nutrition is significant in India, where the regions are experiencing different stages of demographic transition and uneven distribution in socioeconomic and healthcare development. Over time, health system reforms with high-impact interventions help reduce maternal and child deaths, and increases utilization of maternal and child health (MCH) services. With the extension from MDG to SDG, the MCH issue remains a priority under "GOAL 3 – which ensures healthy lives and promotes well-being for all at all ages" to be accomplished by the Year 2030. Though free reproductive, maternity, and childcare services were provided by the state, current models of care and interventions are failing to reach those who living in adverse circumstances that lead to poor MCH outcomes. Despite accelerated progress, many states yet to meet MDG targets in health and nutrition. The reasons for the gaps in achievements in these indicators are complex and uneven across different contexts.

Globally, maternal and child mortality is declining. The South Asian countries relatively fared poorly in meeting the public health challenges, particularly in maternal and child health (Hate and Gannon, 2010). India along with Nigeria, accounts for one-third of global maternal deaths and India still contributes 15% of global maternal mortality (WHO, 2015). Likewise, the likelihood to die among neonates is ten times and nine times more in sub-Saharan Africa and South Asian countries than in high-income countries. India has ranked 12th among 52 lower-middle-income nations (UNICEF, 2018) and ranked 3rd highest (22.7 %) among the South Asian countries after Pakistan and Afghanistan in neonatal mortality (UN IGME, 2019). With regard to nutritional indicators, there has been an improvement; however, progress is slow to achieve global nutrition targets. Global nutrition report (2020) highlights an unacceptably large number of malnourished people, and **India is among 88 countries that are likely to miss global nutrition targets**

DOI: 10.4324/9781003430636-1

by 2025. India alone had 47 million stunted children and 26 million wasted children, the highest in the world in 2018 (Development Initiatives, 2018). The first-ever Comprehensive National Nutrition Survey (CNNS) found that 35% of children under the age of five were stunted, and 17% and 33% were wasted and underweight, respectively, in 2016–2018 (MoHFW & UNICEF, 2019).

The progress in MCH becomes a critical component of India's National Health Mission (NHM). In 2005, the implementation of the National Rural Health Mission (NRHM) led to massive investment in healthcare resources and innovative strategies were implemented, and the Indian health system is making a visible impact on its MCH indicators afterwards. For a successful run towards compliance with SDG goals in MCH, the allocation of resources in the health sector is also increasing over the years. Despite a positive stride, India ranked 143 among 188 countries in the SDG indicators, with widespread heterogeneity across the regions (Panda & Mohanty, 2018; Lim et al., 2015). Given the socio-demographic and economic diversity, the resource-poor states in India recorded relatively higher maternal and child deaths with lesser utilization of services. At the same time, the inequality in MCH indicators not only varies across the states but also between different socioeconomic groups. Addressing such disparities is a matter of concern as it contributes to widening inequalities in healthcare access and outcomes. Alongside such disparities, the public policies of the states are shaped by the regional parties having different ideologies that influence the performance of developmental indicators including health.

There are specific regions in India that figure consistently poor in health indices. In 2001, the Ministry of Health and Family Welfare (MoHFW) identified eight states, including Bihar, Chhattisgarh, Jharkhand, Madhya Pradesh, Odisha, Rajasthan, Uttarakhand, and Uttar Pradesh as empowered action group (EAG) states. The EAG states draw specific attention in maternal and child health and nutrition, as these states share the misfortune of poor MCH and socioeconomic backwardness that goes along with their slow pace of demographic and epidemiological transition than non-EAG states. Maternal and child health and nutrition continue to pose a major challenge in these states. India's performance in achieving the SDG targets of MMR (70) is improving with a decline in MMR from 130 in 2014–15 to 97 in 2018–20. The inter-regional variation in MMR as per the latest SRS report, however, shows MMR is 137 for the EAG state, 49 and 76 for south and other regions. Undeniably, these states perform poorly for a long time; hence, the improvement started from a low base.

The performance of the EAG states in most of the socioeconomic and health indicators is a long way behind that of developed states. Besides health system bottlenecks and unregulated private care, challenges underpinned by poverty, inequality, and marginalization-induced huge inequity in accessing healthcare services render these states vulnerable to realizing desirable levels of performance in MCH indicators. Evidence shows that in India, more than one-fifth of women have low BMI and half of the pregnant women are anaemic, and the share is significantly higher in the EAG states. Nearly half of the children under the age of five are stunted and underweight which has significant implications for human capital development in these states. It would, therefore, be not exaggerated to state that MCH holds the key to developmental transition in the EAG states. There could be a multiplicity of factors responsible for the poor state of health and nutrition of women and children in these regions. But splitting them out and prioritizing them in order can only offer the expected improvement.

With the implementation of the NRHM, the Indian health system has greatly influenced its health and nutritional indicators on a positive note. Though these states are progressing, a performance gap persists in relation to the rest of India. For instance, the infant mortality rate is highest in Madhya Pradesh (43 per 1000), whereas it was only six in Kerala. Among the EAG states, the IMR as mentioned is highest in Madhya Pradesh (43), and it was lowest in Uttarakhand (24) in 2020. These facts show there is a long way to achieve SDGs in health indices in the EAG states. Emphasis on supply-side factors can not overlook the demand-side barriers, and therefore, the policy response has to be implemented in keeping with the community-level needs, if any needs to be context-specific. This will require a laser-sharp focus on addressing both the demand and supply-side barriers. Achieving the SDG's target on MCH thus requires addressing the shortcomings in its regional facet with specific emphasis on the EAG states.

The book offers a brief account of progress in the health and nutritional status of mothers and children in the EAG states along with an exposition of regional disparities. The chapters presented in the book unfolds a range of issues relating to the distribution of health outcomes, inequalities in access to MCH services, mechanisms of poor nutrition, health expenditure and impoverishment, structural bottlenecks of the health system, effective implementation of the programmes, and appropriate strategies for more informed policy. An exploration of such issues is highly desirable for addressing the performance gap and formulation of appropriate policies and programmes. The present edited book has engaged in a discussion on all these dimensions and provides direction to tackle major challenges faced by the health system of the EAG states in realizing improved MCH outcomes. With a background on the significance of studying MCH, the first part of the introduction chapter offers an overview of the status of MCH indicators with a focus on the EAG states. The second part of the chapter elaborates structure of the book and its chapter scheme.

Given the wide range of perspectives to be covered in the volume, the chapters are divided into four sections. Section one will unfold the regional inequalities and correlates between maternal and child health and nutrition and their implications for health policy. Despite an increase in coverage of services, gaps remain. Women and children at different stages from early pregnancy to child care are deprived of accessing care in the continuum. The second section, hence, attempts to showcase the factors serving as barriers to access and utilization of MCH care. The nutritional status of mother and child is alarming in the EAG states given its underperformance. Owing to its contribution to family wellbeing and economic growth, critical assessment of the nutritional status of mother and child is thus a matter of investigation for appropriate state intervention. The third section of the book will pin down the micro and macro realities behind malnutrition and the necessary strategic interventions to curb it. The chapters in the last section are engaged in discussing the major challenges for the health system towards improving the status of MCH in terms of health system functioning, the effectiveness of existing programmes and strategies to be adopted for betterment. Considering the key findings and recommendations from all chapters, a note on the way forward is presented highlighting the critical areas for further investigation and the strategic solutions for accomplishing SDG targets in MCH in the EAG states.

Section I

Regional Pattern, Causes, and Implications

This section of the book focuses on the regional pattern in health and nutritional indicators in the EAG states. The chapters show the distribution of health and nutritional indicators across socioeconomic and demographic attributes and spatial variation among EAG states. The factors contributing to poor health outcomes related to MCH are discussed in this chapter. The evidence presented in this section highlights that there is considerable scope for focused area-specific interventions for improvement in MNCH indicators across EAG states.

The chapter on 'Maternal mortality: Role of EAG states' by Anjali Radkar analyses the status of maternal health in the EAG states and the significance of its reduction for development. The discussion in the chapter highlights the critical areas of intervention gaps in the EAG states, such as addressing antenatal and natal care, strategies to increase the use of contraception to control fertility and higher-order births and to achieve sustainable development goals in maternal mortality.

The risk factors contributing to neonatal mortality in EAG states are discussed in the chapter 'Determinants of neonatal mortality in the EAG states of India'. In this chapter, Bhandari and Yadav using the birth history information from a surviving mother available in National Family Health Survey (NFHS) data examined the role of biodemographic and health system factors in determining neonatal mortality. This study highlights the significance of health intervention that may act as a preventive measure of multiple gestations with short-term birth intervals as it increases the risk of neonatal death.

The third chapter in the group is by Aditya Kumar Patra on 'Disparities in health outcome of empowered action group (EAG) states of India: A panel data approach'. Using the panel data regression model, this chapter has explored the health and non-health-sector determinants of infant mortality. The analysis suggests that states with higher per capita health expenditure and more institutional delivery have a higher chance of better health outcomes. Furthermore, the determinants like safe drinking water, toilets, and female literacy beyond the health sector also affect IMR.

Section II: Access and Utilization

Inequities in MCH care access not only caused poor outcomes but also create challenges towards achieving universal health coverage. Though structural reforms in the health sector are occurring over the last two decades, disparities persist across socioeconomic classes and such inequality appears to be more in the EAG states. Over the MDG period, the key health status indicators in the EAG states have been improved; however, large inequalities yet persist and much is still left to be accomplished. Understanding the drivers of inequity and overcoming the structural and societal barriers is critical to achieve SDG goals in health and nutrition.

Sanghmitra S. Acharya, in the chapter, 'Differential access to maternal and child health across social groups-issues and challenges of discrimination', discusses the key challenges of the health system in attaining equitable access to MCH care. Unfortunately, a large section of maternal and child health seekers is deprived of health care due to their social identities. The author argues it is imperative to understand and explore the perception of the care providers about care seekers and vice versa on the basis of social identity in these poor-performing states.

A continuum of care (CoC) is one of the important sustainable pathways to increase utilization of MCH services and reduce mortality among mothers and newborns. The factors affecting the continuation of receiving care have been rigorously examined in 'Continuum of care for maternal and child health in India and EAG states' by Rinju and Abhisek Sharma. The continuum of care was computed using four healthcare indicators, namely, the use of antenatal care, institutional delivery, and mother and child postnatal care. The findings show the reach of the CoC is considerably low among poor and uneducated women and significantly varies across states. The study advocates some strategic measures, inbuilt with wealth and education facets, for the better utilization of MCH services specifically in the EAG states.

The chapter by Puspendra Singh and Sandhya Mahpaptro assesses the influence of change in place of residence on out-of-pocket expenditure for normal/caesarean section delivery by place of hospitalization and type of healthcare facilities. The findings reveal that caesarean birth is higher in private hospitals and urban areas and increases with the hospitalization of women outside of the place of residence. The urban cost of living, cultural factors, and health system challenges are attributed to higher out-of-pocket expenditures.

The level of maternal healthcare deprivation and associated causes in Bihar has been rigorously analysed in the chapter on the 'Incidence and intensity of maternal healthcare deprivation in Bihar'. In this chapter, using the Alkire-Foster methodology, Brajesh Kumar provides a quantitative assessment of the incidence and intensity of maternal healthcare deprivation. The incidence and intensity of maternal healthcare deprivation in Bihar are mainly associated with the socioeconomic determinants and suggest that focus should be paid more to postnatal care aspect.

Section III: Nutrition and Wellbeing

Poor nutrition is a global concern as it affects productivity, human capital, and health indicators negatively. Evidence shows EAG states represent a gloomy picture in nutritional indicators which might be attributed to the economic performance of the state, household food insecurity, and less utilization of healthcare services. The nutrition-specific interventions under ICDS and various health interventions although brought improvement; challenges still persist. The chapters presented in this section discuss these aspects.

The level of nutrition has a direct bearing on health outcomes. The chapter on 'Determinants and trends in nutrition outcomes of mothers and children on health status' by Neha Yadav and Krishna Choudhary critically examines the linkages of nutrition with MCH outcomes in the EAG states. Furthermore, the chapter also evaluated the nutrition-specific interventions in influencing health and nutrition outcomes. The chapter findings show variations in nutritional outcomes across and within states and are linked to nutrition-specific interventions. The study underscores the importance of state-specific analysis as a one-size-fits-all approach would not work for all contexts.

The migration of parents has a significant influence on the nutritional status of children left behind. Understanding this association is critical for the EAG states as most of these states are experiencing large out-migration. The paper by Chakraborty and Mukherjee on 'Association between parental migration and undernutrition among the children left behind in rural EAG states' using India Human Development Survey data attempts to analyse the effects of parental migration on morbidity and nutritional status of the children. Based on parental migration status, the children were grouped into three mutually exclusive groups: (1) children of non-migrant parent(s) (C-NM); (2) left behind children of returned migrant parents (LBC-RM); and (3) left behind children of currently migrant parents (LBC-CM). The study finds children of return migrants are more likely to be stunted and underweight than other groups.

The chapter by Rudra Narayan Mishra, on the 'Utilisation of Integrated Child Development Services (ICDS) and nutritional outcomes in EAG states of India: Evidence from two national surveys' argues there is a need to strengthen the implementation of the ICDS in the EAG states as the utilization of ICDS is low and increases little among the poor and marginalized in some of the EAG states. Adopting the ICT platforms for grievance redressal, effective monitoring, and community vigilance is key to improving the functioning of the ICDS programmes in the EAG states.

Household food security and dietary diversity have serious implications on the nutritional status of children. The chapter 'Implication of household food security on child health – Evidence from rural Jharkhand' by Neha Shri explored the linkages between food insecurity prevalence and dietary diversity score on children's nutritional status. To determine the status of food insecurity, the average Household Food Insecurity Access Scale (HFIAS) and then household food insecurity access prevalence categories were generated following the method suggested by FANTA. The study was conducted in selected rural villages of Chandankiyari, Bokaro district of Jharkhand. The study shows the risk of undernutrition has increased with an increase in the level of food insecurity. Low land size and high dependence on agriculture have an impact on the nutritional status of the children.

Section IV: Health Governance, Policies, and Programmes

It is well evident that the challenges for improving health indices are more pronounced in EAG states. Many policy initiatives and health system reforms have taken place over the last two decades, and there is still scope for progress in the interventions. Lack of political will, poor governance, and structural bottlenecks in the health system resulted in poor implementation of programmes. It is in this context significant to address the policy gaps and factors contributing to the effective implementation of programmes for improving health service delivery and health outcomes. The chapters in this section discuss the healthcare interventions and governance issues of the health system, in MCH care utilization.

The chapter 'Factors affecting inequity in institutional delivery and choice of providers: the role of Janani Suraksha Yojana (JSY) and community health workers (CHWs) in Bihar' provides a comprehensive assessment of factors influencing institutional delivery and the role of the demand side financing scheme on this. The study finds the lack of CoC although institutional delivery shows an increasing trend. To ensure equitable and universal access to MCH care, particularly safe delivery in Bihar, there is a need to distil the major socioeconomic loopholes from the big deck of health and awareness. Besides, strengthening of Primary Health Centres and Community Health Centres in delivering MCH care is important to achieve Universal Health Coverage.

The second chapter of this group 'Men's role in unpaid activities and maternal health care in India: How far women get support from men?' by Aditi Prasad and Aparajita Chattopadhyay examines critically male involvement and its impact on the utilization of MCH services. The analysis shows gender inequality in unpaid work widens the gender gap in employment, influences their empowerment, and is also linked to their healthcare utilization. The findings recommended a strong need to address the involvement of rural, poor, and illiterate men in maternal health.

The chapter on 'Quality of maternal health care in public hospitals of Uttar Pradesh: A case study of selected facilities of Lucknow district' by Soniya Verma and C S Verma deals with the quality of facility care and its influence on service utilization. Quality of maternal care as observed in the study is compromised due to a shortage of specialist doctors and necessary infrastructure.

The last chapter 'Assessment of Health System Governance (HSG) in EAG states in India' by Pravin Kumar assesses the availability and gap in health-care policy, regulation, finance, health resources, and improvement in health indicators. It attempts to identify the issues and challenges and find possible ways to achieve SDGs and UHC among the EAG states.

References

Development Initiatives (2018). *2018 Global Nutrition Report: Shining a Light to Spur Action on Nutrition*. Bristol, UK: Development Initiatives. Google Scholar.

Global Nutrition Report (2020). *Action on Equity to End Malnutrition*. Bristol, UK: Development Initiatives. Available at: www.globalnutritionreport.org/reports /2020-global-nutrition-report.

Lim, S. S., Allen, K., Bhutta, Z. A., Dandona, L., Forouzanfar, M. H., Fullman, N., ... & Chang, J. C. (2016). Measuring the health-related Sustainable Development Goals in 188 countries: A baseline analysis from the Global Burden of Disease Study 2015. *The Lancet, 388*(10053), 1813–1850.

Ministry of Health and Family Welfare (MoHFW), Government of India, UNICEF et al. (2019). *Comprehensive National Nutrition Survey (CNNS): National Report*. New Delhi: Ministry of Health and Family Welfare (MoHFW), Government of India, UNICEF. Google Scholar.

Panda, B. K., & Mohanty, S. K.. (2018). Progress and prospects of health-related sustainable development goals in India. *Journal of Biosocial Science, 51*(3), 335–352.

World Health Organization (2015). Trends in estimates of maternal mortality ratio 1990–2015. WHO, UNICEF, UNFPA, World Bank Group and the United Nations Population Division estimates

Haté V, Gannon S (2010). Public health in South Asia: a report of the CSIS Global Health policy center. Washington, DC: Center for Strategic and International Studies.

Part I

Regional Pattern, Causes and Implications

1 Maternal Mortality

Role of EAG States

Anjali Radkar

Introduction

International Conference on Population and Development (ICPD) was held in Cairo in 1994 when the world as a whole first voiced about reproductive health. Certain goals related to reproductive health were discussed and set; however, no population in the world met those goals. After ICPD, Cairo, when studied minutely, it was realized that comprehensive reproductive health issues are more and also more acute in developing countries and need immediate attention. Furthermore, to address the development agenda for all participating countries, MDGs were developed out of several commitments set forth in the Millennium Declaration signed in September 2005. Eight set MDGs were about poverty, primary education, maternal and child health, HIV/AIDS, environmentally sustainable development and empowerment of women. After the stipulated period, in continuation with MDGs, a new bunch, a more comprehensive one, came forward in the form of SDGs. SDGs set in 2015 are the blueprint to achieve a better and more sustainable future for all. Seventeen SDGs address global challenges, including those related to hunger, poverty, health, inequality, climate change, environmental degradation, peace and justice.

Maternal mortality, a development indicator, is addressed in both MDGs and SDGs. Maternal mortality indices show a great disparity between developed and developing countries. For developing countries, it is about 42 times higher than the developed countries. In 2017, approximately 810 women died a day due to preventable causes related to pregnancy and childbirth. The MMR in developing countries in 2017 was 462 per 100,000 live births versus 11 per 100,000 live births in developed countries (WHO, 2019). Reduction in maternal mortality at the national level is thus a commitment when India approved MDGs and SDGs. More recently, the target of the SDG sets by the United Nations aims at reducing the global MMR to less than 70 per 100,000 live births. Certain countries have MMR in single digits. Italy, Norway, Poland and Belarus have the lowest MMR of two, while Germany and the United Kingdom have seven. Other countries with low MMR are Canada (10) and the United States (19). India's neighbouring countries, Nepal (186), Bangladesh (173) and Pakistan (140), have

DOI: 10.4324/9781003430636-3

high MMR, whereas MMR for China and Sri Lanka is less than 29 and 36, respectively (World Bank, 2019).

As maternal mortality, the most prominent indicator of development shows wide disparities between developed and developing countries at the global level, and it shows the disparities at the national level also. It is not just about the maternal health, but it also relates to many other dimensions like educational level, the status of women, empowerment of women and maternal nutrition with the backdrop of the utilization of maternal health care.

Maternal Mortality

Maternal mortality ratio, i.e. number of maternal deaths per 100,000 live births, per se does not give any idea on the cause of death or the characteristics of the woman. Each maternal death or complication represents a tragedy. It is estimated that 80% of maternal deaths are preventable and avoidable through effective and affordable actions, even in resource-poor countries (WHO, 2002). It is an outcome of a chain of events and disadvantages throughout women's life (Motashaw, 1997). The determinants of maternal mortality as portrayed by Jejeebhoy (1997) include women's autonomy, role in decision making, mobility, control over economic and other resources, gender and power relations, household economic status, physical accessibility to healthcare services and quality of services. Exactly on similar lines, in the case study of India, Choe and Chen (2006) have come out with determinants of maternal mortality as knowledge of reproductive health, access to and utilization of reproductive as well as medical health care along with the socio-economic and cultural factors associated with knowledge and use of services.

Getting the data on maternal mortality is a challenge. Despite high maternal mortality, very little information about deceased women is available in India. In order to take any specific action for its reduction, more specific information about the associated causes is required but not available. Sample registration system (SRS) publishes estimates of maternal mortality regularly. For the past 20 years, it is available every two years consistently that gives trends in MMR in India and states, and also on the group of states. Understanding the causes of maternal death is a task further. As reflected in the literature, the reasons for maternal death are multi-layered. At the forefront, obviously are medical/clinical causes before, during and after childbirth and abortion. Behind medical causes are logistic causes like not-so-efficient health service delivery and lack of transport facilities and last but not the least the causes are social, cultural and political factors which together determine the status of women, their fertility and health-seeking behaviour.

The distribution of maternal deaths in India by the timing of death was like this: 40.4% of maternal deaths take place when a woman is pregnant, 10% during or after abortion, 15.4% during childbirth and 34.2% after six weeks of childbirth or at the end of pregnancy (Radkar and Parasuraman, 2007). The burden of maternal deaths in India is huge as its share of close to 20%. Women here are about 50 times more likely to die a maternal death than of women in certain developed countries. Global goals about maternal mortality would not be achieved unless India responds. In India, the eight socio-economically backward states of Bihar, Chhattisgarh, Jharkhand, Madhya Pradesh, Odisha, Rajasthan, Uttaranchal and Uttar Pradesh, referred to as the EAG states, lag behind in the demographic transition and have the highest infant mortality rates in the country. These are high-focus states in terms of implementation of special programmes and policies, as all of these continue to have higher levels of fertility, infant mortality and maternal mortality. The EAG states lag behind in demographic transition compared to other Indian states. Among the EAG states, as per Raghuram Rajan Committee Report of 2013, Bihar, Odisha, Uttar Pradesh, and Jharkhand are the four most backward states of India. Odisha is supposed to be the most backward state in India right now (Ministry of Finance, 2013).

Reaching global maternal mortality goals depends on the performance of India because of its large share in maternal deaths. For maternal mortality purposes, Assam is clubbed with the EAG states considering the high MMR there. Therefore, in further discussion, Assam though not an EAG state would be present along with them. These nine states together contribute to 48% of the Indian population. This means that about half the Indian population with a large share of maternal deaths needs more exploration of the maternal mortality scenario.

Objectives

This study tries to shed light on maternal mortality scenarios in the EAG states in India. The objectives of the study include

- To trace the trends in MMR in India vis-à-vis EAG states
- To highlight the share of live births and maternal deaths and its causes in the EAG states
- To explore the possible required actions for reduction in MMR in the EAG states and in India.

Methodology

For getting into maternal mortality scene, it is necessary to quantify maternal mortality. Between the two indicators, Maternal Mortality Ratio (MMR) and Maternal Mortality Rate, MMR is a more robust. It portrays the scenario based on the live births, which is a proxy to number of pregnancies. It is also necessary to explore more on the determinants of MMR so as to propose the necessary action.

The main source of data for this study is SRS. It periodically presents MMR for India and major states. Apart from that, data on the determinants of maternal mortality are compiled from the reports of two major country-wide surveys, National Family Health Survey (NFHS) round 2 and round 5 conducted in 1997–98 and 2019–21, respectively, on a large representative sample. This is also the period when consistent MMR data are available and a lot of change in the values of indicators is observed.

Results

Although India is one of the countries with high MMR, recent estimates show sizeable decline from 1321 in 1957–60 to 398 in 1997–98 to 212 in 2007–09 to 97 in 2018–20 (Table 1.1).

Initially, the decline in MMR was faster compared to the recent period, which is in line with the fact that as the estimates reach lower levels, it is difficult to maintain the same pace to take it down further. In that case, more efforts and attention from planners and policymakers are required. The decline in maternal mortality is also associated with the decline in fertility (Bhat et al., 1995), which highlights that maternal mortality cannot be looked at in isolation. Within India, for both demographically advanced and demographically not-so-advanced states, fertility and mortality also have gone down significantly.

Table 1.1 Maternal Mortality Ratio, India, 1957–20

Year	Maternal Mortality Ratio (MMR)	Source
1957–1960	1321	NSS*
1963–1964	1195	NSS*
1972–1976	853	SRS
1977–1981	810	SRS
1982–1986	580	SRS
1987–1991	519	SRS
1992–1996	440	SRS
1997–1998	398	SRS
1999–2001	327	SRS
2001–2003	301	SRS
2004–2006	254	SRS
2007–2009	212	SRS
2010–2012	178	SRS
2011–2013	167	SRS
2014–2016	130	SRS
2016–2018	113	SRS
2017–2019	103	SRS
2018–2020	97	SRS

*Based on indirect time series estimates

MMR in India is coming down; however, as expected the decline is not uniform across the country. Depending on the stage of demographic transition, different states are behaving differently. Southern states have a very low MMR, and EAG states have the highest. All other states are in-between. Though earlier the difference in MMR figures for different subgroups of the states was visibly high, over the years it is declining. It can be looked at as the beginning of convergence (Figure 1.1).

It is seen that MMR in India is declining fast. Similarly, MMR is associated with fertility. When fertility declines, births at later ages go down. The same has been reflected in the available age distribution of maternal deaths, which shows the change in the pattern (Figure 1.2). Earlier share of maternal deaths used to be relatively high even in the older reproductive ages. However, it has been realized that now the deaths are highest in the ages 20–24 and 25–29 years: the age groups where fertility is the highest. Fertility is declining, and contraceptive use is increasing; hence, births in later ages are declining and so is mortality. Higher age of the mother at the time of birth is one of the determinants of maternal mortality, which has been controlled automatically.

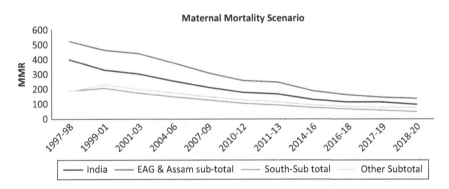

Figure 1.1 Maternal Mortality Ratio, India, and States Subgroups, 1997–98 to 2018–20

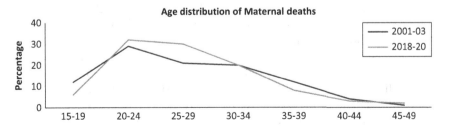

Figure 1.2 Age Distribution of Maternal Deaths, India, 2001–03 and 2018–20

Maternal Mortality in EAG States

To look at the trends in MMR data for the past 22 years have been compiled from various SRS bulletins, specially published to explore the maternal mortality scenarios. This period matches exactly with the period when India adopted the Reproductive and Child Health (RCH) programme, nationally. Among the total maternal deaths, roughly two-thirds of the deaths are from the EAG states, namely Bihar, Jharkhand, Madhya Pradesh, Chhattisgarh, Rajasthan, Uttar Pradesh, Uttaranchal, and Odisha and Assam (SRS, 2006). The geographic distribution of maternal deaths in RCH-2 indicates that 67.8% of deaths are from these regions, almost matching to SRS estimates (Radkar and Parasuraman, 2007); hence, the situation is half the population and two-thirds of maternal deaths.

The extent of maternal deaths is more among rural, backward women with the standards of living, displaying the characteristics that are associated with poverty and rural residence (Radkar and Parasuraman, 2007). A similar finding is recorded by Anandlakshmy and her colleagues (1993). The differentials in maternal deaths are observed by caste and the standard of living of women along with the place of residence, indicating lower socio-economic groups experience more maternal mortality. It has become clear that women residing in rural areas belonging to backward castes and having a low standard of living are the most vulnerable women in terms of maternal mortality. Lesser maternal deaths in urban areas reflect easier access of the city-dwellers to medical services (WHO, 1991). Most of the EAG states relate to lower development-related characteristics and display high MMR.

The EAG states are demographically lagging behind as a consequence of high fertility, high infant mortality and high maternal mortality. In a way, all these indicators are linked; change in one is reflected in the other. Along with the EAG states, it is necessary to look at India and also the three best-performing states of the country as regards maternal mortality. This will facilitate the comparison and understanding where the Indian states can reach.

Table 1.2 and Table 1.3 present the required data for India, the EAG states and the top three states in maternal mortality, viz., Kerala, Maharashtra and Tamil Nadu. It shows that these top three states have achieved particularly low levels of MMR, being a part of the same country; following a similar set of policies and programmes. The EAG states are lagging behind, though each of the EAG states has shown a significant decline in the past 22 years.

At the end of the previous century, MMR was very high, more than 500 for Assam, Bihar/Jharkhand, Rajasthan and Uttar Pradesh/Uttaranchal. However, all the EAG states have worked on it to get the MMR down by 2017–19 and among the group; only Assam now has it over 200. The decline in Bihar/Jharkhand (531 to 130) and Uttar Pradesh/Uttaranchal (606 to 167) is substantial. The same is reflected in the relative change also, where the reduction in Bihar/Jharkhand is 75.5%, in Rajasthan 72.2% and in Uttar Pradesh/Uttaranchal 72.4%. Considering the overall change of the EAG

Table 1.2 Maternal Mortality Ratio, India and EAG States 1997–98 to 2017–19 and 2018–20

Year	India	Assam	Bihar/Jharkhand	Madhya Pradesh/Chhattisgarh	Odisha	Rajasthan	Uttar Pradesh/Uttaranchal	EAG and Assam
1997–1998	398	568	531	441	346	508	606	520
1999–2001	327	398	400	407	424	501	539	461
2001–2003	301	490	371	379	358	445	517	517
2004–2006	254	480	312	335	303	388	440	375
2007–2009	212	390	261	269	258	318	359	308
2010–2012	178	328	219	230	235	255	292	257
2011–2013	167	300	208	221	222	244	285	246
2014–2016	130	237	165	173	180	199	201	188
2016–2018	113	218	149	173	150	164	197	161
2017–2019	103	205	130	163	136	141	167	145
2018–2020	97							137
Change in 22 years	74.1	63.9	75.5	63.0	60.7	72.2	72.4	72.1

Table 1.3 Maternal Mortality Ratio, India and Top Three States 1997–98 to 2018–20

Year	India	Kerala	Maharashtra	Tamil Nadu
1997–1998	398	150	166	131
1999–2001	327	149	169	167
2001–2003	301	110	149	134
2004–2006	254	95	130	111
2007–2009	212	81	104	97
2010–2012	178	66	87	90
2011–2013	167	61	68	79
2014–2016	130	46	61	66
2016–2018	113	43	46	60
2017–2019	103	30	38	58
2018–2020	97	19	33	54
Change in 23 years	75.6	87.3	80.1	58.7

states from 520 in 1997–98 to 137 in 2018–20, the relative decline is 73.6%, while at all India, the change is 75.6%. The EAG states are performing for sure. However, close to 60% change states are Assam, Madhya Pradesh/Chhattisgarh and Odisha. These states need penetrating action.

Obviously, the MMR of the three top-performing states is low. During 1997 to 2020, MMR for Kerala has come down to 19 from 150, Maharashtra 33 from 166 and Tamil Nadu 54 from 131. Relative change during this period for Kerala is 87%; for Maharashtra, it is 80%; and for Tamil Nadu, it is 58.7% (65% from 167 in 1999–00). These states are still faster in reduction. Assam, Madhya Pradesh/Chhattisgarh and Uttar Pradesh/Uttaranchal still could not reach the level of MMR that the top three states achieved in 1997, while remaining states like Bihar/Jharkhand, Odisha and Rajasthan have just managed it. This indicates how much effort is required for these states, for the requisite decline in MMR, so as to reach the SDG goal.

Determinants of Maternal Mortality

To get the MMR further down, it is necessary to have an action plan. One needs to work on the determinants of maternal mortality and see the reflection in the MMR.

Radkar (2018) looked at the MMR figures vis-à-vis certain social, biological, demographic and healthcare utilization-related variables to explore their strength of relationship with each one; that might suggest the strategies to be adopted so as to improve on these variables and in turn the MMR. Radkar (2018) used the data on MMR presented by the SRS and the values of the determinants of MMR as collected in the National Family Health Survey-3. It is seen here that the strong relationship of MMR pertains to all the variables that are related to health systems, and thus, the service delivery including contraceptive use and fertility level followed by the social development-related variables like spousal violence and decision making.

Table 1.4 Correlation Coefficients between MMR and Determinants of Maternal Mortality

Determinants of Maternal Mortality	Coefficient
TFR	0.686**
Sex Ratio	−0.113
Sex ratio at birth	0.237
Current use – Any Modern method	−0.834**
Mothers who had antenatal check-up in the first trimester	−0.729**
Mothers who had at least 4 antenatal visits	−0.817**
Institutional births	−0.806**
Births assisted by health personnel	−0.827**
Mothers who received postnatal care from a doctor/nurse/LHV/ANM/ midwife/other health personnel within 2 days of delivery	−0.852**
Children aged 12–23 months fully immunized	−0.891**
Women whose BMI is below normal	0.483
Pregnant women aged 15–49 years who are anaemic	0.396
Currently married women who usually participate in household decisions	−0.350
Women who worked in the last 12 months who were paid in cash	−0.440
Ever married women who have ever experienced spousal violence	0.558*
Percentage of women who know that HIV/AIDS can be prevented by using condoms	−0.642**
Percentage of women who usually make decisions alone or jointly – own health care	−0.189

As reported in the study by Radkar (2018), the relationship of MMR with different biological, demographic, social and healthcare utilization-related variables is varying. To reduce maternal mortality, apart from maternal healthcare utilization, contraceptive use and fertility reduction, the EAG states should also focus on the status of women, the nutritional status of women and women's workforce participation. Although the strength of the relationship between MMR and anaemia in pregnancy is less, anaemia needs improvement. In India, about half of the women of reproductive ages and two-thirds of pregnant women are anaemic. It is difficult for such women to sustain the haemorrhages, either intra-partum or post-partum, because of anaemia overall immunity goes down and women catch the infections. Anaemia among women in reproductive ages and issues related to their social status also has to be addressed against the backdrop of maternal mortality. It is well known that those who are deprived of maternal care are socio-economically underprivileged, rural, illiterate/less educated and socially deprived women with low standard of living. The share of such women is more in the EAG states implying higher MMR.

To explore further, whether and how the values of the determinants have reduced, data on the selected determinants are compiled from two rounds of NFHS: round 2 and round 5 for India and the EAG states (Table 1.5). Data for the states like Jharkhand, Chhattisgarh and Uttaranchal are not presented because data for these states are not available during NFHS-2.

Table 1.5 Selected Determinants of Maternal Mortality, 1997–98 (NFHS-2) and 2019–21 (NFHS-5), India and EAG States

Determinants	India	Assam	Bihar	Madhya Pradesh	Odisha	Rajasthan	Uttar Pradesh
NFHS-2 – 1997–98							
TFR	2.3	1.5	2.8	2.6	2.2	3.0	2.9
Current use – any modern method	42.8	26.6	22.4	42.6	40.3	38.1	22.0
Mothers who had complete antenatal care	20.0	15.8	6.4	10.9	21.4	8.3	4.4
Institutional births	33.6	17.6	14.6	20.1	22.6	21.5	15.5
Mothers who received postnatal care from a doctor/nurse/LHV/ANM/other health personnel within two days of delivery for their last birth	16.5	21.4	10.0	10.0	19.2	6.4	7.2
All women age 15–49 who are anaemic	51.8	69.7	63.4	54.3	63.0	48.5	48.7
Ever married women who have ever experienced spousal violence (%)	18.8	14.1	24.9	19.7	22.9	9.8	20.8

Determinants	India	Assam	Bihar	Madhya Pradesh	Odisha	Rajasthan	Uttar Pradesh
NFHS-5 – 2019–21							
TFR	2.0	1.9	3.0	2.0	1.8	2.0	2.4
Current use – any modern method	56.5	45.3	44.4	65.5	48.8	62.1	44.5
Mothers who had at least four antenatal visits	58.1	50.7	25.2	57.5	78.1	55.3	42.4
Institutional births	88.6	84.1	76.2	90.7	92.2	94.9	83.4
Mothers who received postnatal care from a doctor/nurse/LHV/ANM/other health personnel within two days of delivery for their last birth	78.0	65.3	57.3	83.5	88.4	85.3	72.0
All women age 15–49 who are anaemic	57.0	65.9	63.5	54.7	64.3	54.4	50.4
Ever married women who have ever experienced spousal violence (%)	29.3	32.0	40.0	28.1	30.6	24.3	34.8
Pregnant women age 15–49 who are anaemic	52.2	54.2	63.1	52.9	61.8	46.3	45.9

The values of all the determinants for the major EAG states have improved sizeably and that is what is reflected in the MMR values. Although institutional births and postnatal care have increased over the period, a little more effort in antenatal care will help get MMR down. The use of contraception also is very low in the EAG states that need attention, though fertility is declining. Anaemia is persistent, and for that, sustained efforts are required.

To get an idea on the share of births and share of maternal deaths in the EAG states and Assam explains the MMR scenario. For the comparison, information about just the best-performing state, Kerala, is presented in Table 1.6.

The share of births in the EAG states and Assam together is much less than the share of maternal deaths. Over the period, both the share of births and the share of maternal deaths have reduced, and the difference between these two, however, is substantial. This indicates the need for reduction in maternal mortality and bridging the gap. Kerala, the best-performing state in terms of MMR, the situation is exactly opposite. The share of births is more and the share of maternal deaths is less and is declining. The EAG states should reduce maternal deaths that in turn will reverse the direction.

Although data presented in Table-1.7 are not recent, it gives an idea about the causes of maternal deaths in different subgroups of states in India. The causes of maternal death for India and in sync with the cause of death for the EAG states, considering their large share in maternal deaths is presented. It is to be noted here that the causes differ substantially for EAG and southern states. Avoidable reasons like haemorrhage and abortion are handled well by

Table 1.6 Share of Births and Maternal Deaths, 1997–98 to 2014–16, EAG States and Kerala

Year	1997–98	2004–06	2014–16
EAG states and Assam			
Share of births	47.08	39.70	39.86
Share of maternal deaths	61.04	57.38	56.29
Kerala			
Share of births	4.01	3.36	3.57
Share of maternal deaths	1.51	1.26	1.26

Table 1.7 Causes of Maternal Deaths from 2001 to 2003 Special Survey of Death (in percentages)

Cause of death	India	EAG and Assam	South	Other
Haemorrhage	38	37	30	40
Sepsis	11	11	17	10
Hypertensive disorders	5	4	13	6
Obstructed labour	5	5	9	4
Abortion	8	10	4	3
Other conditions	34	33	26	37

southern states. If the EAG states take the action and avoid such deaths, their MMR would reduce substantially (National Institute of Public Cooperation and Child Development, 2015).

In order to bring down IMR and MMR, the Ministry of Health and Family Welfare (MoHFW) is supporting all states/Union Territories (UTs) in the implementation of Reproductive, Maternal, New-born, Child, Adolescent Health and Nutrition (RMNCAH+N) strategy under National Health Mission (NHM) based on the Annual Program Implementation Plan (APIP) submitted by states/UTs. The interventions taken up by government are presented in Annexure 1.

Conclusions

It is seen that MMR has reduced substantially in India with the latest figure of 97 so as the MMR for the EAG states and Assam (137). To reduce the MMR further and contribute to reduction of global MMR, there is a strong need to reach out to mothers from the EAG states. In the absence of health services, having accessibility issues, health care-deprived poor women succumb to various morbidities and mortality during pregnancy and childbirth. With all the problems and difficulties in service delivery, unreachable should be reached. The population that is of health services does not demand it strongly, they meet their healthcare requirements in their way, and in the process, a few lives are lost. Maternal deaths assume importance, not just for health reasons but also when the woman dies, there are significant social and economic losses. Children who lose their mothers suffer the most. The risk of death for children under five years increases if the mother dies a maternal death. Maternal mortality thus affects child mortality.

For Global MMR reduction, India should lower its MMR. Exactly in the same way for reduction of Indian MMR, the EAG states should lower their MMR, considering their large share in both births and maternal deaths. When pregnancies and births are more, the requirement of health services is more, and also, the deaths are more. The EAG states, to reduce maternal mortality, apart from, maternal healthcare utilization, contraceptive use and fertility reduction, should also focus more on the status of women, nutritional status of women and women's workforce participation to get long-term results. All these variables depend strongly on development, and thus, acting on them would be the essential step towards reaching sustainable goals around maternal mortality. EAG states are lagging behind here.

References

Abou-Zahr, C. L., Royston, E., & World Health Organization (1991). *Maternal Mortality: A Global Factbook* (No. WHO/MCH/MSM/91.3). Geneva, Switzerland: World Health Organization.

Anandalakshmy, P. N., Talwar, P. P., Buckshee, K., & Hingorani, V. (1993). Demographic, socioeconomic and medical factors affecting maternal mortality-an Indian experience. *Journal of Family Welfare*, 39(3), 1–4.

Bhat, P. M., Navaneetham, K., & Rajan, S. I. (1995). Maternal mortality in India: Estimates from a regression model. *Studies in Family Planning*, Jul-Aug., 26(4), 217–232.

Choe, M. K., & Chen, J. (2006). Potential for reducing child and maternal mortality through reproductive and child health intervention programmes: An illustrative case study from India. *Asia Pacific Population Journal*, 21(1), 13.

India. Office of the Registrar General, & University of Toronto. Centre for Global Health Research. (2006). *Maternal Mortality in India, 1997–2003: Trends, Causes, and Risk Factors*. Office of the Registrar General India.

Interventions (n.d.). https://pib.gov.in/PressReleaseIframePage.aspx?PRID =1796436

Jejeebhoy, S. J. (1997). Maternal mortality and morbidity in India: Priorities for social science research. *Journal of Family Welfare*, 43, 31–52.

Motashaw, N. D. (1997). Root causes of maternal mortality: Infancy to motherhood. *Journal of Family Welfare*, 43, 4–7.

National Institute of Public Cooperation and Child Development (2015). *An Analysis of Levels and Trends in Maternal Health and Maternal Mortality Ratio in India 2015. A Report*. New Delhi: National Institute of Public Cooperation and Child Development.

Office of the Registrar General, Ministry of Home Affairs, Government of India (2011). *Special Bulletin on Maternal Mortality in India 2007–09.*, Sample Registration System, Vital Statistics Division, New Delhi.

Radkar, A. (2018). Correlates of Maternal Mortality: A Macro-level Analysis. *Journal of Health Management*, 20(3), 337–344.

Radkar, A., & Parasuraman, S. (2007). Maternal deaths in India: An exploration. *Economic and Political Weekly*, 4 August, 2007, 42(31), 3259–3263.

Rajan, R., Pandey, T. K., Jayal, N. G., Ramaswami, B., & Gupta, S. (2013). *Report of the Committee for Evolving a Composite Development Index of States*. Ministry of Finance, Govt. of India.

Registrar General of India (2009). *Special Bulletin on Maternal Mortality in India 2004–06*. New Delhi: SRS Office of the Registrar General, India.

Registrar General of India (2013). *Special Bulletin on Maternal Mortality in India 2010–12*.

Registrar General of India (2017). *India: Special bulletin on maternal mortality in India 2007–13*. Sample Registration System bulletin, Vital Statistics Division, New Delhi.

SRS (2022). *Special Bulletin on Maternal Mortality in India, 2017–2019*. New Delhi: Registrar General of India.

UNICEF, I (2009). Maternal and perinatal death inquiry and response. In *Empowering Communities to Avert Maternal Deaths in India*. New Delhi: UNICEF.

WHO (2005). *Reducing Maternal Deaths: The Challenge of the New Millennium in the African Region*. Brazzaville: Congo: WHO Regional Office for Africa.

WHO (2019). https://www.who.int/news-room/fact-sheets/detail/maternal-mortality

World Bank (2019). https://data.worldbank.org/indicator/SH.STA.MMRT

2 Nutritional, Bio-Demographic and Socioeconomic Determinants of Neonatal Mortality in the EAG States of India

Pravat Bhandari and Suryakant Yadav

Introduction

Achieving the lowest number of infant and child death has been a major national health goal in India for several decades. Fortunately, the greater reach of health programmes, especially the maternal and child health (MNCH) programmes in recent decades, has contributed to a decline in postnatal mortality, including infant and child mortality in India; however, reduction of neonatal mortality was substantially lower with respect to infant and child mortality (Kumar et al., 2013). Evidence from several low-income countries suggests that neonatal deaths are the largest burden which contributes to nearly two-thirds of total infant deaths (Kruk et al., 2018; Rajaratnam et al., 2010). As estimated by Liu et al. (2015), worldwide, 5.9 million children under five years of age died in 2015, 45% of whom were neonates. The mortality of children under the age of five fell sharply by 53% between 1990 and 2015; however, the decrease in neonatal mortality during the same period was much lower at an estimated 47% (You et al., 2015). In India, between 1981 and 2011, the share of neonatal deaths to total infant deaths increased by 17% (Saikia et al., 2016). However, being a larger territory, the progress in infant and child mortality is not uniform across the geographical regions of India. There have been remarkable variations in terms of reduction of infant and child mortality between the demographically progressive states (e.g., Kerala and Tamil Nadu) and demographically lagging-behind states (e.g., Uttar Pradesh and Bihar).

The Central Government of India constituted the empowered action group (EAG) in 2001 to implement area-specific health interventions in eight demographically lagging-behind states. This group includes the socio-economically poorer states of Bihar, Madhya Pradesh, Chhattisgarh, Uttarakhand, Jharkhand, Orissa, Rajasthan and Uttar Pradesh. Apparently, the common focus of past studies on infant mortality as a single measure has had a detrimental effect as it disguises the unequal share of neonatal and post-neonatal mortality. Moreover, the determinants of infant mortality tend to vary from that of the relative contribution of bio-demographic, healthcare and socioeconomic determinants on the decomposed components of neonatal mortality.

It has been estimated that, globally, about three-quarters of neonatal deaths could be prevented if currently available interventions were more

DOI: 10.4324/9781003430636-4

effectively followed (Cooper, 2016). Several scholastic articles have suggested that almost three-fourths of infant deaths take place during the neonatal period (i.e., the first 28 days of life) (Akseer et al., 2015; Sankar et al., 2016). Similar to other developing countries, about three-fourths of infants die in the neonatal period in India; this proportion is even higher in the above-mentioned eight EAG states of India. Reduction of these preventable deaths in this period is crucial to meet the targets of Sustainable Development Goals (SDGs) (Rajaratnam et al., 2010). Earlier research from low-income countries, including India, investigated the determinants of early neonatal mortality, infant mortality and under-five mortality (Fottrell et al., 2015; Kumar et al., 2013; Ladusingh, Gupta & Yadav, 2016). A large body of literature has agreed that early neonatal mortality is predominated by multiple neonatal (e.g., gender and birthweight), maternal (e.g., age, birth interval and parity), household (e.g., standard of living) and socio-economic factors (e.g., parental education and occupation). Similar types of risk factors also have been identified for infant and under-five deaths. Recent studies have also argued that poor nutrition status of a mother before and during pregnancy negatively impacts neonatal survival, by increasing the risk of preterm delivery and congenital malformations (Moss et al., 2002). Maternal anaemia during pregnancy increases the risk of intrauterine growth retardation (IUGR), which further adversely impacts neonatal survival.

However, there remains a lack of recent evidence on determinants of neonatal mortality in such an environment where neonatal deaths are very high. This limits our understanding of the neonatal mortality pattern in the EAG states and the associated factors for an evidence-based programming. We made an attempt to identify and fill this existing knowledge gap in Indian EAG states. Here, in this study, we aim to explore the characteristics of neonatal mortality in some of the socio-economically backward Indian states in particular. Our results could be useful in assisting policymakers and researchers to develop efficient strategies to improve survival of the new-borns in some of the economically regressive states of India.

Objectives

The objective of this study is to: (1) assess the levels of neonatal mortality in the EAG states by different nutritional, bio-demographic and socio-economic characteristics and (2) examine the association between neonatal mortality and potential determinants in the EAG states of India.

Data and Methods

Data Source

Eight economically lagging-behind states of India, namely, Bihar, Chhattisgarh, Jharkhand, Madhya Pradesh, Odisha, Rajasthan, Uttar Pradesh and

Uttarakhand, were selected to investigate the determinants of neonatal mortality. We analysed the recent data available from the fourth and fifth rounds of National Family Health Survey (NFHS-4, 5) conducted in 2015–16 and 2019–21, respectively, across all the states and union territories of India. The NFHS data provide demographic and health information based on three different questionnaires: women, men and households employed during the interview. The survey collected a wide range of information on maternal and children's health status, healthcare availabilities and utilizations and other health-related behaviours, and these included child mortality, nutritional status of children and mothers, maternal and childhood morbidities, fertility preferences, antenatal care services, facility delivery, postnatal care and so on (IIPS and ICF, 2017, 2021). Aside from this, common demographic and socio-economic characteristics across child (including age, sex, birth order, etc.), mother (age, marital status, educational attainment, etc.) and household (wealth, location, etc.) are also recorded.

Outcome Event and Other Variables

The outcome variable for this study was neonatal death, defined by a binary variable as the death of a live-born baby within the first 28 days of life. The mothers in the age group 15–49 years were interviewed about the day of death of their children. The independent variables considered in this study consist of biological, demographic and socio-economic characteristics of child, mother and household such as maternal body mass index (BMI) (underweight, normal, overweight and obese), maternal haemoglobin level (anaemic and non-anaemic), birth size (large, average, small and very small), child sex (male and female), birth order (first, second to fourth and fifth or higher), multiple gestation (yes or no), mother's age at birth (less than 18 years, 19–34 years and 35–49 years), birth interval (less than two years and two years or above), desire for pregnancy (wanted then, wanted later and wanted no more), antenatal visits (no visits, less than four and four or above), place of delivery (home and health sector), caesarean delivery (yes and no), delivery assistance (traditional birth assistant and health professionals), mother's educational attainment (none, primary, secondary and higher), household wealth (poorest, poor, middle, rich and richest) and place of residence (urban and rural) and states.

Statistical Analyses

Weighted frequency and percentage were calculated to describe the level of neonatal mortality by selected risk factors for both NFHS-4 and NFHS-5. After assessing the level of neonatal mortality, a probit regression model was used to examine the relationship between selected risk factors and neonatal deaths. For the regression analysis, we used data from NFHS-5. We estimated beta coefficients (from probit regression model) by adding all potential factors into our baseline equation with neonatal mortality as the outcome variable. Analysis was made using STATA 14.2, MP (Stata Corp, Inc.) software package.

Findings

Table 2.1 presents the distribution of selected risk factors for neonatal mortality in the EAG states of India. Numbers and percentages of the analysis were weighted by using the individual sampling weight of the respondent from the NFHS-4 and NFHS-5 data. Among the included 136536 livebirths that took place within five years preceding the NFHS-4, 5597 (4.10%) infants died within the first month of their life. In NFHS-5, of the 118596 livebirths, 3726 (3.14%) infants died during the neonatal period, thereby indicating a decline in neonatal mortality rate among the EAG states. Nearly 71.9% and 72.7% of the infants, respectively, in NFHS-4 and NFHS-5 had average birth size. The result shows that both smaller- and larger-sized births had considerably higher mortality rate than average-sized births. Prevalence of maternal anaemia was widespread in both surveys, and it seems that maternal anaemia played an important role in neonatal deaths. In both surveys, infants born to mothers with anaemic symptoms had a greater risk of dying during the neonatal period compared to those born to mothers with non-anaemic symptoms. The percentage of neonatal deaths was consistently higher among the male children compared to the female children (4.51% vs. 3.65% in NFHS-4; 3.41% vs. 2.85% in NFHS-5). Most of the new-borns were singletons. However, about one-fifth (22.33% in NFHS-4 and 18.3% in NFHS-5) of the twin new-borns died during the neonatal period. A vast majority of mothers were in the middle age group (19–34 years) and experienced significantly lower neonatal deaths compared to younger and older mothers. A significant proportion of mothers gave birth to their child in a short birth interval; this group of children had an increased risk of neonatal mortality in both the surveys (5.51% in NFHS-4 and 3.85% in NFHS-5). Between 2015–16 and 2019–21, the proportion of women receiving 'no antenatal visit' declined dramatically. In NFHS-4, one in four births (24.98%, n = 24101) took place without receiving any antenatal care visit; in NFHS-5, this figure has dropped to 1 in 14 (7.2%, n = 6225). A significant decline was observed in facility-based delivery. Still, about 15% of deliveries were made in the home environment in NFHS-5. Moreover, nearly 14% (n = 16425) of the deliveries were conducted by unskilled birth attendant which tends to be associated with an increased neonatal death in comparison to the deliveries conducted by skilled birth attendants, 3.97% vs. 3.01%. In the NFHS-5, nearly 30% of children's mothers had no formal education, a considerable decrease from the NFHS-4's 43%. The majority of the household heads in our dataset were males, without primary education. Nearly four out of ten infants (35.6%) in NFHS-5 were from the lowest wealth quintile group, followed by the poor (25.1%), middle (17.1%), rich (12.9%) and richest (9.4%) wealth groups.

Table 2.1 Distribution of Selected Risk Factors for Neonatal Mortality in the EAG States of India, 2015–16 and 2019–21

Predictors	2015–16	2019–21
	Yes	Yes
Nutritional Factors		
Birth Size		
Average	3449 (3.51)	2395 (2.78)
Smaller than average	1287 (7.04)	700 (5.51)
Larger than average	862 (4.29)	631 (3.20)
Maternal Nutritional Status		
Normal	1412 (3.72)	2279 (3.04)
Underweight	3402 (4.05)	804 (3.18)
Overweight	454 (3.99)	423 (3.51)
Obese	114 (4.37)	123 (4.34)
Maternal Anaemia Status*		
Non-anaemic	1806 (3.69)	1299 (2.96)
Anaemic	3568 (4.11)	2280 (3.26)
Bio-demographic Factors		
Child Sex		
Male	3209 (4.51)	2107 (3.41)
Female	2389 (3.65)	1619 (2.85)
Multiple Gestation		
No	5068 (3.78)	3370 (2.89)
Yes	530 (22.33)	356 (18.25)
Mother's Age at Child Birth		
≤18 years	368 (6.81)	326 (5.02)
19–34 years	4850 (3.92)	3234 (3.00)
35–49 years	380 (5.10)	166 (3.79)
Birth Order		
First	2162 (4.82)	1554 (3.71)
Second to fourth	2662 (3.47)	1812 (2.67)
Fifth or higher	774 (5.15)	360 (4.06)
Birth Interval**		
<2 years	1440 (5.51)	852 (3.85)
≥2 years	1871 (2.92)	1259 (2.32)
Desire for Pregnancy		
Wanted then	4947 (4.02)	3387 (3.09)
Wanted later	305 (5.00)	190 (4.01)
Wanted no more	314 (4.26)	149 (3.51)
Healthcare Factors		
Antenatal Visits		
No visit	865 (3.59)	209 (3.36)
<4 visit	1169 (2.74)	902 (2.34)
≥4 visit	624 (2.10)	740 (1.79)
Place of Delivery		
Health sector	3822 (3.91)	3034 (3.03)
Home	1775 (4.57)	692 (3.77)
Caesarean Delivery		
No	5111 (4.11)	3280 (3.14)

(*Continued*)

Table 2.1 Continued

Predictors	2015–16	2019–21
	Yes	Yes
Yes	486 (4.04)	446 (3.15)
Delivery Assistance		
Unskilled birth attendant	1668 (4.77)	652 (3.97)
Health professionals	3929 (3.87)	3074 (3.01)
Socio-economic Factors		
Mother's Educational Level		
No schooling	2576 (4.41)	1260 (3.55)
Primary	938 (4.53)	549 (3.33)
Secondary	1786 (3.79)	1625 (3.06)
Higher	297 (2.91)	292 (2.16)
Sex of the household head		
Male	4849 (4.12)	3154 (3.14)
Female	748 (3.98)	572 (3.16)
Education of household head		
No schooling	2957 (4.45)	2281 (4.02)
Primary	557 (4.37)	311 (3.05)
Secondary or higher	2084 (3.63)	1134 (2.33)
Wealth Status		
Lowest	2451 (4.66)	1506 (3.57)
Low	1416 (4.30)	1008 (3.39)
Middle	875 (3.97)	596 (2.94)
High	562 (3.43)	406 (2.66)
Highest	294 (2.34)	210 (1.88)
Regional Characteristics		
Place of Residence		
Urban	831 (3.29)	429 (2.50)
Rural	4768 (4.28)	3297 (3.25)
States		
Bihar	1286 (3.97)	737 (3.50)
Chhattisgarh	284 (4.37)	253 (2.97)
Jharkhand	274 (3.62)	282 (2.81)
Madhya Pradesh	694 (3.96)	489 (3.00)
Odisha	256 (3.05)	249 (2.92)
Rajasthan	490 (3.22)	316 (2.16)
Uttar Pradesh	2250 (4.80)	1296 (3.62)
Uttarakhand	61 (3.04)	104 (2.75)
Total	5597 (4.10)	3726 (3.14)

Source: Authors' calculation from NFHS-4 and NFHS-5 data.
Note: Values in the parentheses present proportions; *Comprises missing cases; **Excluding primigravida

A clear wealth gradient was observed in neonatal deaths, with the highest percentage of deaths occurring in the lowest wealth quintiles and the lowest percentage in the top quintile groups.

Table 2.2 describes the results of the probit model where neonatal mortality was the outcome variable and was controlled by several

Table 2.2 Association between Neonatal Death and Several Risk Factors in the EAG States of India, 2019–21

Determinants	Coeff.	Std. Err.	P>z	95% CI
Nutritional Factors				
Birth Size				
Average	Ref.			
Smaller than average	0.253	0.029	0.000	0.197, 0.309
Larger than average	0.082	0.027	0.003	0.029, 0.134
Mother's BMI				
Normal	Ref.			
Underweight	0.057	0.026	0.030	0.006, 0.109
Overweight	0.218	0.038	0.000	0.144, 0.291
Obese	0.314	0.061	0.000	0.195, 0.434
Mother's Anaemia				
Non-anaemic	Ref.			
Anaemic	0.011	0.022	0.635	−0.032, 0.052
Bio-demographic Factors				
Sex				
Female	Ref.			
Male	0.069	0.021	0.001	0.028, 0.109
Multiple Gestation				
No	Ref.			
Yes	1.166	0.065	0.000	1.040, 1.291
Mother's Age at Birth				
≤18 years	−0.006	0.050	0.897	−0.105, 0.092
19–34 years	Ref.			
35–49 years	0.168	0.069	0.014	0.034, 0.302
Birth Order				
First (Primigravida)	0.317	0.125	0.011	0.071, 0.562
2nd to 4th	Ref.			
5th and above	0.119	0.037	0.001	0.046, 0.192
Birth Interval				
≥2 years	Ref.			
<2 years	0.110	0.029	0.000	0.055, 0.165
Desire for Pregnancy				
Wanted then	Ref.			
Wanted later	0.090	0.048	0.061	−0.005, 0.184
Wanted no more	−0.009	0.051	0.862	−0.108, 0.090
Healthcare Factors				
Antenatal Visit				
No visit	Ref.			
<4 visit	−0.131	0.037	0.000	−0.202, −0.060
≥4 visit	−0.203	0.039	0.000	−0.278, −0.129
Place of Delivery				
Home	Ref.			
Health sector	0.005	0.041	0.908	−0.075, 0.084
Caesarean Birth				
No	Ref.			
Yes	0.121	0.031	0.000	0.062, 0.180

(*Continued*)

Table 2.2 Continued

Determinants	Coeff.	Std. Err.	P>z	95% CI
Delivery Assistance				
Traditional birth attendant	Ref.			
Health professionals	–0.084	0.041	0.039	–0.163, –0.005
Socio-economic Factors				
Mother's Education				
No education	Ref.			
Primary	–0.029	0.034	0.383	–0.094, 0.037
Secondary	–0.070	0.027	0.009	–0.123, –0.018
Higher	–0.204	0.045	0.000	–0.29, –0.118
Sex of the Household Head				
Male	Ref.			
Female	–0.018	0.029	0.528	–0.074, 0.038
Whether Household Head Has Primary Education?				
No	Ref.			
Yes	–0.058	0.053	0.274	–0.163, 0.046
Household Wealth				
Poorest	Ref.			
Poor	0.041	0.027	0.130	–0.012, 0.092
Middle	–0.104	0.034	0.002	–0.169, -0.039
Rich	–0.150	0.040	0.000	–0.227, -0.072
Richest	–0.302	0.053	0.000	–0.404, -0.201
Geographical Factors				
Residence				
Urban	Ref.			
Rural	–0.003	0.034	0.937	–0.069, 0.064
State				
Bihar	Ref.			
Chhattisgarh	0.009	0.046	0.853	–0.082, 0.099
Jharkhand	–0.013	0.044	0.769	–0.098, 0.073
Madhya Pradesh	–0.018	0.040	0.650	–0.095, 0.059
Odisha	–0.052	0.047	0.263	–0.143, 0.039
Rajasthan	–0.075	0.043	0.079	–0.158, 0.009
Uttar Pradesh	0.109	0.031	0.000	0.049, 0.170
Uttarakhand	–0.023	0.067	0.737	–0.154, 0.109
Constant	**–1.519**	**0.147**	**0.000**	**–1.806, –1.232**

Source: Authors' calculation from NFHS-4 (2015-16) data, Ref. = Reference category

nutritional, bio-demographic, maternal, socio-economic and other risk factors. Multivariable adjusted results confirmed that both smaller- ($\beta = 0.253$, 95% CI: 0.197–0.309) and larger-sized births ($\beta = 0.082$, 95% CI: 0.029–0.134) are significantly and positively associated with neonatal mortality. The result also shows that maternal BMI had a significant association with neonatal mortality, indicating a higher mortality risk among those children who were born to overweight (β = 0.218, 95% CI: 0.144–0.291) and obese (β = 0.314, 95% CI: 0.195–0.434) mothers. We observed that multiple gestations had the highest positive coefficient of neonatal mortality (β = 1.166, 95% CI: 1.040–1.291). Birth order was found to be associated with a higher likelihood of mortality among a birth order of five or more (β = 0.119, 95% CI: 0.046–0.192). Children born with a shorter birth interval of less than two years were more likely (β = 0.110, 95% CI: 0.055–0.165) to die than the children delivered with at least two years of birth interval. Older maternal age at birth also had a positive association with neonatal deaths. The association of antenatal care visit of a mother and neonatal death shows a negative direction. Children delivered by the mothers who received less than four (β = –0.131, 95% CI: –0.202 to –0.060) and four and above (β = –0.203, 95% CI: –0.278 to –0.129) antenatal care visits were associated with less likelihood of neonatal mortality than the children delivered by mothers who did not utilize any antenatal care visit. Children delivered by skilled health professionals were associated with less likelihood of neonatal death. Mother's educational attainment also had a significant association with the outcome variable. Infants born with a high household wealth setting had a decreased risk of dying during the neonatal period when compared with the poorest household wealth group.

Discussion

Using a nationally representative cross-sectional data, we investigated the determinants of neonatal mortality in eight EAG states of India and found that smaller birth size, maternal overweight, mother's low level of haemoglobin, multiple gestations, higher birth order, shorter birth interval, caesarean birth and younger (less than 18 years) or older (more than 35 years) maternal age had a strong association with the increased likelihood of neonatal deaths. On the other hand, receiving antenatal care services during pregnancy, delivery by a health professional and maternal education level had a protective effect against neonatal mortality. Our study reasserted the consequence of these potential risk factors for neonatal deaths in the context of high concentration of infant mortality in this region.

Consistent with earlier findings, birth size was an important predictor of neonatal deaths (Mekonnen et al., 2013; Titaley et al., 2008); both smaller-than-average-sized and larger-than-average-sized babies have an increased risk of neonatal mortality. In the absence of adequate birthweight data, we used birth size as a proxy of nutritional status of infants at birth. However, it has widely been evidenced that small-sized births, which may result from premature deliveries, face higher risks of contracting childhood infections and developing other abnormalities, which increases their risk of mortality (Simmons et al, 2010). In contrast, larger-than-average-sized babies have a greater risk of birth injury, congenital malformations and birth asphyxia which could increase the survival risk for neonates (Mekonnen et al., 2013).

We also noted that maternal nutritional status that was measured by BMI had an implication on neonatal mortality; a high maternal BMI was associated with increased risk of neonatal mortality. This may be a result of higher hypertensive disorders in overweight and obese women (Short et al., 2018). Maternal anaemia during pregnancy may cause premature delivery and low birthweight which could increase the risk of neonatal deaths (Young, 2018).

Our results suggest that multiple births are at higher odds of neonatal deaths. A five-year-long prospective study in The Gambia reported that mortality among twins was nearly six times higher than the singletons during the neonatal periods (Miyahara et al., 2016). This may be explained by the fact that infants of multiple gestations have a higher degree of prematurity compared to singletons which increases the mortality risk among them (Kayode et al., 2014). Infants born with shorter birth intervals (less than two years) are positively associated with neonatal deaths in the present study, in line with earlier findings from several low- and middle-income countries (Abdullah et al., 2016; Adewuyi & Zhao, 2017; Nisar & Dibley, 2014). This finding implies that extending the interval between two subsequent pregnancies adds benefits to the mothers preparing for the later pregnancy.

Mother's age at the time of child birth plays a crucial role in neonatal survival. We noted that both younger and older maternal age increase the odds of dying of an infant during the neonatal period. This finding is consistent across several earlier studies in the context of neonatal and post-neonatal mortality (Abdullah et al., 2016; Kibria et al., 2018). The relationship between younger maternal age and neonatal survival becomes crucial perhaps due to the fact that adolescent mothers could not reach their full biological or reproductive potential for pregnancy and childbearing (Sharma et al., 2008). Apart from biological or reproductive immaturity, younger mothers lack experience regarding healthcare knowledge and new-borns' care practices which may act as potential factors for neonatal deaths. On the other side, an older maternal age is associated with increased delivery complications and low birthweight which may significantly elevate the risk of neonatal survival (Jacobsson et al., 2004).

We noted that utilization of antenatal care during pregnancy significantly reduces the risk of death among the neonates. This finding is consistent with previous studies conducted in India and its neighbour countries, suggesting that four or more antenatal care (ANC) visits have a protective effect on neonatal survival (Singh et al., 2013). From regular ANC visits, pregnant women receive treatment for preventive diseases such as anaemia and tetanus and receive counselling regarding institutional delivery practices (Bloom, Lippeveld & Wypij, 1999). Regular antenatal care visits have been one of the key strategies recommended to prevent the maternal and neonatal deaths in many low- and middle-income countries, including India. Due to its effectiveness, it is also considered one of the four main pillars of the 'Safe Motherhood Initiative'. However, our results report that more than one-fourth of pregnant women never visited for an ANC service in the EAG states of India, indicating that ANC service is poorly utilized in this region.

Conclusion and Policy Recommendation

Several nutritional, bio-demographic and socio-economic factors of children and mothers have emerged as highly significant predictors of neonatal mortality in the EAG states of India. Besides, a number of socio-economic and household factors contributed to increasing the number of neonatal deaths in the EAG states of India. While identifying the potential determinants of neonatal deaths in eight highly focussed states of India, we recommend that an integrated or multifaceted approach is needed to address all the potential factors associated with neonatal deaths in the EAG states. From an intervention point of view, it is necessary to consider the modifiable risk factors in designing neonatal survival programmes. Programmes that focus on alleviating maternal anaemia during pregnancy and after childbirth are urgently needed in the EAG states. Reducing maternal anaemia through locally produced iron-rich food distribution has gained renewed attention among the policymakers in sub-Saharan African countries due to its low cost and effectiveness (Pasricha et al., 2013). New strategies such as community outreach programmes could supplement the regular ANC visit. There is an urgent need for community-level monitoring and evaluation on ongoing continuum care services to track the progress in maternal and new-born healthcare utilization at the grassroots level (Kenny et al., 2013). Adopting family planning services can benefit in increasing the birth interval time as well as reducing the proportion of undesirable pregnancies among younger or older mothers. Furthermore, delaying the age of marriage for women, thereby reducing the burden of young age pregnancy and childbearing, could improve the situation of neonatal mortality in the EAG states. More research is needed to identify other unexamined factors in the context of high neonatal deaths in the EAG states.

References

Abdullah, A., Hort, K., Butu, Y., & Simpson, L. (2016). Risk factors associated with neonatal deaths: A matched case–control study in Indonesia. *Global Health Action, 9*(1), 30445.

Adewuyi, E. O., & Zhao, Y. (2017). Determinants of neonatal mortality in rural and urban Nigeria: Evidence from a population-based national survey. *Pediatrics International, 59*(2), 190–200.

Akseer, N., Lawn, J. E., Keenan, W., Konstantopoulos, A., Cooper, P., Ismail, Z.,... & Bhutta, Z. A. (2015). Ending preventable newborn deaths in a generation. *International Journal of Gynecology & Obstetrics, 131*(Supplement 1), S43–S48.

Al Kibria, G. M., Burrowes, V., Choudhury, A., Sharmeen, A., Ghosh, S., Mahmud, A., & Angela, K. C. (2018). Determinants of early neonatal mortality in Afghanistan: An analysis of the Demographic and Health Survey 2015. *Globalization and Health, 14*(1), 47.

Bloom, S. S., Lippeveld, T., & Wypij, D. (1999). Does antenatal care make a difference to safe delivery? A study in urban Uttar Pradesh, India. *Health Policy and Planning*, 14(1), 38–48.

Cooper, P. (2016). Strategies to reduce perinatal mortality. *The Lancet Global Health*, 4(1), e6–e7.

Fottrell, E., Osrin, D., Alcock, G., Azad, K., Bapat, U., Beard, J.,... & Manandhar, D. (2015). Cause-specific neonatal mortality: Analysis of 3772 neonatal deaths in Nepal, Bangladesh, Malawi and India. *Archives of Disease in Childhood-Fetal and Neonatal Edition*, 100(5), F439–F447.

International Institute for Population Sciences (IIPS) and ICF (2017). *National Family Health Survey (NFHS-4), 2015–16: India*. Mumbai: IIPS.

International Institute for Population Sciences (IIPS) and ICF (2021). *National Family Health Survey (NFHS-5), 2019–21: India*. Mumbai: IIPS.

Jacobsson, B., Ladfors, L., & Milsom, I. (2004). Advanced maternal age and adverse perinatal outcome. *Obstetrics & Gynecology*, 104(4), 727–733.

Kayode, G. A., Ansah, E., Agyepong, I. A., Amoakoh-Coleman, M., Grobbee, D. E., & Klipstein-Grobusch, K. (2014). Individual and community determinants of neonatal mortality in Ghana: A multilevel analysis. *BMC Pregnancy and Childbirth*, 14(1), 165.

Kenny, L. C., Lavender, T., McNamee, R., O'Neill, S. M., Mills, T., & Khashan, A. S. (2013). Advanced maternal age and adverse pregnancy outcome: Evidence from a large contemporary cohort. *PloS One*, 8(2), e56583.

Kruk, M. E., Gage, A. D., Joseph, N. T., Danaei, G., García-Saisó, S., & Salomon, J. A. (2018). Mortality due to low-quality health systems in the universal health coverage era: A systematic analysis of amenable deaths in 137 countries. *The Lancet*, 392(10160), 2203–2212.

Kumar, C., Singh, P. K., Rai, R. K., & Singh, L. (2013). Early neonatal mortality in India, 1990–2006. *Journal of Community Health*, 38(1), 120–130.

Ladusingh, L., Gupta, A. K., & Yadav, A. (2016). Ecological context of infant mortality in high-focus states of India. *Epidemiology and Health*, 38, e2016006.

Liu, L., Oza, S., Hogan, D., Chu, Y., Perin, J., Zhu, J.,... & Black, R. E. (2016). Global, regional, and national causes of under-5 mortality in 2000–15: An updated systematic analysis with implications for the Sustainable Development Goals. *The Lancet*, 388(10063), 3027–3035.

Mekonnen, Y., Tensou, B., Telake, D. S., Degefie, T., & Bekele, A. (2013). Neonatal mortality in Ethiopia: Trends and determinants. *BMC Public Health*, 13(1), 483.

Miyahara, R., Jasseh, M., Mackenzie, G. A., Bottomley, C., Hossain, M. J., Greenwood, B. M.,... & Roca, A. (2016). The large contribution of twins to neonatal and post-neonatal mortality in The Gambia, a 5-year prospective study. *BMC Pediatrics*, 16(1), 39.

Moss, W., Darmstadt, G. L., Marsh, D. R., Black, R. E., & Santosham, M. (2002). Research priorities for the reduction of perinatal and neonatal morbidity and mortality in developing country communities. *Journal of Perinatology*, 22(6), 484.

Nisar, Y. B., & Dibley, M. J. (2014). Determinants of neonatal mortality in Pakistan: Secondary analysis of Pakistan Demographic and Health Survey 2006–07. *BMC Public Health*, 14(1), 663.

Pasricha, S. R., Drakesmith, H., Black, J., Hipgrave, D., & Biggs, B. A. (2013). Control of iron deficiency anaemia in low-and middle-income countries. *Blood: The Journal of the American Society of Hematology*, 121(14), 2607–2617.

Rajaratnam, J. K., Marcus, J. R., Flaxman, A. D., Wang, H., Levin-Rector, A., Dwyer, L.,... & Murray, C. J. (2010). Neonatal, postneonatal, childhood, and under-5 mortality for 187 countries, 1970–2010: A systematic analysis of progress towards Millennium Development Goal 4. *The Lancet, 375*(9730), 1988–2008.

Saikia, N., Shkolnikov, V. M., Jasilionis, D., & Chandrashekhar. (2016). Trends and sub-national disparities in neonatal mortality in India from 1981 to 2011. *Asian Population Studies, 12*(1), 88–107.

Sankar, M. J., Natarajan, C. K., Das, R. R., Agarwal, R., Chandrasekaran, A., & Paul, V. K. (2016). When do newborns die? A systematic review of the timing of overall and cause-specific neonatal deaths in developing countries. *Journal of Perinatology, 36*(S1), S1.

Sharma, V., Katz, J., Mullany, L. C., Khatry, S. K., LeClerq, S. C., Shrestha, S. R.,... & Tielsch, J. M. (2008). Young maternal age and the risk of neonatal mortality in rural Nepal. *Archives of Pediatrics & Adolescent Medicine, 162*(9), 828–835.

Short, V. L., Geller, S. E., Moore, J. L., McClure, E. M., Goudar, S. S., Dhaded, S. M.,... & Goldenberg, R. L. (2018). The relationship between body mass index in pregnancy and adverse maternal, perinatal, and neonatal outcomes in Rural India and Pakistan. *American Journal of Perinatology, 35*(09), 844–851.

Simmons, L. E., Rubens, C. E., Darmstadt, G. L., & Gravett, M. G. (2010). Preventing preterm birth and neonatal mortality: Exploring the epidemiology, causes, and interventions. *Seminars in Perinatology, 34*(6), 408–415.

Singh, A., Pallikadavath, S., Ram, F., & Alagarajan, M. (2013). Do antenatal care interventions improve neonatal survival in India?. *Health Policy and Planning, 29*(7), 842–848.

Sinha, S., Aggarwal, A. R., Osmond, C., Fall, C. H., Bhargava, S. K., & Sachdev, H. S. (2016). Maternal age at childbirth and perinatal and under-five mortality in a prospective birth cohort from Delhi. *Indian Pediatrics, 53*(10), 871–877.

Titaley, C. R., Dibley, M. J., Agho, K., Roberts, C. L., & Hall, J. (2008). Determinants of neonatal mortality in Indonesia. *BMC Public Health, 8*(1), 232.

You, D., Hug, L., Ejdemyr, S., Idele, P., Hogan, D., Mathers, C.,... & Alkema, L. (2015). Global, regional, and national levels and trends in under-5 mortality between 1990 and 2015, with scenario-based projections to 2030: A systematic analysis by the UN Inter-agency Group for Child Mortality Estimation. *The Lancet, 386*(10010), 2275–2286.

Young, M. F. (2018). Maternal anaemia and risk of mortality: A call for action. *The Lancet Global Health, 6*(5), e479–e480.

3 Disparities in Health Outcome of Empowered Action Group States of India

A Panel Data Approach

Aditya Kumar Patra

Introduction

Infant and child mortality have traditionally been considered the most significant indicator of health. Children are important assets of a nation; hence, reduction in infant and child mortality is the prime objective of the Millennium Development Goals (MDGs), which were recently redesigned and rechristened as Sustainable Development Goals (SDGs), and Goal 3: Target 3.2 of SDG proclaims 'by 2030, end preventable deaths of newborns and children under 5 years of age, with all countries aiming to reduce neo-natal mortality to at least as low as 12 per 1,000 live births and under-five mortalities to at least as low as 25 per 1,000 live births'.

There is remarkable progress in the decline in child mortality across the globe. The global under-five mortality rate (U5MR) dropped from 93 per 1,000 live births in 1990 to 41 per 1,000 live births in 2016. The latest figure for India shows that the infant mortality rate (IMR) is 28 and U5MR is 32 (SRS, 2020), but there exists inter-state variation regarding IMR and U5MR in India. IMR records are high in northern states such as Madhya Pradesh (43), Uttar Pradesh (38), and Chhattisgarh (38) and low in southern states such as Kerala (6), Tamil Nadu (12), and Karnataka (19). Likewise, U5MR ranges from a high of 51 in Madhya Pradesh, 43 in Uttar Pradesh, 41 in Chhattisgarh, and 40 in Rajasthan to as low as 8 in Kerala, 13 in Tamil Nadu, 18 in Maharashtra, 21 in Karnataka, and 22 in West Bengal.

It has been evident from various studies that infant mortality is negatively associated with the level of child immunisation, better socio-economic status, and better nutritional status of mother and child. Studies found the health status of an infant is determined by environmental factors, income, and education (Auster et al. 1969; Hadley, 1982). Culyer (1991) pointed out that income, public expenditure on health and literacy rate influences health status significantly; the World Bank (1993) mentioned that, in less developed economies, income and female literacy affect the health status significantly, while in advanced economies, income distribution plays a dominant role on health status; John Hobcraft (1993) analysed the importance of women's education for child health, especially child survival in the Third World countries. Link B.G. and Jo Phelan (1995) highlighted the role of female education

DOI: 10.4324/9781003430636-5

to reduce the disease burden of the society. Krieger J. and Donna L. Higgins (2002) examined the importance of social determinants of health including housing conditions, viz., safe drinking water facility, waste disposal, toilet facility and sanitation, on the health of the people, while examining the biological determinants, Khadka et al. (2015) observed that size of a baby at birth, birth order, and birth interval or spacing are important biological determinants of infant mortality rate. Genowska et al. (2015) found that poor working environments and industrial pollution cause high infant mortality. The study by Kiross et al. (2021) emphasises community-level factors, viz. place and region of residence, access to improved water and sanitation, decision-making autonomy of females, and multidimensional poverty index, which needs to be considered to control infant mortality. Researchers very often mentioned the importance of female education and per capita GDP/ GSDP as key determinants of infant mortality (Schell et al., 2007; Mukherjee et al., 2019; Dutta et al., 2020). Research undertaken by Tang (2019) and Patel et al. (2021) concluded that public healthcare spending, governance system and utilisation of healthcare services by people determine the extent of infant death.

The studies documented above suggest progress in the field of health outcomes in terms of reduction in child mortality hinges on the availability and accessibility of healthcare facilities or infrastructure. Further, it is worth mentioning that few studies in the Indian context specifically emphasises the empowered action group (EAG) states and the associated factors of IMR in these states.

Against this backdrop, an attempt has been made in this chapter to examine two important aspects of health sector, viz. (1) to trace out the regional disparity that exists with regard to health infrastructure and some controllable non-health-system variables and (2) mapping of the EAG of states vis-a-vis other states of India in the field of health outcome, more particularly infant mortality rate and its associated components.

The State of Infant and Child Mortality in India and States

The latest figure for India shows that IMR is 28 and U5MR is 32 for the Year 2020 (SRS, 2020). However, there exists inter-state variation regarding IMR and U5MR. Among the major states of India, the IMR and U5MR are high for Uttar Pradesh, Madhya Pradesh, Rajasthan, Bihar, Chhattisgarh, Odisha, and Assam and low in Kerala, Tamil Nadu, Maharashtra, and Delhi. As evidenced by the sample registration system (SRS), the trend in mortality level for India and its bigger states has stagnated since the late 1990s (Saikia et al., 2010; Claeson et al., 2000). Further, it is observed from the SRS data, the rate of decline in infant mortality stagnated for a brief period during 1981–97 and was then followed by a subsequent rapid decline (Figure 3.1). However, during the period 1999–06, the reduction in infant and child mortality rates slowed down considerably (Saikia et al., 2010).

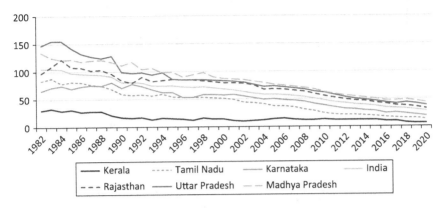

Figure 3.1 Infant Mortality Rate in Six Major States of India

The decline in infant and child mortality is not uniform across time and region. This can be verified from the table given below (Table 3.1).

Literature suggests that infant mortality is negatively associated with the level of child immunisation, better socio-economic status, and better nutritional status of mother and child. For analytical purpose, it is useful to categorise different conditions and causes of infant deaths as antenatal care, conditions of delivery and birth, immunisation, early diagnosis and treatment of fevers, coughs, acute respiratory infection, diarrhoea and other infectious diseases, and safe drinking water and sanitation (Mosley and Chen, 1984; Martin et al., 1983; Mishra et al., 2005; Fotso et al., 2007). Different states of India are not uniformly placed across these variables. This causes inter-state disparity with respect to IMR and U5MR.

It is observed that although progress in some states is satisfactory, poor performance in some other states, particularly Bihar, Uttar Pradesh, Madhya Pradesh, Rajasthan, and Odisha, is proving to be a drag on national achievement. Unless urgent and focused interventions are undertaken to address the issues of reproductive and child healthcare in these states, the attainment of demographic goals seems unlikely.

In tune with this, the Prime Minister of India in his address to the National Population Commission announced the creation of the EAG in the Ministry of Health and Family Welfare for undertaking measures for population stabilisation and intersectoral convergence. Accordingly, on 20 March 2001, the EAG was constituted as an administrative mechanism for the purpose of closely monitoring the implementation of the Family Welfare Programme in the EAG states, viz. Bihar, Jharkhand, Madhya Pradesh, Chhattisgarh, Uttar Pradesh, Uttarakhand, Rajasthan, and Odisha to facilitate the preparation of area-specific programme to address unmet needs. In India, these eight socio-economically backward states are referred to as the EAG states. The EAG is a high-powered window clearance mechanism for approving schemes to

Table 3.1 Childhood Mortality Rate among the States of India

State	NFHS II (1998–99)		NFHS III (2005–06)		NFHS IV (2015–16)		NFHS V (2019–21)	
	IMR ($_1q_0$)	USMR ($_5q_0$)	IMR ($_1q_0$)	USMR ($_5q_0$)	IMR ($_1q_0$)	USMR ($_5q_0$)	IMR ($_1q_0$)	USMR ($_5q_0$)
EAG States								
Bihar	72.9	105.1	61.7	84.8	48.1	58.1	46.8	56.4
Chhattisgarh			70.8	90.3	54.0	64.3	44.3	50.4
Jharkhand			68.7	93.0	43.8	54.3	37.9	45.4
Madhya Pradesh	86.1	137.6	69.5	94.2	51.2	64.6	41.3	49.2
Odisha	81.0	104.4	64.7	90.6	39.6	48.1	36.3	41.1
Rajasthan	80.4	114.9	65.3	85.4	41.3	50.7	30.3	37.6
Uttarakhand			41.9	56.8	39.7	46.5	39.1	45.6
Uttar Pradesh	86.7	122.5	72.7	96.4	63.5	78.1	50.4	59.8
Non-EAG States								
Andhra Pradesh	65.8	85.5	53.5	63.2	34.9	40.8	30.3	35.2
Assam	69.5	89.5	66.1	85.0	47.6	56.5	31.9	39.1
Goa	36.7	46.8	15.3	20.3	12.9	12.9	5.6	10.6
Gujarat	62.6	85.1	49.7	60.9	34.2	43.5	31.2	37.6
Haryana	56.8	76.8	41.7	52.3	32.8	41.1	33.3	38.7
Karnataka	51.5	69.8	43.2	54.7	26.9	31.5	25.4	29.5
Kerala	16.3	18.8	15.3	16.3	5.6	7.1	4.4	5.2
Maharashtra	43.7	58.1	37.5	46.7	23.7	28.7	23.2	28.0
Punjab	57.1	72.1	41.7	52.0	29.2	33.2	28.0	32.7
Tamil Nadu	48.2	63.3	30.4	35.5	20.2	26.8	18.6	22.3
West Bengal	48.7	67.6	48.0	59.6	27.5	31.8	22.0	25.4
India	67.6	94.9	57.0	74.3	40.7	49.7	35.2	41.9

Source: National Family Health Survey

finalise strategies and addressing the gaps in the ongoing programmes, and to facilitate intersectoral convergence. It provides a specific focus on the concerned states and helps them to plan, implement, and monitor interventions that are aimed at raising performance indicators.

Data and Method

To examine the objectives stated above, we have used data from secondary sources, viz. National Family Health Survey 2nd, 3rd, 4th, and 5th rounds. The period of reference is 1998–99, 2005–06, 2015–16, and 2019–21. The study concentrates on examining the situation of 18 states of India. These are Andhra Pradesh, Assam, Bihar, Chhattisgarh, Gujarat, Haryana, Jharkhand, Karnataka, Kerala, Maharashtra, Madhya Pradesh, Odisha, Punjab, Rajasthan, Tamil Nadu, Uttarakhand, Uttar Pradesh, and West Bengal.

To examine the inter-state disparity of Health Sector Development in India, this article focuses on the relative efficiency of the public health system in improving the health outcome (in terms of IMR) of different states in India. An efficient health service system is one that achieves the best result with the lowest cost. Farrell (1957) initiated the concept of modern efficiency measurement for any decision-making unit. The economic efficiency of any unit is the product of technical efficiency (TE) and allocative efficiency (AE). The former reflects the ability of a unit to obtain maximum output from a given set of inputs and technology, whereas the latter shows the ability of a unit to use inputs in optimal proportions given their respective prices. The prime concern in technical efficiency is whether the actual outcome could be achieved with fewer inputs or if the same set of inputs could produce better outcomes. Broadly, there are two approaches to estimating efficiency: The parametric approach known as 'stochastic frontier analysis' and non-parametric approach popularly known as 'data envelopment analysis'.

Empirical studies using the stochastic frontier approach analysed health sector efficiency at both country- and state-specific levels (Schmacker and McKay, 2008; Kontodimopoulos, Nanos and Niakas, 2003; Farsi, Filippini and Lunati, 2008; Sankar and Kathuria, 2004;, Mathiyazhgan (2006), Purohit (2008) for India and states; Wang, Zhao, and Mahmood (2006).

In this study, we employ the stochastic frontier approach for panel data to measure the technical efficiency of health outcomes (in terms of IMR) in 18 major states of India. Following the works of Murray and Frank (1999) and Evans et al. (2001) as a theoretical backdrop for the estimation of health system performance, i.e., efficiency of different states is explained below (Figure 3.2).

In the figure, the goal of the health sector is shown on the vertical axis and the inputs that require to achieve the goal are shown on the horizontal axis. The upper line represents the frontier or the maximum possible level that could be obtained for a given level of inputs, and the lower line reflects the level that would occur in the absence of the system, assuming that a society is

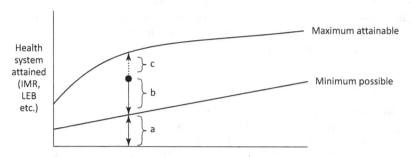

Figure 3.2 Investment in Health System Resources and Other Health Determinants

Source: Adapted from Murray and Frenk (1999)

observed to have achieved (a+b) units against the maximum possible (a+b+c) units. Therefore, the system performance in the present scenario will be b/(b+c). The above ratio indicates the level of achievement vis-a-vis the potential. The ratio of actual and potential performance is nothing but a measure of 'technical efficiency.' The system could have achieved better outcomes with the resources that it has invested in the health system along with other determinants of the health outcome.

Therefore, the pertinent question is how we can measure the maximum potential level of health outcome a society can achieve with the available inputs. Under the 'stochastic frontier approach', we start with a simple production function as:

$$Y_{it} = A_i f(X_{kit}) \tag{1}$$

where Y denotes the health outcome; X denotes the health sector inputs; i subscript shows cross-section; t subscript shows time; k shows number of inputs; and A_i is the level of productivity, which is assumed to vary across states as each state is a distinct unit and utilises different infrastructures in a unique way even with similar circumstance to achieve the health outcome.

The empirical model can be written as:

$$y_{it} = \alpha + X'_{it}\beta + v_{it} - u_i \tag{2}$$

Here, y_{it} is output (say IMR) for state i in time period t; X_{it} is a vector of k inputs; v_{it} is the stochastic (white noise) error term; and u_i is a one-sided error term representing the technical (in)efficiency of health system of the state, which differ across states. Both v_i and u_i are assumed to be independently and identically distributed (iid) with variances σ_v^2 and σ_u^2, respectively.

Most earlier studies on frontier estimation have been cross-sectional, but now with the availability of panel data, the need for strong distributional assumptions about the error term becomes obviates. This facilitates the estimation of state-specific technical efficiency. In panel data analysis, u_i is an unobservable time-invariant state-specific effect that can be measured either by fixed-effects model (FEM) or random-effects model (REM). In the literature of econometrics, the choice of FEM or REM is settled through the 'Hausman test'.

Now the earlier model represented in equation (2) can be rewritten as:

$$y_{it} = \alpha_i + X'_{it}\beta + v_{it} \tag{3}$$

where $\alpha_i = (\alpha - u_i)$ is the efficiency level of the ith state. If the maximum of α_i is the health performance of the most efficient state (MES), then the relative efficiency of ith state would be:

$$E_i = |\alpha_i - \alpha| \tag{4}$$

A high value of E_i in absolute term implies that the state i is very inefficient relative to the most efficient state, and if the efficiency level of MES is 100 per cent, then each state's estimated productivity efficiency in relation to MES can be calculated as:

$$S_i = E_i / \alpha \tag{5}$$

The analytical approach of this article is twofold: 1) to find out the most efficient state with respect to health performance (in terms of IMR) and map out the position of other states and 2) to ascertain the impact of non-health parameters on the efficiency level.

Tracking Health and Non-Health Sector Infrastructure Facilities

Government Medical Institution

Table 3.2 describes the state-wise population served per 'government medical institution' and 'Number of Government Medical Institutions' per lakh of population in the years 2005 and 2015. The table also describes the change in the status of the state in this regard. It is observed from the table that in four out of eighteen states, the situation has deteriorated. These states are Andhra Pradesh, Karnataka, Gujarat, and Maharashtra. Even though the absolute number of medical institutions in these states has increased, yet with the increase in population, 'population served per government medical institution' and 'number of government medical institution per lakh of population' has been reduced. All other states have improved their position in this respect. Rajasthan and Uttarakhand top the list with 4.35 medical institutions per lakh of population, so the number of population served per medical institution has been reduced from 120176 to 22288 and 247917 to 22824, respectively. On the contrary, Haryana is at the bottom with 0.60 institutions per lakh of population and a high of 165198 populations served per medical institution.

Table 3.2 Population Served per Medical Facility

States	Population Served per Government Medical Institution		Change of Status over the period	Government Medical Institution per lakh of Population	
	2005	2015		2005	2015
Andhra Pradesh	154376	190772	D	1.30	1.06
Assam	280500	27545	I	0.36	3.48
Bihar	869406	69839	I	0.11	1.30
Chhattisgarh	159500	39104	I	0.62	2.35
Gujarat	108974	156106	D	0.93	0.61
Haryana	170444	165198	I	0.59	0.60
Jharkhand	602191	59825	I	0.16	1.59
Karnataka	76744	101377	D	1.31	0.94
Kerala	177614	27392	I	0.58	3.76
Madhya Pradesh	186373	174022	I	0.50	0.56
Maharashtra	86560	109874	D	1.14	0.90
Odisha	96190	23688	I	1.05	4.02
Punjab	158350	117828	I	0.62	0.83
Rajasthan	120176	22288	I	0.84	4.35
Tamil Nadu	153917	86630	I	0.66	1.06
Uttar Pradesh	601241	222688	I	0.16	0.46
Uttarakhand	247917	22824	I	0.40	4.35
West Bengal	131924	58188	I	0.77	1.66
ALL INDIA	156556	61011	I	0.64	1.60

Source: National Health Profile, 2005, CBHI, MoH and FW, GoI
Notes: 'I' stands for improvement, and 'D' stands for deterioration

Non-Health Sector Parameters

It has been observed from the literature that non-health sector parameters play a crucial role in the development of healthcare services. Table 3.3 displays several non-health sector variables like drinking water, toilet facility, female literacy rate, and per capita income across states of India in 2005-06, 2015-16, and 2019-21 as per NFHS III, NFHS IV, and NFHS V, respectively. In every indicator, it is observed that there is an improvement over time, irrespective of the economic status of the states. With regard to drinking water facilities, most of the states achieved more than 90 per cent coverage. Two states, Jharkhand and Madhya Pradesh, recorded low achievements of 86.8 and 88.9 per cent, respectively. However, in the field of toilet facility data are not so encouraging. Kerala tops the list with 99.8 per cent followed by Punjab with 97.3 per cent. Economically backward states depict a very dismal picture in toilet facilities. Bihar recorded the lowest position in the toilet facility with 61.7 per cent preceded by Odisha with 71.3 per cent. The female literacy rate is concerned that Kerala and Tamil Nadu achieved more than 90 per cent, and most of the states record more than 60 per cent. The female literacy rate in undivided Bihar and Rajasthan is 53.3 and 52.6, respectively. The disparity in per capita income is very high in Indian states, and it

Table 3.3 Non-Health Sector Parameters

State	NFHS-3 Drinking Water	NFHS-4 Drinking Water	NFHS-5 Drinking Water	NFHS-3 Toilet Facility	NFHS-4 Toilet Facility	NFHS-5 Toilet Facility	2001 Female Literacy	2011 Female Literacy	2005–06 Per Capita Income	2015–16 Per Capita Income
Andhra Pradesh	94	72.7	99.1	42.4	61.3	85.3	50.43	59.74	25959	43694
Assam	72.4	83.8	86.4	76.4	88.9	95.9	54.61	67.27	16782	24729
Bihar	96.1	98.2	99.1	25.2	33.5	61.7	33.12	53.33	7914	12816
Chhattisgarh	77.9	91.1	95.6	18.7	41.3	85.9	51.85	60.59	18559	33745
Gujarat	89.8	96.9	97.5	54.6	71	81.9	57.8	70.73	32021	61462
Haryana	95.6	91.6	98.6	52.4	89.8	96.8	55.73	66.77	37972	68599
Jharkhand	57	77.7	86.8	22.6	30	69.6	38.87	56.21	18510	26921
Karnataka	86.2	89.3	95.6	46.5	65.8	83.1	56.87	68.13	26882	58332
Kerala	69.1	94.3	94.9	96.1	99.2	99.8	87.72	91.98	32351	62055
Madhya Pradesh	77.9	84.7	88.9	18.7	42.8	76.2	50.29	60.02	15442	24468
Maharashtra	92.7	91.5	93.8	52.9	71.2	87.6	67.03	75.48	36077	63328
Odisha	78.4	88.8	90.8	19.3	35	71.3	50.51	64.36	17650	29918
Punjab	99.5	99.1	98.8	70.8	92.9	97.3	63.36	71.34	33103	52874
Rajasthan	81.8	85.5	96.4	30.8	54	78.7	43.85	52.66	18565	35608
Tamil Nadu	93.5	90.6	98.6	42.9	61.7	81.5	64.43	93.86	30062	58603
Uttar Pradesh	93.7	96.4	99.2	59.6	45.8	78.4	42.22	59.26	12950	19086
Uttarakhand	87.4	92.9	95.5	56.8	82.9	93.8	59.63	70.7	24726	65556
West Bengal	93.7	94.6	97.5	59.6	74.9		59.61	71.16	22649	30088
ALL INDIA	77.9	89.9	95.9	36	61.1	89.0	53.67	65.46	24095	47818

Source: NFHS Rounds 3 and 4, Census Report, Government of India, and RBI Data Base

accentuates over time. The list of per capita income in 2015-16 is headed by Haryana with Rs. 68599 and ended by Bihar with Rs. 12816. Therefore, the ratio of the highest and lowest per capita income stands at 5.35:1.

Maternal Healthcare Indicators

Maternal healthcare indicators play a very crucial role in lowering the maternal mortality ratio and infant mortality rate. We have selected four maternal care indicators in the analysis. It includes percentage of pregnant women who had full antenatal care visits (full ANC includes having received at least four ANC visits, at least one TT injection, and taken IFA tablets or syrup for 100 or more days), percentage of births delivered in a health facility (institutional delivery), percentage of deliveries assisted by a skilled health provider (a skilled provider includes a doctor, ANM, nurse, midwife, lady health visitor, and other health personnel), and percentage of deliveries with a postnatal check for the mother in first two days of birth (DPNC2). Table 3.4 displays data on these variables across eighteen states and all India levels in 2005–06, 2015–16, and 2019–21. Data reveal that maternal healthcare indicators have shown an improvement in all states over time.

With regard to pregnant women who had full antenatal care visits, it is noticed that the performance of the states is not encouraging. Several states, viz. Bihar, Jharkhand, and Uttar Pradesh, recorded less than 50 per cent. At the all-India level, it is only 58.1 per cent. Tamil Nadu spearheaded the list with only 89.9 per cent. However, in the field of institutional delivery, states are in a comfortable position. At the all-India level, it is 88.6 per cent. Twelve out of eighteen states recorded more than 90 per cent points, and most of them are more than 95 per cent. The list is headed by Kerala (99.8 per cent), and Jharkhand (75.8 per cent) is at the nethermost position.

So far as percentage of deliveries assisted by a skilled provider (DASHP) is concerned, the result is more or less the same as that of institutional delivery. The minimum percentage is registered in Bihar at 78.9. The all-India average stands at 89.4 per cent and Kerala marked a record value of 100 per cent.

A major portion of maternal and neonatal death occurs within forty-eight hours of delivery. Therefore, percentage of deliveries with a postnatal check for the mother in the first two days of birth (DPNC2) is very important. Kerala, where 93.3 per cent of deliveries have a postnatal check for the mother in the first two days of birth, tops the list followed by Haryana with 93.1 per cent. On the contrary, Bihar reported a low of 64.2 per cent and stands at the lowest ebb.

An analysis of physical and service inputs clearly shows that there exists inequality in the availability and accessibility of public healthcare services at the state level. Moreover, southern states like Kerala, Karnataka, and Tamil Nadu perform very encouraging results, whereas undivided Bihar, Madhya Pradesh, Odisha, Rajasthan, and Uttar Pradesh depict disquieting features. Economically advanced states like Haryana, Gujarat, and Maharashtra do

Table 3.4 Maternal Healthcare Indicators

States	NFHS-3 All ANC	NFHS-4 All ANC	NFHS-5 All ANC	NFHS-3 Ins Del	NFHS-4 Ins Del	NFHS-5 Ins Del	NFHS-3 DASHP	NFHS-4 DASHP	NFHS-5 DASHP	NFHS-3 DPNC2	NFHS-4 DPNC2	NFHS-5 DPNC2
Andhra Pradesh	28.2	43.9	67.5	64.4	91.5	96.5	74.9	92.1	96.1	64.1	80.5	91.0
Assam	9.6	18.1	50.7	22.4	70.6	84.1	31	74.3	86.1	13.9	57.6	69.4
Bihar	5.8	3.3	25.2	19.9	63.8	76.2	29.3	69.9	78.9	15.9	45.9	64.2
Chhattisgarh	11.3	21.7	60.1	14.3	70.2	85.7	41.6	78	88.8	28.4	69	89.1
Gujarat	25.6	30.7	76.9	52.7	88.5	94.3	63	87.1	93.2	56.5	66	91.1
Haryana	14.7	19.5	60.4	35.7	80.4	94.9	48.9	84.6	94.4	55.9	70.8	93.1
Jharkhand	7.5	8	38.6	18.3	61.9	75.8	27.8	69.6	82.5	17	48.5	76.7
Karnataka	29.6	32.8	70.8	64.7	94	97.0	69.7	93.7	93.8	58.5	65.8	87.9
Kerala	63.6	61.2	78.6	99.3	99.8	99.8	99.4	99.9	100	84.9	88.8	93.2
Madhya Pradesh	7.2	11.4	57.5	26.2	80.8	90.7	32.7	78	89.3	28.5	56.9	86.4
Maharashtra	21.6	32.4	70.3	64.6	90.3	94.7	68.7	91.1	93.8	58.7	79.7	85.9
Odisha	18.4	23	78.1	35.6	85.3	92.2	44	86.5	91.8	33.3	78.5	92.2
Punjab	19.6	30.7	59.3	51.3	90.5	94.3	68.2	94.1	95.6	62	89.3	88.1
Rajasthan	8.6	9.7	55.3	29.6	84	94.9	41	86.5	95.6	28.9	64.9	86.1
Tamil Nadu	34	45	89.9	87.8	98.9	99.6	90.6	99.2	99.8	87.2	74.2	92.4
Uttar Pradesh	4.1	5.9	42.4	20.6	67.8	83.4	27.2	70.4	84.8	13.3	58.8	79.0
Uttarakhand	16.1	11.5	61.8	32.6	68.6	83.2	38.5	71.2	83.7	32.4	58.4	84.1
West Bengal	12.3	21.8	75.8	42	75.2	91.7	47.6	81.6	94.1	40.7	63.7	69.6
ALL INDIA	15	20.9	58.1	38.7	78.9	88.6	46.6	81.4	89.4	37.3	65.1	69.6

Source: National Family Health Survey Round III, IV, and V

not pay sufficient attention to the creation of service infrastructure in the field of the health sector; therefore, in many respects, the results are not commensurate with the level of development. The newly created state Uttarakhand carved a respectable position in the health scenario of the country. Barring Kerala and Bihar, no other state maintains its position in the hierarchy of ranking with respect to different health indicators.

Empirical Result

In the present article, we have chosen IMR as the outcome variable and its associated components antenatal care, conditions of delivery and birth, immunisation, early diagnosis and treatment of fevers, coughs, acute respiratory infection, and diarrhoea as the process indicators; health system inputs like the number of medical institutions, number of beds in medical institutions, number of doctors, and other health personnel that contribute to producing the output as input variable; and some controllable non-health-system variables like per capita healthcare expenditure, female literacy rate, provision of safe drinking water, and sanitation as the other determinants of health.

Accessibility and availability of public healthcare services by the residents determine the health performance of the state. The above two facts depend on the number of medical institutions, number of beds in the medical, number of doctors, and other health personnel. But unfortunately, state-wise information is not available for these variables at the reference period. Hence, we select per capita state health expenditure (PCSHE) as one proxy variable to cover these parameters. Further, institutional delivery (ID) and delivery assisted by health personnel are important process variables for lowering the value of IMR. However, these two variables are highly correlated, so we opt for institutional delivery.

In our stochastic model, IMR is the output variable, and per capita state health expenditure and institutional delivery are input variables for 18 states at three different time periods. The results of the fixed-effects model, random-effects model, and Hausman test are reported in Table 3.5. The Hausman test prescribes using the FEM towards the calculation of state-level 'technical efficiency' in the health sector.

The result of the estimation reveals that the input variables, per capita state health expenditure, and institutional delivery are statistically significant and also have correct signs. This implies that the states with higher per capita health expenditure and more institutional delivery have a higher chance of better health outcomes in the form of lower infant mortality rates.

Now, by employing α's (constants) from the stochastic production frontier estimated under the fixed-effects model, we can calculate the relative efficiency indices for different states. Table 3.6 reports the estimated efficiency scores along with the health outcomes. The second column reports the relative efficiency of different states under FEM, the actual IMR for the year

Table 3.5 FEM and REM Estimation of Stochastic Frontier Analysis

Dependent Variable: Infant Mortality Rate

Variable	Fixed-Effects Model		Random-Effects Model	
	Coefficient	Significance (p)	Coefficient	Significance (p)
Constant	108.1798	0.0000	93.4087	0.0000
PCSHE	−7.7766	0.0044	−3.1886	0.1266
ID	−0.2387	0.0250	−0.4485	0.0000
R^2	0.9360		0.7883	
Hausman test: χ^2 = 10.4841 (2 df, P value 0.0053)				

Source: Author's estimates

Table 3.6 Relative Efficiency Score (in %) and Rank

State	Relative Efficiency Score	Actual IMR	Potential IMR	Efficiency Rank
EAG States				
Bihar	81.24	48.1	39.1	8
Chhattisgarh	70.04	54	37.8	17
Jharkhand	77.97	43.8	34.2	12
Madhya Pradesh	70.56	51.2	36.1	16
Odisha	75.40	39.6	29.9	14
Rajasthan	73.58	41.3	30.4	15
Uttarakhand	78.84	39.7	31.3	10
Uttar Pradesh	69.02	63.5	43.8	18
Non-EAG States				
Andhra Pradesh	77.84	34.9	27.2	13
Assam	78.02	47.6	37.1	11
Gujarat	80.23	34.2	27.4	9
Haryana	87.54	32.8	28.7	4
Karnataka	87.15	26.9	23.4	5
Kerala	100.00	5.6	5.6	1
Maharashtra	90.52	23.7	21.5	2
Punjab	84.87	29.2	24.8	7
Tamil Nadu	86.90	20.2	17.6	6
West Bengal	88.63	27.5	24.4	3

Source: Author's estimates

2015–16 is shown in the next column, the fourth column depicts potential IMR, and the last column exhibits the rank of the state in terms of efficiency. Potential IMR is calculated on the basis of the relative efficiency score and the current IMR level. Relative efficiency shows how efficiently a particular state performed in the health sector as compared to the most efficient state.

In the second stage of our analysis, we try to understand the effect of non-health sector parameters on the differences in the technical efficiency of the health system. For this, we posit a model that runs as: dispersion in technical

Table 3.7 Efficiency Dispersion Analysis

Dependent Variable: Efficiency Index			
Variable	Coefficient	t-statistics	P value
Constant	79.034	3.423	0.0039
Safe drinking water facility	0.082	0.376	0.7120
Toilet facility	0.081	0.773	0.4520
Females not attending school	−0.402	−1.910	0.0767
$R^2 = 0.5584$			

Source: Author's estimates

efficiency = f(safe drinking water facility, availability of toilet facility, females not attended school). Hence, the efficiency index is regressed against safe drinking water facilities, availability of toilet facilities, and females not attending school. The result of the analysis is presented in Table 3.7. The estimate indicates that the coefficients of these variables have correct sign, but only one variable is significant.

Conclusion

At the present juncture, many Indian states are far behind SDG with regard to the targeted infant mortality rate and U5MRs. In this chapter, we focus on the efficiency of the healthcare system at the state level to achieve the target. The stochastic frontier approach has been employed towards this end. Our result reveals that EAG states are lagging behind their non-EAG counterparts. So far as the efficiency of the healthcare system is considered, Kerala tops the list followed by Maharashtra and West Bengal, whereas Uttar Pradesh preceded by Chhattisgarh is at the tail end. The result of the panel data estimation shows that states with higher per capita health expenditure and more institutional delivery have a higher chance of better health outcomes. Further, among the non-health sector determinant of healthcare facilities, the important items are safe drinking water facilities, availability of toilet facilities, and female literacy rate. Hence, efforts should be geared up to improve the level of above-mentioned factors to achieve the target. The approaches followed by the efficient states for provisioning of different healthcare facilities and non-health sector parameters be considered as role models and others, more particularly the least efficient states, should adopt them in their policy framework. Distal determinants, like drinking water facilities, sanitation and female literacy, and proximal elements like high public healthcare expenditure, institutional delivery, availability of health personnel, and neonatal services, are emphasised for the reduction of infant mortality rate and U5MRs.

To sum up, it may be suggested that the EAG states should take every effort to avail adequate healthcare facilities for the benefit of the public and due attention be paid to the betterment of different non-health sector parameters, viz. safe drinking water facilities, toilet facilities, and female education to improve the efficiency of the healthcare system.

References

Auster, R., Levenson, I., & Sarachek, D. (1969). The production of health: An exploratory study. *Journal of Human Resources, 4*, 411–436.

Claeson, M, Bos, E. R., Mawji, T., & Pathmanathan, I. (2000). Reducing child mortality in India in the new millennium. *Bulletin of the World Health Organisation, 78*(10), 1192–1199.

Culyer, A. J. (1991). Health care systems in transition: The search for efficiency. In *Social Policy Studies, 7*, Paris: OECD.

Dutta, U. P., Gupta, H., Sarkar, A. K., & Sengupta, P. P. (2020). Some determinants of infant mortality rate in SAARC countries: An empirical assessment through panel data analysis. *Child Indicators Research, 13*(6), 2093–2116.

Farrell, M. J. (1957). The measurement of productive efficiency. *Journal of the Royal Statistical Society Series A, 120*(3), 253–278.

Farsi, M., Filippini, M., & Lunati, D. (2008). *Economies of Scale and Efficiency Measurement in Switzerland's Nursing Homes.* Department of Economics Working Paper 08-01. Switzerland: University of Lugano.

Fotso, J.-C., Ezeh, A. C., Madise, N. J., & Ciera, J. (2007). Progress towards the child mortality millennium development goal in Urban Sub-Saharan Africa: The dynamics of population growth, immunisation, and access to clean water. *BMC Public Health, 7*, 218.

Genowska, A., Jamiołkowski, J., Szafraniec, K., Stepaniak, U., Szpak, A., & Pająk, A. (2015). Environmental and socio-economic determinants of infant mortality in Poland: An ecological study. *Environmental Health, 14*(1), 1–9.

Hadley, J. (1982). *More Medical Care, Better Health.* Washington, DC: The Urban Institute.

Hobcraft, J. (1993). Women's education, child welfare and child survival: A review of the evidence. *Health Transition Review, 3*(2), 159–175.

Kelvin, A. A., & Halperin, S. (2020). COVID-19 in children: The link in the Transmission chain. *Lancet Infect Dis, 20*, 633–634.

Khadka, K. B., Lieberman, L. S., Giedraitis, V., Bhatta, L., & Pandey, G. (2015). The socio-economic determinants of infant mortality in Nepal: Analysis of Nepal demographic health survey, 2011. *BMC Pediatrics, 15*(1), 1–11.

Kiross, G. T., Chojenta, C., Barker, D., & Loxton, D. (2021). Individual-, household- and community-level determinants of infant mortality in Ethiopia. *PloS One, 16*(3), e0248501.

Kontodimopoulos, N., Nanos, P., & Niakas, D. (2003). Balancing efficiency of health services and equity of access in remote areas in Greece. *Health Policy, 76*(1), 49–57.

Krieger, J., & Higgins, D. L. (2002). Housing and health: Time for public health action. *American Journal of Public Health, 92*(5), 758–768. Retrieved from https://doi.org/10.2105/ajph.92.5.758

Link, B. G., & Phelan, J. C. (1995). Social conditions as fundamental causes of disease. *Journal of Health and Social Behaviour, 35*, 80–94.

Martin, L. G., Trussell, J., Salvail, F. R., & Shah, N. M. (1983). Co-variates of child mortality in the Philippines, Indonesia, and Pakistan: An analysis based on hazard models. *Population Studies*, 37(3), 417–432.

Mathiyazhgan, M. K. (2006). *Cost Efficiency of Public and Private Hospitals: Evidence from Karnataka State in India*, Institute of South Asian Studies Working Paper 8. National University of Singapore.

Mishra, V., Roy, T. K., & Retherford, R. D. (2005). Sex differentials in childhood feeding, healthcare, and nutritional status in India. *Population and Development Review*, 30(2), 269–295.

Mosley, W. H., & Chen, L. C. (1984). An analytical framework for the study of child survival in developing Countries. *Population and Development Review*, 10, 25–45.

Mukherjee, A., Bhattacherjee, S., & Dasgupta, S. (2019). Determinants of infant mortality in rural India: An ecological study. *Indian Journal of Public Health*, 63(1), 27.

Murray, C. J. L. and Frenk, J. (1999). *A WHO Framework for Health System Performance Assessment: Global Programme on Evidence and Information for Policy*. Washington, DC: World Bank.

National Family Health Survey (NFHS-2), India, 1998–99 (2007). Mumbai: IIPS.

National Family Health Survey (NFHS-3), India, 2005–06 (2007). Mumbai: IIPS.

National Family Health Survey (NFHS-4), India, 2015–16 (2017). Mumbai: IIPS.

National Family Health Survey (NFHS-5), India, 2020–21 (2021). Mumbai: IIPS.

Patel, K. K., Rai, R., & Rai, A. K. (2021). Determinants of infant mortality in Pakistan: Evidence from Pakistan demographic and health survey 2017–18. *Journal of Public Health*, 29, 693–701.

Purohit, B. C. (2008). Efficiency of healthcare system: A sub-state level analysis for West Bengal (India). *Review of Urban and Regional Development Studies*, 20(3), 212–225.

Saikia et al. (2010). Has child mortality in India really increased in the last two decades? *Economic and Political Weekly*, 45(51) December, 2002, 62–70.

Sankar, D., & Kathuria, V. (2004). Health system performance in rural India: Efficiency estimates across states. *Economic & Political Weekly*, 39(13), 1427–1433.

Schell, C. O., Reilly, M., Rosling, H., Peterson, S., & Mia Ekström, A. (2007). Socioeconomic determinants of infant mortality: A worldwide study of 152 low-, middle-, and high-income countries. *Scandinavian Journal of Public Health*, 35(3), 288–297.

Schmacker, E. R., & McKay, N. L. (2008). Factors affecting productive efficiency in primary care clinics. *Health Services Management Research*, 21(1), 60–70.

Tang, C. F. (2019). Determinants of infant mortality rate in Malaysia: Evidence from dynamic panel data study. *Journal of Health Management*, 21(4), 443–450.

Wang, J., Zhao, Z., & Mahmood, A. (2006). Relative efficiency, scale effect, and scope effect of public hospitals: Evidence from Australia. *IZA Discussion Paper*, 2520. Available at: http://ssrn.com/abstract=956386

3.A Appendix Table

State	Institutional Delivery				Per Capita State Public Health Expenditure		
	1998–99	2005–06	2015–16	2019–21	1998–99	2005–06	2015–16
EAG States							
Bihar	14.6	19.9	63.8	76.2	75.54	122.25	393.80
Chhattisgarh	20.1	14.3	70.2	85.7	147.74	175.16	985.54
Jharkhand	14.6	18.3	61.9	75.8	75.54	334.18	611.53
Madhya Pradesh	20.1	26.2	80.8	90.7	147.74	160.18	702.47
Odisha	22.6	35.6	85.3	92.2	114.26	137.96	837.19
Rajasthan	21.5	29.6	84.0	94.9	162.06	203.63	1059.75
Uttarakhand	15.5	32.6	68.6	83.2	82.23	403.49	1365.27
Uttar Pradesh	15.5	20.6	67.8	83.4	82.23	182.86	627.90
Non- EAG States							
Andhra Pradesh	49.8	64.4	91.5	96.5	139.79	211.05	1025.82
Assam	17.6	22.4	70.6	84.1	91.09	155.79	864.66
Gujarat	46.3	52.7	88.5	94.3	185.58	202.48	1109.85
Haryana	22.4	35.7	80.4	94.9	155.28	211.54	933.76
Karnataka	51.1	64.7	94.0	97.0	75.76	212.44	908.00
Kerala	93.0	99.3	99.8	99.8	184.52	312.33	1397.04
Maharashtra	52.6	64.6	90.3	94.7	128.13	218.53	843.55
Punjab	37.5	51.3	90.5	94.3	221.43	270.18	885.05
Tamil Nadu	79.3	87.8	98.9	99.6	191.82	261.30	1108.69
West Bengal	40.1	42.0	75.2	91.7	147.70	193.67	854.96

Source: Author's Compilation

Part II
Access and Utilisation
Gaps and Challenges

4 Differential Access to Maternal and Child Health Across Social Groups

Issues and Challenges of Discrimination

Sanghmitra S. Acharya

Introduction

There is an intricate relationship between development, women, and health. In this trajectory, utilization of resources and services pertaining to health, by women, is determined by three factors: access, availability, and perception of self. These factors reflect the disparity in utilization and are relevant in addressing the social inclusion of vulnerable populations in the large health system. Thus, it becomes extremely relevant, to examine the determinants of utilization and their interplay with social discrimination and consequent access to health care across population groups. Health, especially maternal and child, has been recognized as an important development indicator. Ensuring healthcare access among vulnerable populations is the prerogative of the state. The financial burden of curative care is higher among lower socio-economic groups. Pathways towards the development goals, the SDGs, and bettering the performance of the EAG states, for instance, align with lowering the burden of curative care among the poor. Although India has achieved considerable improvement in the health of its people in recent times, the gap across social groups remains wide. There is an evident association of low health status with poor, female gender, rural place of residence, tribal ethnicity, scheduled castes (SCs), and specific minority groups. Therefore, the need is to revisit the policy implementation regimes and environment to ensure health equity.

It is imperative to understand the perception of the care providers about care seekers and vice versa on the basis of social identity. While the social determinant framework has given direction to explore beyond economic factors, it does not elaborate on the 'social class'. In the Indian context, given the plurality, or the segmented layers in which the population is grouped, the concept needs to be unpacked accordingly. There are social factors which promote or undermine health, and there are social processes underlying unequal distribution of these factors between groups which occupy unequal positions in the social hierarchy. This paper, therefore, aims at understanding maternal and child health issues in the light of the challenges posed by the selected indicators of social identity, poverty, and illness-induced expenditure across social groups; and the policy suggestions through the index of

DOI: 10.4324/9781003430636-7

maternal and child health using a descriptive analysis approach. It draws from secondary data and the primary data that gathered from the field – a slum colony in Delhi to reflect on the paradox of poor socio-demographic conditions of EAG, despite being a 'metropolitan'.

Development and Women of Different Hues

The development narrative concentrates on gender parity and positions women evenly across strata. It often homogenizes experiences and contexts and does not delve deeper into women's life experiences. It has accounted women as beneficiaries more than participants in development. It has also not explored the complex socio-political, cultural, and economic dynamics that women live through every day. There are about 33 million women in Self Health Groups (SHGs); 1.3 million women elected representatives in our panchayats[1]; and we also have 20,000 homemakers committing suicide annually.[2] Significantly higher than that farmer suicides, which form a big part of our country's developmental and political discourse, this remains devoid of explicit concern despite the fact that they host and nurture future generations.

Development narrative focuses either on the productive role of women and their bodies or on their economic role as workers. The category of 'women' is itself pluralistic. Treating women as a homogenous group has yielded erroneous frameworks for any enquiry about them. Women as the homogenized group have hidden more than revealed the realities about them across social groups. Thus, the discourse on women in the context of development and health needs to be disaggregated keeping aside the fear of fracturing the 'unity'. The gendered consciousness requires to be independent of any commitment to patriarchy (Burton, 2014). As development reflects itself through a spectrum of indicators, women, by gender disaggregation, begin to slip down the ladder of gender justice.[3] Among women, Dalit women bear the larger burden in spaces within and outside the household. Rather than making marginalised women objects of enquiry, they need to be engaged as the primary agents of enquiry (Rege, 2004; Kapadia, 2017), particularly for access to health care. A large section of maternal and child health care seekers is deprived of or are denied access to healthcare resources owing to their social identities. This calls for an understanding of discrimination in access to health care in general before focusing on maternal and child health.

Defining the Concept of Discrimination in Healthcare Access

Social discrimination is related to a lack of access to services and goods offered by societies. Social and religious groups appear to accentuate social discrimination by denying certain opportunities pertaining to social and religious practices and access to services to some and not to others. Caste-based discrimination is permanent in nature and differs from exclusion that is created and recreated by the operations of social and economic forces. It focuses directly on the nature of the lives people live and the disadvantages they experience (Kundu and Thorat, 2006). It is a part of the basic institutional framework and institutional arrangement within a nation and refers to institutions and rules that enable and constrain human interaction. Public goods and services which should be available to all are limited to a select few based on the caste hierarchy. They are isolated, lack social ties to the local community, voluntary associations, trade unions or even nations. They are disadvantaged in their ability to use their legal rights and constitutional provisions effectively. They are unable to overcome both consumption and work-related disadvantage. Forced inclusion or exclusion, partial or complete, amounts to discrimination (Thorat, 2002).

On the basis of the foregoing understanding, discrimination in accessing health care can be understood as the complete exclusion of *Dalits* from accessing health care. There is denial of certain services and selective inclusion or partial denial of services to reflect access to some and not to others. There can be unequal care access in terms of time spent with; tone and use of derogatory words for; dispensing of the medicine via a medium to; and not touching the discriminated groups by the provider. Unfavourable or forced inclusion in providing certain services such as health camps and exclusion from certain service provisioning such as health camps, health education programmes, water supply, electricity, and infrastructure too can be understood as caste-based social exclusion. As an attribute of individuals, caste-based discrimination focuses directly on the health status of *Dalits* and disadvantages they experience.

The state healthcare system entails the provision of services to all without any discrimination. However, if a group of people are completely excluded from availing some services for whatever reasons, it may be termed as *complete exclusion*. Many times some people have access to some services and not to others. Also, they may be discriminated against by the service providers and co-users at the place of service delivery in terms of priority and proximity. They may have access to some services and not to others. This is *partial denial or selected exclusion*. This can be visualized in two ways – differential treatment by the health providers and differential treatment by the co-users of the care. There are different types of care providers, public sector, private sector, non-profit/Non government Organisation (NGO) sector. The providers are from different streams of care – allopathic, homeopathic, and indigenous/traditional. The treatment can be differential in terms of providing no, less, or wrong information; providing discriminatory treatment at the place of delivery of care; involuntary inclusion or exclusion in some schemes; discriminatory treatment during the emergency and home visits; and behaviour and attitude of the provider.

The co-users of the care can discriminate in the use of space for waiting. Their behaviour and attitude can be derogatory, dominating, and suppressing. They may be surpassing rules to use the services when it is actually due to the people from the discriminated groups (pushing them back in the queue). In access to water and electricity too, there is evidence of such discrimination. There can also be differential treatment for certain services. There can be forceful inclusion in certain services for some specific groups. There could be some forceful inclusion to participate in health camps; sanitation and cleaning of the village; local self-governing bodies like Panchayats, in the case of mothers. There are also chances that some people are forced to avail of some services in spite of their unwillingness. This may be considered as *unfavourable or forced inclusion*.

Discrimination in access to health care is mostly observed in the disparity in care provisioning at the healthcare centre by the providers – doctors and supporting staff, and at home during the visit by the health worker. Discrimination in access and utilization of health at the health centre is likely to be practised during diagnosis and counselling, dispensing of medicine, and laboratory tests, while waiting in the health centre, and in paying the user fee. Discrimination during diagnosis may be measured in terms of time spent asking about the problem, and touching the user during diagnosis. Discrimination during dispensing of the medicine can be measured in terms of the way medicine is given to the user – kept on the palm, kept on the window sill/floor, and someone else is asked to give it. Discrimination in the laboratory can be measured in terms of direct touching of the user for the tests and x-ray. Discrimination while waiting and payment of user fee can be measured in terms of duration of waiting, space for waiting, waiting till the other dominant castes have been provided care, and attitude of the paramedics towards them while they wait. Discrimination during payment of user fee, if any, can be measured in terms of the actual amount being paid, time spent waiting to pay, space for waiting, and a separate queue for payment.

Discrimination at home during the visit by the health worker may occur while entering the house, touching the user, sitting, drinking/eating in the user's house, and while giving medicine and information regarding health camps/programmes to them. Selective dissemination of information regarding health camps and programmes, and exclusion of *Dalits* in accessing certain types of services where touch is involved (such as vaccination) also reflect on the traditional notion of polluted and pure and the consequent discrimination.

Thus, discrimination can be practised by different providers across spheres and forms. Present policies and programmes for health care and against discrimination; awareness regarding them and ability to use them culminate in the experience of discrimination, expressed as complete or partial exclusion; and forced inclusion in access to healthcare services

Disparity, Disadvantage, and Discrimination

Existing discrimination across social groups has been an outcome of historical disadvantage experienced by vulnerable groups like SCs and scheduled tribes (STs). This has also maintained the disparities defeating the objective of the state policies envisioned under affirmative action to ensure equity. As evident from the locational disadvantage in accessing healthcare facilities, there are more ST and SC women as compared to those from advantaged social groups (Others) for whom distance has been a barrier to access care. Consequently, the difference between advantaged (Others) and disadvantaged groups (ST, SC, and OBC) also decreases in that order. Similar is the situation in the case of availability of the care providers. It is noteworthy that despite the persistent differences between the two broad groups, the quantum difference has reduced between NFHS-3 and NFHS-4 (Table 4.1).

As regards women aged 15–49 years who received antenatal care (ANC) by different types of providers during pregnancy for the most recent live birth, there were more than 70% of women from advantaged groups who received ANC from a doctor as compared to 55% SC and 48% ST women. Similarly, skilled providers (including doctors, Auxiliary Nurse Midwife (ANM), nurses, midwives, and lady health visitor) provided ANC to 86% of women from advantaged groups as compared to 78% of SC and 73% of ST women. Following the same pattern, fewer women from the advantaged group (46%) used public sector facilities for delivery as compared to SC (60%) and ST (56%) women (Table 4.2).

Table 4.1 Problems in Accessing Health Care Across Social Groups

Social Groups	Problems in Accessing Health Care							
	Distance to Health Facility				No Provider Available			
	NFHS-3	Diff	NFHS-4	Diff	NFHS-3	Diff	NFHS-4	Diff
Scheduled Caste	27.3	18.5	32.5	8.3	23.9	5.7	46.3	4.3
Scheduled Tribe	44.0	35.5	42.0	17.8	35.2	17.0	54.9	12.9
Other Backward Castes	26.0	17.5	29.4	5.2	23.2	5.0	43.9	1.9
Others	8.5	00	24.2	00	18.2	00	42.0	00
Don't Know	–	–	38.5	–	–	–	45.8	–
Total	–	–	29.9	–	–	–	44.9	–

Note: Diff= Absolute difference between 'Others' and other social groups in each NFHS Round (Calculated by the Author); NFHS-3 =2005–06; NFHS-4=2015–16
Source: Table 11.21 Problems in Accessing Health Care, IIPS and ICF, 2017

Table 4.2 Healthcare Providers and Access to Public Institutions for Child Delivery

Social Group	Doctor	Skilled Providers	Place of Delivery: Public Institution
Scheduled Caste	54.6	77.5	59.9
Scheduled Tribe	47.9	72.9	55.9
Other Backward Castes	57.2	78.2	50.4
Others	70.3	85.6	46.1
Don't Know	57.8	73.4	54.7
Total	–	–	52.1

Source: Table 8.3; and Table 8.13 ANC Providers and Place of Delivery, IIPS and ICF, 2017

Infant and Child Mortality

As regards infant mortality, a wide range of policies and programmes have been put in place to improve health outcomes. It is noteworthy that Infant Mortality Rate (IMR) has improved from 1992–93 to 2015–16, but the difference between the privileged (Others) and the under privileged groups (SCs and STs) has remained consistent. Although the gap has reduced over the period, the persistent gap continues. Even in the case of child mortality, the gap between advantaged and disadvantaged groups follows a similar pattern (Table 4.3). It is evident that while there has been an overall improvement in health indicators, the current policies have failed to achieve the expected outcomes among marginalized communities such as *Dalits* and tribes (Diwakar, 2015).

The disadvantaged status of the SCs has led to *Dalit* women's comparatively shorter life span. They live 14.6 years lesser than advantaged caste women. The average age at death is 39.5 years for SC women and 54.1 years for privileged (or advantaged) caste women is evident from the NFHS-4 (**IIPS and ICF, 2017**).

Illustration from Kusumpur Pahadi

This disadvantage experienced by SCs and STs is illustrated by Kusumpur Pahadi, a notified slum, located behind the CBI colony in Vasant Vihar, SW Delhi, alongside the remnants of the endangered Delhi Ridge Area Social composition of the population suggests that about one-fourth belong to other backward classes (OBC); more than half are from privileged caste; about 17% belong to SCs and about 8% are STs. The slum is divided into five blocks A, B, C, D, and E based on the socio-cultural identity of people from Haryana, Uttar Pradesh, Rajasthan, southern states, and eastern states, respectively. One of the largest slums in Delhi is inhabited by more than two lakh migrants. Considering the fluidity of the population and the physical space, there are varied figures available to suggest its population size. Approximately there are around 15,000 to 20,000 households in the area.

A microstudy[4] conducted in this area on 101 households reflected that more SC households were semi-pucca compared to pucca houses, which was reversed for the advantaged groups (Others). It was notable that out of 74 households with electricity, 42 were SC. More SCs lived in rented houses as compared to owned ones. Fewer of them (12) could afford and therefore use cooking gas as compared to the advantaged caste groups (20). The average number of rooms in her household ranged room 1.5 among SCs to 2.75 among advantaged castes (Acharya, 2020).

In contrast to the larger socio-demographic characteristics of the Slum, the composition of study households (study participants) comprised of more SC (78%) households followed by the advantaged castes (17%), OBCs (6%), and the ST (2%). Only about 12 percent of the study participants were in

Table 4.3 Trends in Infant and Child Mortality Difference across Social Groups

Social Groups	Infant Mortality Rate and Differences between NFHS Rounds								Child Mortality (1-5 years)
	NFHS-1	Diff	NFHS-2	Diff	NFHS-3	Diff	NFHS-4	Diff	
Scheduled Caste	107.6	25.4	83.0	21.2	66.4	17.5	45.2	4.3	11.1
Scheduled Tribe	90.5	8.3	82.2	20.4	62.1	13.2	44.4	3.5	13.4
Other Backward Castes	–	–	76.0	14.2	56.6	7.7	42.1	1.2	9.0
Others	82.2	00	61.8	00	48.9	00	40.9	00	6.6
Total	86.3	–	73.0	–	57.0	–	40.7	–	11.6

Note: Diff= Absolute difference between 'Others' and other social groups in each NFHS Round (calculated by the Author); NFHS-1=1992-92; NFHS-2=1998-99; NFHS-3 =2005-06; NFHS-4=2015-16 Source: IIPS and ICF, 2017

Table 4.4 House Type and Facilities and Amenities across Social Groups (in percentage)

House Type and Facilities and Amenities	Households across Social Groups					Percent to Total
	SC	ST	OBC	Other	Total	
Pucca	12	1	6	16	35	34.55
Semi-pucca	28	1	5	6	30	39.60
Kachcha	24	0	1	1	26	25.74
Own House	22	2	8	15	47	46.53
Rented House	42	0	4	8	54	53.47
HH with Electricity	**42**	**2**	**11**	**20**	**75**	**74.26**
Average No. of Rooms	1.5	2.0	3.0	3.0	2.75	–
Use Cooking Gas (LPG)	12	2	4	20	38	37.62
Kerosene for Cooking	38	0	6	3	47	46.53
Other Medium for Cooking	14		2	0	16	15.84
Total HHs	**64**	**02**	**12**	**23**	**101**	100

Source: Acharya, 2020

public sector occupation, although at lower ranks. Most of them were in informal sector (61%) engaging in petty jobs as electrician, plumber, rag-picker, domestic help, watchman, etc. (Figure 4.1).

For the majority of the poor in the study area, the priority for health was last after ensuring livelihood followed by shelter. There is a mix of voluntary, government, and private sector functioning for providing education and healthcare services. There are two health centres run by voluntary organisations. These centres mostly focus on immunization of children, supplementary nutrition, and antenatal care. There is a weekly mobile homoeopathic clinic that comes to the slum every Monday from 9.30 am to 4.40 pm (Figure 4.2).

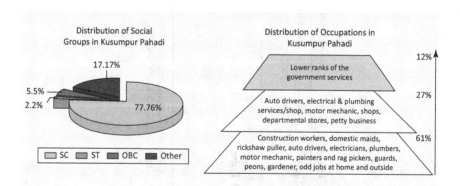

Figure 4.1 Social and Occupational Composition of Study Population

Source: Acharya, 2020

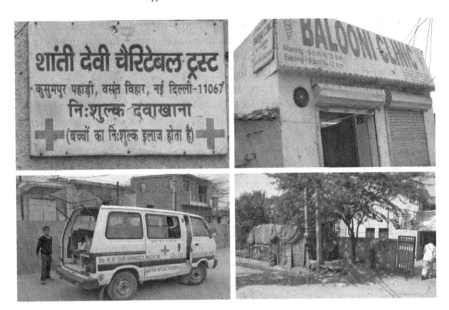

Figure 4.2 Plurality of Healthcare Services in Kusumpur Pahadi

Source: Acharya, 2020

In addition, there are a number of 'clinics' operated by 'doctors', most of whom are trained informally. Only two of them were formally trained, one in allopathic and the other in Ayurveda, and were serving through the charitable trust hospital. There are grocery and/or chemist shops selling medicines for fever, vomiting, headache, and pain. Informal local healthcare service providers mostly affiliated with local healing traditions are often called *Bengali* doctors. Use of injection played an important role in deciding the 'qualification' and 'skill' of the doctor.

The Reproductive and Child Health (RCH) programme was launched in October 1997. Since then, promotion of maternal and child health, particularly of the vulnerable population like the ones in the slum areas, has been one of the most important objectives of the family welfare programme in Delhi.[5] The RCH programme incorporated the components covered under the child survival and safe motherhood (CSSM) programme and also included an additional component relating to reproductive tract infection and sexually transmitted infections. In order to improve maternal and child health in the urban slums, the Government of Delhi established a Health Post or Family Welfare Centre for every 50,000 slum population.[6]

Maternal and Child Health in Kusumpur Pahadi

The study consolidated the importance of reproductive and child healthcare services being provided in the slum. They expressed their discontent with some services, while they also appreciated some other services, particularly provided by the trust. A discussion on antenatal care, child delivery, and post-natal care reflects on the differential access across social groups despite the efforts of the government machinery.

When the access to services for maternal and child health is disaggregated by social groups, it is evident that access is better among OBC and the Others as compared to SC and ST. Even registration for ANC in public sector health facilities (which are free of cost with a minimal user fee, if at all) is two to three times less than that of OBC and 'Others' – socially advantaged groups. Similar differentials are evident in the case of antenatal and post-natal care. Across social groups, more SCs resorted to home delivery as compared to other groups (Table 4.5).

It was also important to understand the beneficiaries' satisfaction level with the RCH services to understand the quality of the services provided in the study slum areas. The users' satisfaction is an important indicator to assess the quality of RCH. They are, more often than not, unaware of whether any standards are followed by the healthcare providers for pro-visioning of care services. Therefore, their perception of 'good service' is reflected in their level of satisfaction with services they availed or want to avail (Table 4.6). About 25.54 per cent of men and women of reproductive ages were fully satisfied with RCH services in the slum, while about 61 per cent of respondents were partially satisfied with these services. It implies that the quality of the RCH services is not perceived to be in a bad condition by the users in the study slums in Kusumpur Pahadi. It is noteworthy that

Table 4.5 Distribution of Services Ever Used in Last Five Years across Social Groups

RCH Services Ever Used in Last Five Years	Per cent Accessing Services to Total Cases across Social Groups				
	Total	SC	ST	OBC	Others
ANC Registration in Government Health Centre	58.02	32	50	65	85
ANC Registration in Private Hospital/Clinic	33.02	8	50	12	31
Received 3 ANC Check-up with IFA Tab 100 and 2 TT	96.69	35	100	89	83
Immunizations done for Children	100	100	100	100	100
Institutional Delivery	97.57	73.5	100	85.1	96.3
Home Delivery Assisted by Trained Health Workers	13.12	26.5	00	14.9	3.7
PNC Services Provided by Health Workers/ANM	62.14	57.5	61.8.	87.5	95.8
Contraceptives Used/Using (Women)	49.52	39.4	73.8	73.8	86.9

Source: Acharya, 2020

Table 4.6 Level of Satisfaction on RCH Services Availed

Level of Satisfaction	Total Population (15–49 years)		Distribution across Social Groups (%)			
	Number	Percentage	SC	ST	OBC	Others
Fully Satisfied	58	25.54	12.61	4.10	3.64	5.19
Partially Satisfied	138	60.61	14.50	6.10	18.41	21.61
Not Satisfied	32	13.85	3.46	00	5.18	5.21
Total	228*	100	30.57	10.20	27.23	32.01

Source: Fieldwork
Note: *includes 117 men and 111 women

among those fully satisfied, nearly half are SC and about one-fifth are HC Hindus (or Others). Perhaps the assertion to question the quality is more among the HC, and therefore, the consequent satisfaction is less. In contrast, the assertion to question the quality is less among the SC, and therefore, the consequent satisfaction is more. Corroborating this is the distribution of those 'not satisfied', wherein lesser SCs as compared to OBC and Others are 'not satisfied'.

People resort to diverse sources of health care for antenatal care, child delivery, and post-natal care. Although this slum is located in the heart of the city, access to services is still a major concern and is evident in the number of women opting for home deliveries mostly with the help of dais with minimal and even no antenatal care or vaccination of the children under the age of five years. This is reflective not only of the structural constraints but also of the socio-cultural norms which influence utilization of certain services with variation across social groups (Ram, Pathak and Anamma, 1998; Kulkarni and Bariak, 2003, Acharya, 2011).

Reliance on government facilities for delivery is prominent in the area as going to the private facility will mean very high expenditure. Sometimes, though, women go to private hospitals for childbirth as they are not satisfied with the functioning of government services. Sometimes, they felt they could afford 'better' services, so they opted for the private, clearly indicating the misconception that the government sector is 'poor' and the private sector is 'good'. Women mostly felt that the waiting time was very high if they went to Safdarjung Hospital. They were not happy with the kind of services they got there. They also pointed out at the language and derogatory words used by the hospital staff for them. One of the women (petty shop owner, widowed aged 32, Muslim) narrated her experience as follows:

These doctors get money from the government. They treat us as if we are coming from the streets. They give the same medicine for cold, cough, fever etc. I really wonder that how can they write the medicine for us without checking us properly, didi. It's all about the game of money and power. If we can look "nice" (like other women) they will talk to us nicely. (IDI, 14)

Health-seeking behaviour for maternal and child health to a large extent was determined by income and socio-cultural norms. But social identity based on caste, religion, and ethnicity was also a strong propeller. Certain cultural norms also influenced the utilization of MCH services, and it was evident in the case of immunization of children, use of Integrated Child Development Scheme (ICDS) services, and assistance during time of delivery.

Utilization of Services

The utilization of care and counselling services depended on their availability and propensity to access. In the study area, availability was poor. Some of those available were used, while others were not for reasons as varied as distance, time, availability of the provider, and awareness regarding the availability of the service(s). The women considered the services at the nearest health facility as satisfactory despite the references made to the 'shortage of medicines' due to which they often had to buy the prescribed drugs. Some also preferred going to private doctors since they were nearer to their residence as compared to the hospital.

There have been instances where the person could not be reached to the health facility because no means of transport was available when needed. They also pointed out that the doctors do not come to the centre regularly and on time. A young adult said, *"after coming so far to the Centre, when the doctor is not there then, we have no other option but to go to the private doctor"* (IDI 10).

For pregnancy and childbirth, there is a preference for private practitioners. An important reason for this decision was the lack of identity documents which obstructed the use of public sector facilities. The household often took loans for meeting the healthcare expenditure. Generally, the very poor go to the government hospital and those who are a little well-off, go to private practitioners. Therefore, the registration of births is not being effectively covered. The Traditional Birth Attendant (TBA) and the private doctor ask for Rs. 1500 and the request to reduce the charges invites displeasure and demeaning attitude reflected as follows:

everybody becomes poor when it comes to giving money for "safe" deliveries... "enjoyment" during the act of procreation is forgotten.[7] (IDI 12)

Quite often the women go for check-ups only after four months of pregnancy when there is stomach ache or vomiting and the work starts getting affected:

Doctor told me I was in my fifth month... I was thinking it was just the beginning of the fourth month... so I registered for ANC. (IDI12)

Although the women seem to be fairly conscious about the immunization of their children, they do not appear to be very regular in taking medicines, weight, and blood pressure for themselves as an expectant mother. So, most of them are contacting healthcare service providers or visiting the facilities almost halfway through the pregnancy. The economic factor is essentially impacting the health behaviour of the vulnerable population. However, there is a marked difference between women across income quintiles as it is between SC and the advantaged castes (Others).

The study also reported that 49.8% of women got married at an age of less than 18 years leading to early deliveries, multiple pregnancies, and abortions. The prevalence of social health determinants such as early marriage, multiple pregnancies and abortions, substance abuse, and domestic violence indicated lower access to services available. As per WHO, about 5.7% of maternal deaths in Asia occur due to unsafe abortion. The present study also revealed a higher rate of abortions (13.2%) among women which may be largely due to lower awareness of birth control measures (as only 39.8% reported to be using them). This percentage of women using birth control measures was similar to findings reported in "The state of Urban Health in Delhi" with about one-third (34.8%) of urban poor women practising any modern contraceptive method in comparison with the urban average of 64%.

Nutritional Status of the Children

In Kusumpur Pahadi, the mean BMI of women of reproductive ages was found to be 21.51 ±1.5 Kg/m^2 (Zehra, 2012). BMI is being increasingly used as a measure of nutritional adequacy in adults and is considered to be a better indicator of chronic energy deficiency. Though the normal mean BMI could be attributed to the representation of pooled data of pregnant, lactating, and non-pregnant non-lactating women, however, within the population, there are vulnerable groups who are more marginalized than others. As per NFHS-4 data, 36% of women are below the BMI cut-off point of 18.5. In the study group of 2088 women, 13.9% of women were found to be having BMI less than 18.5. As per NFHS-3 data for urban poor, 44.7% of the infants were exclusively breastfed. The study data in the Kusumpur Pahadi slums presented similar results with 47.2% of infants being exclusively breastfed for the first six months. Also, the prevalence of infants being breastfed within an hour of birth was only 51% revealing a lower awareness level among the study group. 44.3 per cent of lactating women were feeding their child some other food besides milk such as tea, *saunf ka paani*, sugar water, and water to the child in the first 6 months.

Experience of Caste Discrimination in Accessing Health Services

Respondents in the study area have reported accounts of caste discrimination prevalent in the ICDS centres. One of the respondents said that children from the *Dalit* community are seated separately from those belonging to other castes for mid-day meal programme.

The ANMs and other health workers often visit the *Dalit* households. It was observed that the *Dalit* women hesitate to sit on the benches available in the healthcare centres both public and private. In other provisions of public health like water and sanitation, there is some evidence of caste discrimination, mostly in the form of subtle use of words.

Spheres and Forms of Discrimination

In health sector, spheres and forms of discrimination can be understood in various interactions with the health care service provider, and the way interactions happen. What kind of interactions happen (spheres) and how they happen (forms) are the crux of understanding discrimination in health. In some spheres of discrimination in access to health, such as dispensing of medicine, counselling, waiting, conduct of pathological tests, no evident experiences were reported by the study participants. However, subtle comments such as *"tumko toh sab kuch muft mein milta hai"*[8] was reported by one of the users in context of the caste status and affirmative action for education and job. Dispensing of medicine (by the pharmacist, for instance) was perceived as the most discriminating sphere by most users. Consulting the care providers (usually doctors and specialists) for referral was the sphere where the least discrimination was perceived as well as experienced.

As regards the forms of discrimination, physical immediate expressions of interaction – touch (touch roughly/do not touch) and conversation (speak gently/rudely) – appear to be the areas perceived as most discriminating. Discrimination can also be practised by the providers of healthcare services. Those at the grassroots are perceived as most discriminating by most users, as compared to those who are at the higher hierarchy of work. Also, evident is that the public sector providers are more discriminating.

Index of Maternal and Child Health and Well-Being

Based on the foregoing analysis, an Index of Maternal and Child Health and Well-being (IMCH and WB) was developed. It is derived from the composite index of interconnected domains that measures trends in well-being at a given time point. Well-being is conceptualized as "presence of the highest possible quality of life reflected through good living standards, healthy population, sustainable environment, dynamic communities, educated population, balanced time use, high levels of democratic participation, and access to and participation in leisure and cultural activities" (CIW, 2012). An understanding of well-being through a series of objective and subjective indicators feeds into the knowledge base of policymakers and academics who advocate for change to promote well-being for all. This index has been constructed on the basis of social indicators of maternal and child health. It assumes that multiple, interrelated social and environmental factors contribute to the health and well-being of mothers and children, especially those living in vulnerable spaces. The following criteria were considered for selecting the indicators:

1. Extent to which indicator was directly related to health and well-being as evidenced in the literature, reflecting on validity.
2. The second criterion was whether an indicator could be derived from reliable sources, and simplicity of defining and understanding the concept.
3. Measurement of the indicator was drawn from available literature and reflected on reliability.
4. The fourth criterion was feasibility in terms of availability and accessibility of data.

With these criteria in mind, indicators to represent their specific domain were selected. Indicators could be either positive or negative. For a positive indicator, an increase in numerical value indicated an increase in that aspect of health and well-being; for a negative indicator, an increase in numerical value reflected a decrease in some aspect of health well-being. The number of indicators ranged from two to nine for each domain, totalling to 28, spreading across eight domains. With the indicators having specified, data were compiled to prepare the respective indicators into a composite index for each domain. A simple mean score was used to aggregate the standardized values for the indicators within each domain. The overall mean score for the domain allowed comparison to other domains, as well as examining the extent to which well-being in each domain may be better or worse relative to overall well-being especially in the context of slums. All of the indicators in each domain were assigned with an equal weight as suggested by Michalos et al. (2011). This index is a composite of the mean scores for each domain. The mean composite scores for the eight domains are summed and then divided by eight. This yielded an overall measure of maternal and child health and well-being.

The aim of an index of health and well-being is to ensure that an effective approach for assessing, reporting on, and promoting well-being is evolved. Continuous validation is important considering the floating population in the slums. It draws upon an array of indicators, equally distributed, and weighted within eight interconnected domains: Community Participation, Democratic Engagement, Education, Environment, Healthy Populations, Leisure and Culture, Living Standards, and Time Use (Table 4.7).

The scores for each of these are combined into a composite index to produce a single figure that enabled comparisons between interconnected domains to foster an understanding of how policies and legislation affect maternal and child health and well-being, and which areas require more attention (Table 4.8). It, thus, provides an easily understandable comparison of well-being beyond an economic perspective.

Table 4.7 Domains and Indicators of Index of Maternal and Child Health and Well-Being

Domain	Indicators
Community Participation	Membership of local clubs/groups; participation in community activities, interaction between residents through these activities
Democratic Engagement	Voting; membership of democratically elected bodies; mobilization for elections
Education	Number of girls going to school; the number of dropouts from schools (both boys and girls); number of literate mothers; educational level of men
Environment	Safe drinking water; covered drains; garbage collection frequency; garbage disposal practice;
Health	Life expectancy and conditions that influence maternal and child health; and access to public health services for MCH; perceptions of personal health and the quality of public healthcare services for MCH; public health initiatives for MCH, prevalence (reporting) of diseases/illness during pregnancy
Leisure and Culture	Visit to relatives/friends; visit malls; viewing cinema; celebrating festivals; inviting persons other than those belonging to own social group [during pregnancy]
Living Standards	Nature of work; average household income; assets; house ownership; type of house; civic amenities access (electricity, safe drinking water, toilet)
Time Use	Part-time education; part-time work; activities of the household, community, vocational course

Source: Acharya, 2020

Table 4.8 Standardized Scores for Domains of Well-Being Across Social Groups

Domains	SC	ST	OBC	Others	Total
Community Participation	19.49	3.39	23.72	53.39	100
Democratic Engagement	26.56	1.21	34.06	37.15	100
Education	41.94	1.61	18.55	38.71	100
Health	49.5	1.38	27.68	23.08	100
Environment	13.99	3.13	30.22	36.47	100
Leisure and Culture	30.39	2.44	33.41	33.41	100
Living Standard I	22.58	1.29	30.65	45.48	100
Living Standard II	14.14	3.03	39.40	43.43	100
Access to Resources	23.98	3.51	32.16	40.35	100
Time Use	33.91	0.05	3.19	30.43	100
Composite Score	25.22	2.21	27.26	58.28	100

Source: Acharya, 2020

It is evident from the analysis of Index of Wellbeing (IWB), that across domains, the SC population is consistently far poorer than their non-SC counterparts. The ST fares slightly better than the SCs. The high caste Hindus (Others) appear to be doing best followed by the OBCs. The non-scheduled groups are doing much better in all selected domains as compared to SC and ST (Figure 4.3).

Since there are only two ST households in the study sample, they have not been included for further analysis. While community participation is about 20 points for SC, it is slightly more for OBC by almost double for the HC Hindus (Others). The health domain represented by (negative) variables of morbidity, access to health care and mortality, has the most points 49.5 for SCs and around half for OBC and Others (Table 7.2). Thus, access to health is about two times better for the non-SCs as compared to SCs. As regards leisure and cultural activities, the position on the Composite Index of Wellbeing (CIWB) appears to be fairly similar for all three groups ranging from 30 to 33 points. It is noteworthy, however, that time use denoted by engagement with part-time education and work, vocational courses, and community activities, and value for OBC is far lower than both SC and Others (Figure 4.4). The overall composite index of all selected domains reflects the poor position of the SCs as compared to the OBCs and the Others.

There are no simple solutions for addressing healthcare needs in the study areas across social groups. Standardized service delivery models will work only when flexibility to infuse local needs is considered. Services need to be provided even if the facilities are yet to be built. Service delivery needs to be

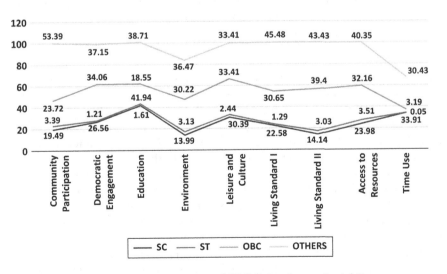

Figure 4.3 Composite Score on Factors of Well-Being Across Social Groups

Source: Acharya, 2020

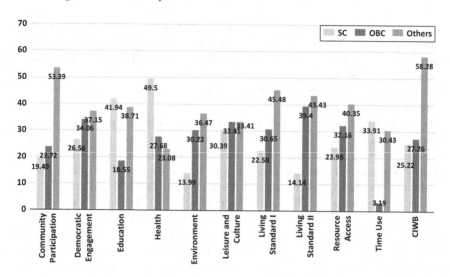

Figure 4.4 Composite Index of Well-Being: Across Domains and Social Groups
Source: Acharya, 2020

started early on with outreach activities. There is a need to focus on critical services and monitor their delivery. Limited curative care is important. To address the needs, fixed days for services, special clinics, providers' accountability, and incentives for their activities are important. The opportunity to partner with community-based organizations as well as the private sector for the provisioning of services needs to be expanded.

Way Forward

As evident from the foregoing analysis, health is not prioritized as it should be. One of the reasons was that the healthcare service system was perceived as highly bureaucratic, and created more obstacles than facilitated the utilization of services. Therefore, the preference was for the trust hospital. They avoided using public sector healthcare services until the situation was unmanageable. The state of healthcare services highlight the following:

The present study reflects that the health-seeking behaviour of low-income households is different from that of middle- and high-income households as is the difference between SC and non-SC households. It is noteworthy that most low-income households are also SCs. The private sector which is easily accessible and is perceived as delivering better quality services is much more expensive and is largely supported by direct out-of-pocket payments. These expenditures accentuate the burden on the poor and poor *Dalits* (SCs) far more than the non-poor and non-*Dalits* (SCs). Slum households having lower per capita income show preference for the health services provided by the government hospitals and health centres. Private hospitals, however, are being frequented mostly by high-income households, since these are completely out of reach of the poorer people. Most of the households which did not seek care were SCs. The most reported reason for not seeking care was lack of money and most among them were SCs. Some households could not receive any medication for their ailment. Many women and girls in the households do not get the treatment because of the apathy from the family due to low priority to their health. Most of the women and girls get treated with 'locally available treatments' which include home remedies and over-the-counter medicines from the shops including groceries.

The government hospitals are major healthcare providers for all slums located in Delhi, and Kusumpur Pahadi is no exception. The doctors provide medical services. A mobile medical van also comes to the slums periodically. The private medical service providers are most likely to be non-qualified practitioners. The reason for choosing private clinics and hospitals is the proximity. But the major reason for opting for government facilities is financial constraints. The household does not have enough money to bear the out-of-pocket expenditure. But sometimes due to constraints of time and lack of required services, a sizeable section of the population seeks care from the private sector. This clearly points to the need to strengthen public healthcare services. The levels of satisfaction with healthcare services are very low. Interestingly, satisfaction levels are better among the SCs as compared to the non-SCs. This could probably be due to the higher aspirations for getting the right kind of services among the non-SCs. Service which was considered as 'good' by the SCs was not perceived the same by the non-SCs. The perceptions of the people regarding public health facilities and the services provided therein are insufficient. Thus, more health facilities and the services provided therein are needed for the slums. Most of the persons across social groups think that the medicines should be given by providers in the health centres. Distance to healthcare facilities plays a major role in the level of utilisation of healthcare facilities. Most SCs are located in the areas which are in the periphery of the Kusumpur Pahadi, while the health facilities are in the spots within the central part of the slums where most non-SCs reside. Therefore, distance too poses a barrier to the use of the services by the marginalized SC population of the study sites.

It is evident that those at the lower level of the social ladder are worse off than those who are positioned at higher rungs of the ladder in access to health care in general and maternal and child health care in particular. Therefore, if the differential unmet needs of the slum dwellers across social groups are not catered to with commitment, parity in access to healthcare resources across social groups will remain a distant dream and restrict the Sustainable Development Goals' achievement which propagates leaving no one behind. Therefore, health issues, particularly maternal and child health in the slums, need to be given high priority.

76 *Sanghmitra S. Acharya*

Notes

1 http://mofapp.nic.in:8080/economicsurvey/pdf/167-185_Chapter_10_Economic _Survey_2017-18.pdf
2 Biswas, Soutik, Why are India's housewives killing themselves? Delhi correspondent. Published 12 April 2016https://www.bbc.com/news/world-asia-india -35994601
3 Iyengar, Sushma https://idronline.org/the-development-discourse-in-india-neglects -women/
4 Acharya, Sanghmitra S (2020) Sustainable Health and Differential Access – Emerging Issues from A Delhi Slum, SRF Report, ICSSR, New Delhi [Unpublished].
5 RCH Phase II – National Programme Implementation Plan (2005-2012), Ministry of Health and Family Welfare, Government of India; Government of India (2006). National Guidelines on Prevention, Management, and Control of Reproductive Tract Infections including Sexually Transmitted Infections, Maternal Health Division and National AIDS Control Organization, Ministry of Health and Family Welfare, Government of India; Government of India (2010). Operational Guidelines on Maternal and Newborn Health, GOI.
6 Government of Delhi (2013). Annual Report of Health Post, Rotary Club, South Delhi.
7 This is a modest translation of the Hindi version of the narrative given during the interview. It had foul words and cannot be put verbatim. The closest attempt could be as follows: "*sex karte waqt to bahut mazaa aata hain, par paise dete waqt dum nikal jata hai... gharib ho jate hai*".
8 When translated, literally means that the one being spoken to gets everything free of cost. The reference is being made to the perception of high caste of the reservation policy which enable the vulnIerable population to access certain resources and services. This was evident from one of the in-depth interviews.

References

Acharya, S. S. (2011). *Understanding access to maternal and child health care and issues of discrimination in a selected slum of Delhi. Report.* Programme for the Study of Social Discrimination and Exclusion, School of Social Sciences, Jawaharlal Nehru University.
Acharya Burton, C. (2014). *Subordination: Feminism and social theory.* Routledge.
Canadian Index of Wellbeing (2012). *How are Canadians really doing?* The 2012 CIW report. Canadian Index of Wellbeing and University of Waterloo.
Iips, I. (2017). *National family health survey (NFHS-4), 2015–16* (pp. 791–846). International Institute for Population Sciences (IIPS).
Kapadia, K. (2017). Introduction we ask you to rethink: Different Dalit women and their subaltern politics. In *Dalit women* (pp. 1–50). Routledge.
Kulkarni, P. M., & Baraik, V. K. (2003). *Utilisation of healthcare services by scheduled castes in India.* Working Paper IIDS.
Kundu, D., & Thorat, S. K. (2006). *Inter-social group disparities in the ownership of private enterprise in India-1998-99.* Indian Institute of Dalit Studies.
Michalos, A. C., Smale, B., Labonté, R., Muharjarine, N., Scott, K., Moore, K., Swystun, L., Holden, B., Bernardin, H., Dunning, B., Graham, P., Guhn, M., Gadermann, A.M., Zumbo, B.D., Morgan, A., Brooker, A.-S., & Hyman, I. (2011). *The Canadian Index of Wellbeing.* Technical Report 1.0. Waterloo, ON: Canadian Index of Wellbeing and University of Waterloo.

NUHM (2010). http://mohfw.nic.in/NRHM/Documents/Urban_Health/UH_Frame workFinal.pdf

Raphael, D. (Ed.). (2009). *Social determinants of health: Canadian perspectives.* Canadian Scholars' Press.

Ram, F., Pathak, K. B., & Annamma, K. I. (1998). Utilisation of health care services by the underprivileged section of population in India-Results from NFHS. *IASSIST Q, 16,* 128–147.

Rege, S. (2004). *Women Writing Caste: Testimonies of Dalit Women in Maharashtra.* Zubaan

Sanghmitra, S. (2020). *Sustainable health and differential access: Emerging issues from a Delhi slum, SRF report.* ICSSR [Unpublished].

Thorat, S. (2002). Oppression and denial: Dalit discrimination in the 1990s. *Economic and Political Weekly,* 572–578.

5 Continuum of Care for Maternal and Child Health in India and EAG States

Rinju and Abhishek Sharma

Introduction

The continuum of care (CoC) has recently received considerable attention in the arena of maternal and child health (Shibanuma et al., 2018). In India, women and children are not receiving all recommended care from pregnancy to post-delivery. In the country, it is not possible to ensure that every woman and her child receive timely and appropriate health services related to maternal and child health (Kumar et al., 2013; Tanahashi, 1978).

The performance of maternal and child health services is evaluated in terms of the coverage of antenatal visits, institutional delivery, postnatal visits, etc. In Indian states, such service coverage has substantially improved over the last few decades, but the adverse pregnancy outcomes have not come down as desired by health professionals (McDougal et al., 2017). It means that ensuring higher levels of utilization of these services alone does not reflect that every woman and her children are receiving all the necessary care (Shibanuma et al., 2018; James et al., 2022). In developing countries, most of the deaths occur during labour or delivery or in the immediate postpartum period. These deaths are mostly avoidable (Iqbal et al., 2017) with timely intervention/care. The appropriate concept to be adopted in this domain of maternal and child health relates to the CoC for maternal and child health, and it must be promoted for improving healthcare service delivery (Mothupi et al., 2018; Chopra et al., 2009).

The 21st century has seen these factors forming part of the policy agenda primarily through the Millennium Development Goals (MDGs) 4 and 5 and its successor the Sustainable Development Goal (SDG) 3. Both MDG 4, 5 and SDG 3 were internationally accepted targets to bring the worldwide maternal mortality ratio (MMR) to less than 70 per 100,000 live births (the current level being MMR is 216/100,000) and neonatal mortality rate (NMR) to under 12 per 1000 live births or lower (current level NMR being 19/1000). To achieve this, there is a wide consensus that the concept of CoC is the way forward.

A CoC throughout pregnancy and the postpartum period is critically important in India where both mothers and children are vulnerable to a range of health risks resulting from the vicious cycle of malnutrition and

DOI: 10.4324/9781003430636-8

poverty. These issues need to be addressed in EAG states as these states are more deprived of socio-cultural and health indicators. The EAG states are experiencing MMR of 161 per 100,000 live births (SRS, 2018). According to an AHS report, infant mortality rates are higher in Madhya Pradesh and Assam. The EAG states together account for over 55% of India's total population living below the poverty line. While the relation between this and the indicators is addressed in the next sections, it should be noted here how the EAG states alone accounted for over half of the maternal deaths in the year 2007–08 (Singh et al., 2012). Moreover, despite a recent decline in infant mortality rates, there is only a little subsequent improvement in most Indian states (Singh et al., 2012, 2014).

Given the prevailing poor conditions of CoC in these states, the main objective of this study is to understand the role of maternal and socio-economic factors in determining continuum care in the EAG states.

Economic Reasons

The economic deprivation of the EAG states is coupled with social issues like low education, low media exposure, early and even child marriages, and customary norms. These ultimately have a bearing on communities availing any kind of institutional care in a sustained manner, thus defeating any CoC aspect. Studies show to improve CoC, initiatives like the Conditional transfer of Janani Suraksha Yojana (JSY) launched by the government of India provide the incentive of Rs. 1400 for institutional delivery that contributes to better health and maternal healthcare utilization (Mukherjee & Singh, 2018; Thongkong et al., 2017).

Socio-Cultural Reasons

The net effect of education on maternal healthcare service utilization among rural adolescent women is significantly interlinked with early-age marriages and early childbearing. Despite several governmental and non-governmental efforts to delay age at marriage, nearly 50% of Indian women in the age group 20–24 were married by 18 years of age, and this proportion is observed to be as high as one in two to three in five in several states (Singh et al., 2012; Kumar et al., 2013). However, it remains to be explored on the ground if low education levels are the primary reasons for limited access to health care.

A study based in Bihar captures the gist of the social norms at play in availing healthcare support. The Ananya programme is an outreach mechanism that focuses on ensuring Reproductive, Maternal, and New-born Health (RMNH) CoC is affected majorly by gender-based issues (Karvande et al., 2016). The programme intends to sustain contact with the family for 1000 days throughout the antenatal and postnatal and intrapartum period, basically from the conception of the child to one year from it. Hence, these programmes go into detailed interventions and measures like ensuring clean cord, skin-to-skin care, use of safe postpartum contraception, immunization, etc. Various studies show how the programme was a success in RMNH CoC (Karvande et al., 2016 & Saxena et al., 2018).

Data and Methodology

The study uses NFHS-4 for analysis purposes. It is a nationally representative survey conducted with a representative sample of the household. NFHS is the largest survey in India covering approximately 6 lakh households and 7 lakh women in the age group of 15–49 and men in the age group of 15–54. It provides an estimate of 29 states, seven union territories, and 640 districts in India using multistage sampling. NFHS survey provides reliable and comparable data at national- and state-level estimates on several health topics such as family planning, unmet need, sexual and reproductive health, and non-communicable and communicable disease, domestic violence, attitude towards people living with HIV/AIDS and HIV prevalence, quality of health and family welfare services, and socio-economic condition and mortality information. We analysed information on maternal and child health, i.e. women who had experienced childbirth preceding the survey. Of 6,99,686 samples of women, 1,90,898 women experienced childbirth in the preceding survey. However, the present study is focused on the EAG states because of their low performance in certain health indicators, meaning that these states are experiencing high maternal deaths and infant deaths. The sample size is limited to 1,12,518 women.

Correlates

The CoC elements for maternal and child health services in this study are included antenatal care (ANC), postnatal care for the mother (PNC-M) and child vaccination 12-23 month. All These services all provided by health professional or ASHA or traditional birth attendant. Those who had ANC are considered as ANC recipients. If a woman had her postnatal check-up within two days of delivery, she is considered as a postnatal care (PNC-M) recipient, and children receiving full vaccination considered at the age of 12–23 months who received specific vaccines at any time before the survey (according to a vaccination card or the mother's report). Children receiving all basic vaccinations, at least one dose of bacille calmette-guérin (BCG) vaccine, which protects against tuberculosis; three doses of diphtheria-tetanus-pertussis (DPT) vaccine, which protects against diphtheria, pertussis (whooping cough), and tetanus; three doses of polio vaccine; and one dose of measles vaccine are referred to as full vaccination recipients.

Mother CoC is considered if women received all services as full CoC, partial is atleast attained on services considered and women received none of the services considered as No CoC. Further, we have correlate with does full

CoC of women also influence children full vaccination, birth order of the child, place of residence, mother level of education and wealth status of the household.

Statistical Analyses

We performed descriptive statistics to show the distribution of CoC of mothers' and children's full immunization. A multinomial logistic regression model was fitted to determine the effect of factors on the dependent variable; CoC of maternal and child health model fitness was checked using a RRR.

The CoC is a system that guides women and children to pursue various services starting from pregnancy to child immunization (Table 5.1). It is observed that only a few women are utilizing all the services during the pregnancy. The majority of women avail of two or three services and discontinue having the rest of the services. Only 81.71 % of eligible women in the EAG states registered their pregnancy during their gestation period. Among them, 88.02% have MCH cards. Followed by the ANC services, 77.43% of women who had visited for ANC received less than four ANC and 44.74% visited the > 4 ANC. The women who are utilizing service pregnancy registration, MCH card, and ANC are also going for institutional delivery. The utilization of MCH services was declined in the case of the use of PNC for mothers and children.

Table 5.1 represents CoC with respect to different combinations of services taken by women during pregnancy and utilization of the services in the EAG states. Among all the women, 9% did not avail of any kind of services. Only 23.9% of women avail all the three services provide to mother (ANC, institutional Delivery and PNC-M). Moreover, along with their service and child postnatal care avail by 23% of maternal and child health services.

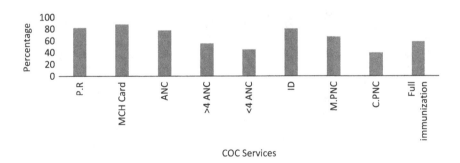

Figure 5.1 Percentage of CoC Maternal and Child Health in the EAG States, NFHS-4
PR: Pregnancy Registration, MCH Card: Maternal and Child Health Card, ANC: Antenatal Care, ID: Institutional Delivery, M-PNC: Mother Postnatal Care, C-PNC: Child Postnatal Care

Table 5.1 Proportion of CoC Services Examine by Maternal and Child in the EAG States

Services	Percentage	Total Sample
Nil	8.62	9,312
ANC	0.65	726
ID	0.56	589
M-PNC	0.63	694
C-PNC	5.69	6,007
M-PNC and C-PNC	0.37	389
ANC, M-PNC, and C-PNC	4.38	4,866
ANC and M-PNC	1.67	1,891
ANC and ID	8.63	9,826
ID and M-PNC	2.26	2,646
ID and C-PNC	1.17	1,346
ANC, M-PNC, and C-PNC	3.16	3,731
ID, M-PNC, and C-PNC	13.16	14,433
ANC, ID, and C-PNC	2.13	2,447
ANC, ID, and M-PNC	23.94	27,116
ANC, ID, M-PNC, and C-PNC	22.98	26,499
Total	100	112,518

Figure 5.2 illustrates child immunization status according to women availing any services, i.e. either ANC or PNC or institutional delivery defined as any MCH services avail by women. The distribution of child full immunization according to accessibility of any MCH services is presented in Figure 5.2. Data presented in the figure show that full immunization is relatively lower (54%) than women availing any MCH services (77%) in the EAG states.

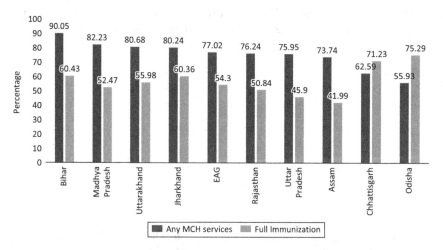

Figure 5.2 Percentage of any MCH Services and Child Full Immunization in the EAG states, NFHS-4

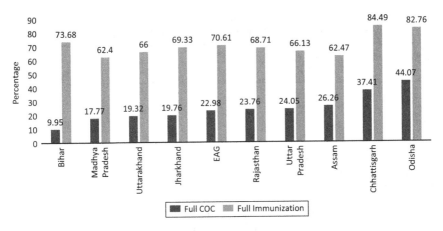

Figure 5.3 Percentage of Full CoC Services and Child Full Immunization in the EAG States, NFHS-4

It shows that mothers who avail of only one service or two services are higher than their children's immunization in all the EAG states except Chhattisgarh and Odisha. For instance, in Bihar women who avail only any MCH services are 90% and full immunization among their children is 60%. In Figure 5.3, it is clearly observed that children's immunization is high among women availing full CoC. As represented in the figure, CoC is higher in Chhattisgarh and Odisha as compared to other EAG states. The pattern is similar to full immunization. Therefore, CoC not only improved mother services but also improved children's services.

Table 5.2 shows that multinomial logistic model is applied to examine the relative significance of suggested correlates between CoC deliveries. The results are presented in terms of RRR for partial CoC and full CoC against no CoC. RRR of having full CoC significantly increases with an increase in education and wealth quintile, while it decreases for the partial CoC. The RRR for the richest wealth quintile is 1.71 for the full continuum, while this is 0.58 for the partial continuum. The RRR of having full CoC increases among those who received MCH benefits than those who have not received them. The RRRs for Odisha and Chhattisgarh have the higher RRR as compared to other states, while this is lower in the case of the partial continuum. We do not find any significant difference in the case of birth order.

Conclusion

The study revealed that the coverage of CoC for maternal and child health in the EAG states is low, with only 23% of mothers receiving essential MCH care. This is despite significant improvements in child immunization across the EAG states. The study found that wealth status, education, place of

Table 5.2 Multinomial Regression Model Predicting the Relative Risk Ratio of a Women Continuum of Care of Maternal and Child Health

Variable/Category	Full CoC (RRR)	95% CI		Partial CoC 95% CI (RRR)		
Urban (ref)	1.00			1.00		
Rural	1.12***	1.08	1.18	0.88***	0.85	0.93
Education level						
No Education (ref)	1.00			1.00		
Primary	1.10***	1.05	1.16	0.90***	0.86	0.95
Secondary	1.04*	1.00	1.09	0.95*	0.92	1.00
Higher	1.09**	1.02	1.16	0.91***	0.86	0.98
Wealth index						
Poorest(ref)	1.00					
Poorer	1.10***	1.12	1.22	0.85***	0.82	0.89
Middle	1.29***	1.23	1.36	0.77***	0.74	0.81
Richer	1.42***	1.35	1.51	0.70***	0.66	0.74
Richest	1.71***	1.60	1.83	0.58***	0.55	0.62
EAG state						
Assam(ref)	1.00			1.00		
Bihar	0.35***	0.33	0.39	2.78***	0.33	0.39
Chhattisgarh	1.70***	1.58	1.85	.58***	1.58	1.85
Jharkhand	0.74***	0.69	0.80	1.34***	0.69	0.80
Madhya Pradesh	0.45***	0.43	0.49	2.17***	0.43	0.49
Odisha	2.04***	1.91	2.19	0.48***	1.91	2.19
Rajasthan	0.62***	0.58	0.67	1.60***	0.58	0.67
Uttar Pradesh	0.92*	0.87	0.98	1.07*	0.87	0.98
Uttarakhand	0.52***	0.47	0.58	1.91***	0.47	0.58
MCH benefit						
Not received(ref)	1.00			1.00		
Received	1.10***	1.06	1.14	0.90***	0.88	0.94
Birth order						
1st order(ref)	1.00			1.00		
2nd order	1.02	0.99	1.06	0.98	0.95	1.01
3rd order	1.06	0.97	1.15	0.95	0.87	1.03
4th and more order	0.91	0.66	1.26	1.10	0.79	1.51

Note: $*p < 0.001$, $**p < 0.05$, $***p < 0.1$

residence, and birth order are strong determinants of healthcare utilization, and that wealth status is a predictor of differentials in CoC for MCH services in India (Kulkarni, 1992; Singh et al., 2012). However, to increase the level of CoC among the poor, the public healthcare system must be strengthened, along with community awareness of the importance of taking all CoC services. Women living in urban areas, with better wealth status and education, are more likely to utilize all MCH services (Guliani et al., 2012; Titaley et al., 2009; Pallikadavath et al., 2004; Johar et al., 2018). Promoting the coverage of antenatal care would make a significant impact on the further utilization of CoC in the EAG states, especially in Bihar, where the coverage is much lower. Women's exposure to antenatal care is a key determinant of the further use of services in the CoC. However, women's perception of service delivery also influences the coverage of maternal healthcare services like ANC and institutional delivery. This suggests the need for behavioral change interventions to overcome the challenges (Bhattacharyya et al. 2015; Bhattacharyya et al., 2018).

Promoting the coverage of antenatal care would make more impact on the further utilization of CoC in the EAG states specifically in Bihar as it is much lower in the state. Previous studies have found that women's exposure to antenatal care would determine the further use of services in the CoC. Nevertheless, women's perception of service delivery influences the coverage of maternal healthcare services like ANC and institutional delivery (Bloom et al., 1999; Magadi et al., 2003; Bhutta et al., 2010). This suggests the implementation of behavioural change intervention to overcome the challenges.

Policy Recommendations

The need for continuum of care approach: This study signifies the need for CoC for maternal and child health services in India's underdeveloped region. Merely taking the coverage of antenatal care or institutional delivery or any other indicators would not suffice to guarantee a reduction in adverse outcomes in the maternal and child health domain in the country. In other words, the statistics of coverage of any singular MCH service may not reflect maternal and child well-being at large.

Strengthen public healthcare system: This recommendation is based on the findings that the CoC among the poor is considerably low in the EAG states. A higher proportion of poor women from rural setting in the EAG states are usually uneducated or less educated. This further aggravates the disqualification of the CoC in maternal and child health services. This observation hints at the promotion of CoC against all odds among the poor and the marginalized to reap the dividend in maternal and child health outcomes.

State governance on public health: The extent of efficiency of the healthcare system significantly differs across the states, and consequently, the CoC also varies. Even though health-related matter belongs in the concurrent list of the Constitution of India, the implementation of all central government programmes rests on the state governments (Balakrishnan et al., 2016; Lingam et al., 2011). The governance of public healthcare institutions in the states is crucial in the matter of healthcare utilization and the CoC particularly among the poor.

Limitations of the Study

The interpretation of levels and patterns of CoC must be taken based on its definition. In this study, the CoC was assessed by the three indicators. The number of indicators taken to define would also affect the levels and patterns of CoC. If more indicators are taken for the evaluation, the probability of this level coming down is very high. In such a situation, we opt for the optimum number of relevant indicators available in the NFHS-4 dataset for the present study. This study only considered women using an allopathic system of medicine, whereas in many parts of the country, especially in tribal areas, the use of Indian systems of medicine like Ayurveda is very common for maternal and child health.

References

Alcock, G., Das, S., More, N. S., Hate, K., More, S., Pantvaidya, S., ... & Houweling, T. A. J. (2015). Examining inequalities in uptake of maternal health care and choice of provider in underserved urban areas of Mumbai, India: A mixed methods study. *BMC Pregnancy and Childbirth*, 15(1), 1–11. https://doi.org/10.1186/s12884-015-0661-6

Balakrishnan, R., Gopichandran, V., Chaturvedi, S., Chatterjee, R., Mahapatra, T., & Chaudhuri, I. (2016). Continuum of care services for maternal and child health using mobile technology: A health system strengthening strategy in low and middle income countries. *BMC Medical Informatics and Decision Making*, 16(1), 1–8. https://doi.org/10.1186/s12911-016-0326-z

Bhattacharyya, S., Srivastava, A., Saxena, M., Gogoi, M., Dwivedi, P., & Giessler, K. (2018). Do women's perspectives of quality of care during childbirth match with those of providers? A qualitative study in Uttar Pradesh, India. *Global Health Action*, 11(1), 1527971.

Bhattacharyya, S., Issac, A., Rajbangshi, P., Srivastava, A., & Avan, B. I. (2015). "Neither we are satisfied nor they" -users and provider's perspective : A qualitative study of maternity care in secondary level public health facilities, Uttar Pradesh, India. *BMC Health Services Research*, 1–13. https://doi.org/10.1186/s12913-015-1077-8

Bhutta, Z. A., Chopra, M., Axelson, H., Berman, P., Boerma, T., Bryce, J., ... others (2010). Countdown to 2015 decade report (2000–10): Taking stock of maternal, newborn, and child survival. *The Lancet*, 375(9730), 2032–2044.

Bloom, S. S., Lippeveld, T., & Wypij, D. (1999). Does antenatal care make a difference to safe delivery? A study in urban Uttar Pradesh, India. *Health Policy and Planning*, 14(1), 38–48.

Bryce, J., Arnold, F., Blanc, A., Hancioglu, A., Newby, H., Requejo, J., ... others (2013). Measuring coverage in MNCH: New findings, new strategies, and recommendations for action. *PLoS Medicine*, 10(5), e1001423.

Chopra, M., Daviaud, E., Pattinson, R., Fonn, S., & Lawn, J. E. (2009). Saving the lives of South Africa's mothers, babies, and children: Can the health system deliver? *The Lancet*, 374(9692), 835–846.

Desai, S., & Wu, L. (2010). Structured inequalities: Factors associated with spatial disparities in maternity care in India. *Margin: The Journal of Applied Economic Research*, 4(3), 293–319.

Guliani, H., Sepehri, A., & Serieux, J. (2012). What impact does contact with the prenatal care system have on women's use of facility delivery? evidence from low-income countries. *Social Science & Medicine*, 74(12), 1882–1890.

IIPS. (2017). *National Family Health Survey 2015–16 (nfhs-4): India Factsheet, India*. Mumbai: IIPS.

Iqbal, S., Maqsood, S., Zakar, R., Zakar, M. Z., & Fischer, F. (2017). Continuum of care in maternal, newborn and child health in Pakistan: Analysis of trends and determinants from 2006 to 2012. *BMC Health Services Research*, 17(1), 189.

James, K., Mishra, U. R., & Pallikadavath, S. (2022). Sequential impact of components of maternal and child health care services on the continuum of care in India. *Journal of Biosocial Science*, 54(3), 450–472. https://doi.org/10.1017/S002193202100016X

Johar, M., Soewondo, P., Pujisubekti, R., Satrio, H. K., & Adji, A. (2018). Inequality in access to health care, health insurance and the role of supply factors. *Social Science & Medicine*, 213, 134–145.

Karvande, S., Sonawane, D., Chavan, S., & Mistry, N. (2016). What does quality of care mean for maternal health providers from two vulnerable states of India? Case study of Bihar and Jharkhand. *Journal of Health, Population and Nutrition*, 1–10. https://doi.org/10.1186/s41043-016-0043-3

Kulkarni, M. N. (1992). Universal immunisation programme in India: Issues of sustainability. *Economic and Political Weekly*, 1431–1437.

Kumar, C., Rai, R. K., Singh, P. K., & Singh, L. (2013). Socioeconomic disparities in maternity care among Indian adolescents, 1990–2006, 8(7), 1–10. https://doi.org/10.1371/journal.pone.0069094 Manuscript, A. (2014). NIH Public Access, 4(3), 1–23. https://doi.org/10.1177/097380101000400303.Structured

Kumar, C., Rai, R. K., Singh, P. K., & Singh, L. (2013). Socioeconomic disparities in maternity care among Indian adolescents, 1990–2006. *PLoS One*, 8(7), e69094.

Lingam, L., & Yelamanchili, V. (2011). Reproductive rights and exclusionary wrongs: Maternity benefits. *Economic & Political Weekly*, 46(43), 94–103.

Magadi, M. A., Zulu, E. M., & Brockerhoff, M. (2003). The inequality of maternal health care in Urban Sub-Saharan Africa in the 1990s. *Population Studies*, 57(3), 347–366.

McDougal, L., Atmavilas, Y., Hay, K., Silverman, J. G., Tarigopula, U. K., & Raj, A. (2017). Making the continuum of care work for mothers and infants: Does gender equity matter? Findings from a quasi-experimental study in Bihar, India. *PLoS ONE*, 12(2), 1–19. https://doi.org/10.1371/journal.pone.0171002

Mothupi, M. C., Knight, L., & Tabana, H. (2018). Measurement approaches in continuum of care for maternal health: A critical interpretive synthesis of evidence from LMICs and its implications for the south African context. *BMC Health Services Research*, 18(1), 539.

Mukherjee, S., & Singh, A. (2018). Has the Janani Suraksha Yojana (a conditional maternity benefit transfer scheme) succeeded in reducing the economic burden of maternity in rural India? Evidence from the Varanasi district of Uttar Pradesh. *Journal of Public Health Research*, 7(1), 1–8. https://doi.org/10.4081/jphr.2018.957

Neogi, S. B., Khanna, R., Chauhan, M., Sharma, J., Gupta, G., Srivastava, R., ... & Paul, V. K. (2016). Inpatient care of small and sick newborns in healthcare facilities. *Nature Publishing Group*, 36(s3), S18–S23. https://doi.org/10.1038/jp.2016.186

Pallikadavath, S., Foss, M., & Stones, R. W. (2004). Antenatal care: Provision and inequality in rural north India. *Social Science & Medicine*, 59(6), 1147–1158.

Patel, A. B., Prakash, A. A., Raynes-Greenow, C., Pusdekar, Y. V., & Hibberd, P. L. (2017). Description of inter-institutional referrals after admission for labor and delivery: A prospective population based cohort study in rural Maharashtra, India.

BMC Health Services Research, 17(1), 1–8. https://doi.org/10.1186/s12913-017-2302-4

Saxena, M., Srivastava, A., Dwivedi, P., & Id, S. B. (2018). Is quality of care during childbirth consistent from admission to discharge? A qualitative study of delivery care in Uttar Pradesh, India, 1–20.

Shibanuma, A., Yeji, F., Okawa, S., Mahama, E., Kikuchi, K., Narh, C., ... others (2018). The coverage of continuum of care in maternal, newborn and child health: A cross-sectional study of woman-child pairs in Ghana. *BMJ Global Health*, 3(4), e000786.

Singh, A., Kumar, A., & Pranjali, P. (2014). Utilization of maternal healthcare among adolescent mothers in urban India: Evidence from DLHS-3, 1–29. https://doi.org/10.7717/peerj.592

Singh, A., Kumar, A., &Pranjali, P. (2014). Utilization of maternal healthcare among adolescent mothers in urban India: Evidence from DLHS-3. *PeerJ*, 2, e592.

Singh, A., Padmadas, S. S., Mishra, U. S., Pallikadavath, S., & Johnson, F. A. (2012). Socio-economic inequalities in the use of postnatal care in India. 7(5). https://doi.org/10.1371/journal.pone.0037037

Singh, P. K., Rai, R. K., Alagarajan, M., & Singh, L. (2012). Determinants of maternity care services utilization among married adolescents in rural India. *PLoS ONE*, 7(2). https://doi.org/10.1371/journal.pone.0031666

SRS (2020). *SRS Special Bulletin on Maternal Mortality in India 2016–2018. Office of the Registrar General of India, Census Commissioner*. New Delhi, India: Government of India.

Tanahashi, T (1978). Health service coverage and its evaluation. *Bulletin of the World Health Organization*, 56(2), 295.

Thongkong, N., Van De Poel, E., Roy, S. S., Rath, S., &Houweling, T. A. J. (2017). How equitable is the uptake of conditional cash transfers for maternity care in India? Evidence from the Janani Suraksha Yojana scheme in Odisha and Jharkhand. *International Journal for Equity in Health*, 16(1), 1–9. https://doi.org/10.1186/s12939-017-0539-5

Titaley, C. R., Dibley, M. J., & Roberts, C. L. (2009). Factors associated with non-utilization of postnatal care services in Indonesia. *Journal of Epidemiology & Community Health*, 63(10), 827–831. https://doi.org/10.1136/jech.2008.081604.

6 Place of Hospitalization and Residence, and Their Effect on Caesarean Section Out-of-Pocket Expenditure in India

Pushpendra Singh and Sandhya Mahapatro

Introduction

The childbirth experience is a profound and powerful human feeling (Oweis & Abushaikha, 2004), and healthcare services are there to provide safe maternal delivery to minimize complication risk for the mother and child (Lundgern & Berg, 2007). With continuous government efforts and various interventions, the health indicators of the country are improving. In 2005, National Rural Health Mission (NRHM) was launched to bring health sector reform including achieving faster and more equitable growth in maternal and child health. Institutional deliveries, in both government and private hospitals, have increased rapidly since the implementation of NRHM (2005) with 4.1 times more chances of institutional deliveries during the post-NRHM period (Pund et al., 2017). Demand-side financing schemes have been initiated to reduce maternal mortality and expand access to safe deliveries. With such efforts, institutional delivery which was 43 percent in 2004 increased to 93.8 percent by 2020 and the substantial increase was in the public sector (NFHS, 2019-20). Along with the increase in facility delivery, the cost of care is also increasing. Even though basic maternal and child health services are meant to be provided free of cost in government hospitals and accredited private hospitals, there still a significant share of the population faces out-of-pocket expenditure. Previous studies have shown that the delivery care expenses were higher for C-section than vaginal delivery (Douangvichit et al., 2012), and hence, an increasing trend in C-section may be attributed to this. The prevalence of the C-section in India was 8.5% in NFHS-3, while it has increased to 32% in NFHS-5, almost four times increase during this period.

The caesarean section has become widely accepted as a safe intervention to minimize maternal delivery risk and reduce maternal and newborn mortality. Caesarean section is required, when there is a significant risk of adverse outcomes for the mother or baby at the time of delivery (Penna & Arulkumaran, 2003). However, medically the use of caesarean section is a vague indication of medical treatment in case of failure of foetus progress and presumed foetal compromise, while non-medically caesarean sections performed for other than the adverse risk of the outcome, which may personally benefit a patient (to avoid physical or psychological trauma) and financially benefited to the

DOI: 10.4324/9781003430636-9

hospital (Lavender et al., 2012; Ryding, 1993). Hence, all these medical and non-medical reasons led the caesarean birth over a period across the globe.

Around 3,00,000 women die every year during childbirth across the globe and almost 99% are from low-income and middle-income countries (WHO, 2019). It has been argued that universal access to caesarean section is a key requisite to improve maternal and perinatal outcomes (Bailey et al., 2009; Sobhy et al., 2019). Often, caesarean sections are performed 'too little, too late', or 'too many, too soon'; both are having adverse outcomes in terms of over and underuse of caesarean sections (Esteves-Pereira et al., 2016; Ologunde, 2014). World Health Organisation (WHO) proposed C-section birth should be 10-15% of birth and if the use of caesarean section is more than 20% of the birth, it will not affect the improvement of maternal and perinatal outcomes (Betrán et al., 2016; Molina, 2015). Since, from the past two decades, the use of caesarean section has been continuously increasing. An increase in caesarean sections beyond a limit will adversely affect them in terms of financial distress among the poor and drag them into impoverishment.

Access to maternal healthcare services is not always free in lower-middle-income countries and carries a risk of financial catastrophe (Schieber, 2007). Globally, each year around 150 million cases of catastrophic medical expenditure have resulted from surgery, including caesarean sections (Shrime, 2015). The National Health Account (NHA) 2016–17 shows that 68.7% of all health expenditure is financed from household revenues. In contrast, only 15.8% is supported by the state governments and 8.7% by the union government, which clearly explains the catastrophic burden on households. Moreover, the increasing caesarean section deliveries in India put an adverse effect on the household economy by increasing medical expenditure. To cope with the financial burden, households especially in the low-income quintile, divert their savings, borrows, mortgage, or sell assets for the ongoing treatment (Govil et al., 2020; Mishra & Mohanty, 2019).

Various studies explore the economic impact of caesarean delivery on individuals as well as on households (Kim et al., 2017) and find caesarean section expenditure affected households' financial condition negatively. India witnessed an increase in institutional birth with the successful implementation of child and reproductive health policies. Within a period of five-year intervals from NFHS-4 to NFHS-5, there is an increase in C-section delivery from 17.2% to 32.3% in India. The increase is more significant in public health facilities from 11.9% to 22.7% between 2015–16 and 2019–20, while the increase was 40.9% to 49% in private facilities for the same period.

As much the institutional birth is increasing, maternal expenditure increases with an upsurge in caesarean section, although caesarean birth is not uniform across India and may vary based on the availability of the state/regional medical facilities. Figure 6.1 reveals in all the EAG states there is more than a two-fold increase in C-section delivery despite the lack of health infrastructure and low economic conditions of people.

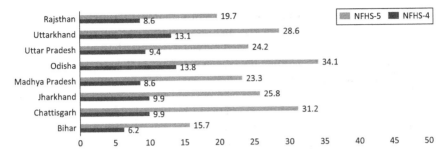

Figure 6.1 Percentage of Caesarean Delivery in EAG States

The prevalence of C-section delivery is more than 30% in Odisha and Chhattisgarh (Figure 6.1). Although maternal factors were attributed to C-section delivery, the increase in institutional birth also would be responsible for C-section delivery even among the poor that may lead to financial hardship on them.

Of the various causes, the vulnerability of increasing maternal expenditure could be on the deficit of the healthcare facilities at the doorstep. The lack of facilities in nearby areas forces women to change their place of residence for delivering the baby, which would lead to an increase in the cost of institutional delivery. Though there are a few studies on caesarean OOPE in India, more studies are needed on the accessibility of maternal care if the place of hospitalization is outside the place of a woman's usual residence and its impact on caesarean OOPE using the national representative dataset.

As a result of these concerns, the major objective of this paper is: 1) to estimate the current prevalence of caesarean/normal delivery by place and type of hospitalization; 2) to assess the influence of change in place of residence on OOPE for normal/caesarean section delivery by place of hospitalization and type of healthcare facilities.

Data and Methods

Data

The present study has used the data from the primary-based unit-level survey from the 75th round (schedule 25.0) of the National Sample Survey Organization (NSSO, 2017–18). The primary aim of the survey was to generate necessary quantitative information on the health sector, such as determining the prevalence rate at the state and national level of general morbidity. The survey has also provided estimates of the incidence and nature of prenatal, post-natal, and place/type of childbirth including normal delivery and the caesarean section as well as the expenditure incurred on childbirth or maternal care, among the women who had experienced pregnancy during the last 365 days.

This study has been restricted to currently married women aged 15–49 years, who delivered a baby in the 365 days before the survey. A total of *148,239* women have been interviewed between the age of 15–49, and out of the total women, 32,215 women have been pregnant in the last 365 days, and about *27,447* women had reported institutional delivery in public and private healthcare facilities during the reference period. The information on normal and caesarean delivery expenditure incurred by households was collected at a disaggregated level as inpatient medical care cost containing sub-components such as bed charges, doctor's/surgeon's fees, the total amount paid for medicines, diagnostic tests, attendant charges, physiotherapy, personal medical appliances, blood, oxygen, etc., during the stay at the hospital in the period of last 365 days. However, the non-medical expenses on the transportation and food of the patient have been estimated separately. Furthermore, to estimate the OOPE for the case of hospitalization, the amount of medical expenses that might be reimbursed by employers or by insurance companies is subtracted from the overall medical expenditure.

Statistical Estimates

This study applied both bivariate and multivariate analysis to fulfil the objectives. First, the proportion and OOPE for the normal/caesarean delivery along with the place of hospitalization have been estimated. Furthermore, the multivariate analysis has been applied to estimate the factors affecting normal/caesarean birth and OOPE separately.

The dependent variable is related to normal and caesarean proportion, out-of-pocket expenditure from the place of residence, and hospital characteristics. On the basis of the practical importance of childbearing costs in India, the study has considered the place of hospitalization as the key explanatory variable (Singh et al., 2016; Govil et al., 2020; Mohanty et al., 2019). The place of hospitalization has been asked as same district (rural area) – 1; same district (urban area) – 2; within-state different districts (rural area) – 3; within-state different districts (urban area) – 4; and other states – 5.

Result

This section will present the pattern and cost of delivery by type of delivery according to the place of hospitalization and type of hospitalization. Such analysis will throw light on the role of distance on the cost of delivery, especially C-section.

Distribution of Normal and Caesarean Birth and Expenditure by Place of Hospitalization

Table 1 shows the distribution of caesarean section delivery and their expenditure by the level of care and place of hospitalization. Of the total women living in urban areas who had delivered in rural areas of same district, 27.5% of them had gone for C-section delivery, whereas 34.7% did C-section who have delivered in urban areas of same district. Similarly, those urban women preferred to deliver in the same place. Almost half of them (49.9%) had delivered through caesarean birth in a private hospital, while only 19.8% of C-section deliveries were conducted in a government hospital. Among women of urban areas who had moved to rural areas of other districts and delivered in private hospitals, 60.9% had a baby born by caesarean, while only 12.6% of deliveries in a government hospital were through caesarean. The proportion of C-sections in public hospitals is higher for urban areas of different districts where 38% of deliveries were C-section. Of the people who live in urban areas and visited other states for maternal delivery, of these all those who visited private hospitals (33.1%) had a caesarean delivery, whereas in government hospitals, it was 21.1%.

Similarly, people who live in the countryside generally consult government hospitals for delivering the baby, however, some opt for private hospitals in the same locality. Of rural women who have delivered in rural areas of same district, only 8.2% delivered through C-section, the share is higher in private (34.6%) than government facilities (4.6%). However, those who are more concerned with safe delivery choose the urban areas for better facilities in the same district, 21% of them had C-section deliveries, and it is significantly higher in the private facility (48.8%) than public (10.8%), while it increases to 21.3% for those delivered in urban areas of same district. Irrespective of the place of birth, the proportion of C-section is higher in private hospitals and relatively more in urban areas.

Despite various efforts to improve the health system, the country is experiencing inadequate health facilities and the lack of healthcare services is more prevalent in rural areas. In that case, people living in rural places may visit other rural areas of nearby districts for availing health facilities. Among them, for those who visited government hospitals, 19.1% have caesarean delivery, while in the private hospitals, it is much higher at 71.4%. Not everyone can afford private hospital charges and visit government hospitals for delivery. Of these, 25.2% have caesarean delivery in government hospitals, and their number is doubled in private hospitals with 52.5% having a caesarean delivery. Their rate of caesarean delivery in the private and government hospitals followed a similar pattern in the other states. The proportion of C-section is higher for inter-state (43.6%) than inter-district movement (32.5% in rural and 37.2% in urban). The table explained that women visited other states for maternal delivery due to many socio-economic reasons whether it is private or government hospitals; only 25.9% have caesarean delivery in government hospitals and 60.8% in private hospitals.

Out-of-Pocket Expenditure for the Maternal Care

Furthermore, Table 6.1 explains the OOPE for both types of institutional delivery. The overall OOPE is higher for the urban residents in all the

Table 6.1 Percentage Distribution of Place of Hospitalization for Normal and Caesarean Section Birth and Delivery Expenditure by Level of Care in India, 2018–19

Area of Residence	Place of Hospitalization	Level of Care	ND (%)	CSD (%)	OOPE [95% CI] (ND)	OOPE [95% CI] (CSD)	ND (N)	CSD (N)	Total (N)
Urban	Same district (rural area)	Govt. Hospital	87.0	13.0	2544.9[2079.3-3010.5]	6656.0[4290.7-9021.2]	225	31	256
		Pvt. Hospital	45.8	54.2	17480.1[14749.7-20210.4]	41629.8[35263.2-47996.4]	62	57	119
		Total	72.5	27.5	5851.4[4851.3-6851.6]	30886.4[25393.0-36379.7]	287	88	375
	Same district (urban area)	Govt. Hospital	80.2	19.8	2362.5[2241.5-2483.6]	5048.1[4755.1-5341.0]	3,999	1,012	5,011
		Pvt. Hospital	50.2	49.9	17614.1[16964.7-18263.5]	37119.2[36275.5-37962.9]	2,249	2,412	4,661
		Total	65.3	34.7	8163.3[7851.5-8475.1]	27894.8[27119.3-28670.3]	6,248	3,424	9,672
	Within-state different districts (rural area)	Govt. Hospital	87.5	12.6	3193.5[1148.0-5239.1]	8232.1[1134.9-15329.3]	33	12	45
		Pvt. Hospital	39.1	60.9	31057.5[21238.1-40876.8]	38078.1[25811.5-50344.6]	9	15	24
		Total	74.8	25.2	7028.1[3260.6-10795.6]	27119.1[17762.1-36476.2]	42	27	69
	Within-state different districts (urban area)	Govt. Hospital	61.9	38.1	3756.3[3306.3-4206.2]	7659.8[6488.5-8831.0]	220	143	363
		Pvt. Hospital	45.9	54.1	19221.8[17199.5-21244.1]	39052.2[36495.8-41608.6]	196	332	528
		Total	53.3	46.7	10982.6[9753.3-12211.9]	27509.0[25289.8-29728.2]	416	475	891
	Other states	Govt. Hospital	78.5	21.5	3024.8[1878.5-4171.1]	9855.4[6151.3-13559.5]	127	29	156
		Pvt. Hospital	66.9	33.1	22402.3[18451.8-26352.8]	41239.6[36650.6-45828.6]	88	126	214
		Total	71.0	29.0	12787.1[10489.4-15084.8]	33157.5[28913.2-37401.9]	215	155	370

Rural									
Same district (rural area)	Govt. Hospital	95.4	4.6	1781.8-[1723.4-1840.3]	4262.3[3601.9-4922.8]	3,989	296	4,285
	Pvt. Hospital	65.9	34.1	12080.3[11183.2-12977.4]	25585.6[23682.8-27488.4]	392	269	661
	Total	91.8	8.2	2686.1[2557.171-2814.965]	15067.8[13742.2-16393.4]	4,381	565	4,946
Same district (urban area)	Govt. Hospital	89.2	10.8	2170.5[2117.7-2223.3]	5470.5[5151.7-5789.3]	5,943	1,070	7,013
	Pvt. Hospital	51.2	48.8	12698.7[12201.7-13195.7]	28649.2[27889.6-29408.9]	1,270	1,316	2,586
	Total	78.7	21.3	4053.8[3918.6-4189.1]	20183.2[19535.7-20830.7]	7,213	2,386	9,599
Within-state different districts (rural area)	Govt. Hospital	80.9	19.1	2320.0[1884.2-2755.8]	5025.9[3428.0-6623.9]	128	34	162
	Pvt. Hospital	28.6	71.4	14289.4[11632.2-16946.6]	40401.9[34401.8-46401.9]	33	37	70
	Total	67.5	32.5	3647.2[2852.9-4441.5]	24934.7[19635.6-30233.8]	161	71	232
Within-state different districts (urban area)	Govt. Hospital	74.8	25.2	3879.2[3422.7-4335.8]	7083.6[6231.6-7935.6]	458	184	642
	Pvt. Hospital	47.5	52.5	16588.7[14879.4-18298.0]	34761.3[32007.2-37515.5]	165	243	408
	Total	62.8	37.2	8091.4[7330.8-8852.1]	24215.3[22114.8-26315.8]	623	427	1,050
Other states	Govt. Hospital	74.1	25.9	3689.8[2185.9-5193.6]	6355.4[4286.2-8424.6]	79	33	112
	Pvt. Hospital	39.2	60.8	13101.0[10744.3-15457.7]	33838.9[29275.5-38402.3]	67	64	131
	Total	56.4	43.6	7037.8[5551.4-8524.1]	25906.3[21862.9-29949.7]	146	97	243

Note: ND: normal delivery; CSD: caesarean section delivery; OOPE: out-of-pocket expenditure

categories of delivery compared to the rural counterpart. However, it has been found that the OOPE for the people residing in the urban areas and for the delivery they have opted for private hospitals in rural areas of the same district is Rs. 41, 629.8, whereas the government hospital OOPE is almost six times lower than Rs. 6,656.0. On the contrary, the OOPE for the same district (urban area) in a private hospital is Rs. 37119.2 as compared to a government hospital is only 5048.1. Similarly, the OOPE is very high for people who prefer other states for maternal delivery.

Furthermore, for those who live in a rural area and are delivered in the same district (rural) and visited government hospitals, the OOPE is Rs. 4262.3 as compared to private hospitals (Rs. 25585.6) for caesarean delivery. In contrast, if they visited the same district (urban) in the government hospital, the OOPE is 5470.5 compared with a private hospital, which is 28649.2 for a caesarean. However, if the caesarean delivery is taking place within the state of different districts, both rural and urban areas, then the OOPE is very high. Finally, if the rural household visits other states primarily in a private hospital, the OOPE is Rs. 33,838.9 as compared to a government hospital is 6355.4 for caesarean delivery.

Correlates between Caesarean Births in India

Table 6.2 presents the adjusted odds ratio (AOR) of factors associated with caesarean births in the rural/urban area of government and private hospitals in India. In government hospitals in rural areas, the odds of caesarean births are increasing as the distance of hospitalization is increasing as compared to the same district (rural area). Similarly, in the private hospital odds ratio of caesarean birth is 1.70 for the same district (urban area) and 2.11 for those within the state but different districts (urban area). Furthermore, if the person lives in an urban area and prefers government hospitals for maternal delivery, the odds ratio of caesarean births are increasing as the place of delivery changes as compared to same district (rural areas). However, the odds ratios are higher (1.99 times) for caesarean births, who get delivered a baby within the state of different districts (urban area) in a private hospital.

Effect of Place of Hospitalization on OOPE in India

Table 6.3 presents the coefficients along with a 95% confidence interval estimated from log-linear regression controlling all the socio-economic variables to estimate the effect of place of hospitalization on caesarean OOPE. For rural areas who choose government hospitals, and had a caesarean birth, the probability of higher OOPE is increasing as the distance of the place of hospitalization is increasing compared to those who had caesarean births in the same district of rural area. However, births associated with a private hospital within a state but different district (urban area) 26.8% (95% CI 17.0%, 37.0%) have a higher probability for higher OOPE as compared to those

Table 6.2 Adjusted Odds Ratio and 95% Confidence Interval (CI) of Caesarean Births Associated With Place of Hospitalization Among the Rural/Urban Area

Place of Hospitalization	Rural		Urban	
	Govt. Hospital aOR [95% CI]	Pvt. Hospital aOR [95% CI]	Govt. Hospital aOR [95% CI]	Pvt. Hospital aOR [95% CI]
Same district® (Rural area)				
Same district (Urban area)	2.05***[1.77–2.36]	1.70***[1.41–2.07]	1.62**[1.08–2.44]	1.36[0.91–2.03]
Within-state different districts (Rural area)	2.40***[1.57–3.67]	2.10 [1.19–3.70]	2.61**[1.11–6.12]	1.34[0.52–3.42]
Within-state different districts (Urban area)	3.35***[2.67–4.19]	2.11***[1.59–2.79]	3.28***[2.06–5.21]	1.99***[1.27–3.10]
Other states	4.12***[2.57–6.60]	1.66[1.08–2.55]	1.45[0.79–2.64]	1.85[1.11–3.06]
Cons	0.01***[0.00–0.01]	0.03***[0.02–0.05]	0.01***[0.00–0.01]	0.04***[0.02–0.09]

Note: *** p<0.01, ** p<0.05, * p<0.10; ®=Reference

Table 6.3 Coefficient of Log-Linear Regression and 95% Confidence Interval (CI) of OOPE on Caesarean Delivery with Place of Hospitalization Among the Rural/Urban Area

Place of Hospitalization	Rural		Urban	
	Govt. Hospital	Pvt. Hospital	Govt. Hospital	Pvt. Hospital
	Coef. [95% CI]	Coef. [95% CI]	Coef. [95% CI]	Coef. [95% CI]
Same district® **(Rural area)**				
Same district (Urban area)	0.200**[0.081–0.320]	0.137**[0.06–0.21]	−0.298[−0.662–0.067]	0.239*[0.057–0.421]
Within-state different **districts (Rural area)**	0.526**[0.201–0.850]	0.207[0.00–0.41]	0.454[−0.230–1.139]	0.269[−0.124–0.662]
Within-state different **districts (Urban areas)**	0.607***[0.438–0.777]	0.268***[0.17–0.37]	0.046[−0.351–0.443]	0.316**[0.121–0.510]
Other states	0.259[−0.071–0.589]	0.247**[0.09–0.41]	0.465[−0.062–0.992]	0.425***[0.208–0.642]
Cons	6.94***[6.59–7.29]	9.09***[8.85–9.34]	7.355***[6.741–7.969]	9.10***[8.79–9.41]

Note: *** p<0.01, ** p<0.05, * p<0.10; ®=Reference

who had caesarean births in the same district of rural area. Contrary to that, for those who live in urban areas and choose private hospitals within the state but different districts (urban area), OOPE is 31.6% (95% CI 12.1%, 51.0%) as compared to those who had caesarean births in the same district of rural areas. Similarly, OOPE is 42.6% (95% CI 20.8%, 64.2%) higher for those who have chosen other states as compared to the reference group.

This shows irrespective of rural and urban locality, as the place of residence changes and with increase in distance, the likelihood of caesarean birth and its cost is increasing.

Discussion

The implementation of the central government flagship program National Rural Health Mission (NRHM) and incentive-based schemes such as Janani Suraksha Yojana (JSY) and Janani Shishu Suraksha Karyakram (JSSK) attributed to a large extent for institutional delivery in India (Joe et al., 2018; Singh et al., 2018). The inclination towards institutional birth is necessary for safe delivery and improvement in health outcomes. This transition towards institutional delivery also increases caesarean section delivery, which may cause long-term health hazards for the mother and child (WHO, 2009). The existing studies have reported increasing trends of caesarean birth with extensive heterogeneity in the incidence (Ghosh & James, 2010; Singh et al., 2018; Ajeet & Nandkishore, 2013; Mohanty et al., 2019). Thus, the increasing caesarean birth creates new public health challenges such as the burden of catastrophic expenditure on the household, malpractices of private health care for making a profit, which led to long-term health consequences for both mother and children.

The study reveals that caesarean birth is lower in public hospitals, while in private hospitals, it is very high and increases with the patient hospitalized outside of the place of residence. The absence of an effective government surgical infrastructure in rural areas forced people towards private maternal healthcare providers, especially the rural elite who can afford the private health facility expenditure are moving to urban medical markets for maternal care (Qadeer, 2011). The popularity of caesarean births remains a preferable option for non-complicated deliveries by the majority of younger generation women at any cost of expenditure either living in rural or urban areas (Bruce et al., 2015). Furthermore, the study shows that some urban living people are used to prefer rural health facilities because of their lower socio-economic background, and they cannot afford maternal care in urban settings. Hence, the people who live in the urban area and prefer rural healthcare services for maternal care are the migrants, who sent their pregnant wives to their native villages where other family members live.

The financing of healthcare expenditure is a key driver of maternal care, and it could be a significant factor to contribute poor care in the long term

(Saini, 2017). Hence, the next part of the study reveals a plausible explanation of OOPE in institutional delivery.

First, those who have been living in rural areas have made less OOPE as compared to urban areas in all categories of hospitalization and level of care. The urban cost of living, changing lifestyle, cultural factors, and commercial pressure may increase the OOPE (Divyamol et al., 2016). Second, the normal delivery in a private hospital is highly expensive as compared to the same delivery in a public hospital. In contrast, the caesarean OOPE is doubled and tripled in the private hospital as compared to the normal delivery, which may cause a higher financial burden on the household. The financing of maternal care for the public and private is widely different. India has adopted the mixed method for maternal financing, which is primarily government-led financing through schemes whereby the mass population is entitled to uniform health coverage in the rural area and on the other a market-based system for the urban, who rely on the private insurers and self-financing. However, both method shows financing are not able to cater for the catastrophic OOPE. The study shows that the OOPE is exceptionally high among private hospitals both in rural and urban areas. It is quite clear that private expenditure dominates the maternal health expenditure in which the individual consumer bears the cost of their own materiality care. The inadequate government financing and neglect of public provision of health services have led to excessive private sector dominance (Tung & Bennett, 2014; Stallworthy, 2014; Mackintosh, 2016). The price of admission to hospitals has doubled in the past 15 years, and that is expanding much faster than in the government sector (Selvaraj & Karan, 2009). This overpayment later converts into the patient's catastrophic OOPE and forces them towards impoverishment. Recent studies have suggested that the higher caesarean section in private healthcare institutions is mainly due to profit motivation (Govil et al., 2020; Mohanty et al., 2019). Finally, the study finds that if the place of hospitalization is at the same place of residents for maternal delivery, then the OOPE is comparatively lower than among other categories of hospitalization. This signifies distance of the hospitalization causes the catastrophic OOP expenditure on maternal delivery, and the probability of caesarean delivery has also increased.

Conclusion

It has always been a challenge for the government to provide accessible and affordable healthcare services to all their citizens as there are many demand and supply-side barriers restricting effective implementation of the schemes. Despite that, the policymakers are trying to facilitate and protect the people from OOPE due to maternal health care through providing health insurance schemes along with investing in health infrastructure continuously to enhance the availability of healthcare services. The nation's newly launched flagship program 'Ayushman Bharat Pradhan Mantri Jan Arogya Yojana' provides free access to health care for 40% of people in the country that should adopt an integrative and multi-sectoral approach that extends beyond the insurance and health financing to cater household from the maternal OOPE. In a way, the country would be able to achieve the targets of the Sustainable Development Goals (SDGs), in maternal and child health.

References

Ajeet, S., & Nandkishore, K. (2013). The boom in unnecessary caesarean surgeries is jeopardizing women's health. *Health Care for Women International, 34*(6), 513–521.

Bailey, P., Lobis, S., Maine, D., & Fortney, J. A. (2009). *Monitoring Emergency Obstetric Care: A Handbook*. World Health Organization.

Betrán, A. P., Ye, J., Moller, A. B., Zhang, J., Gülmezoglu, A. M., & Torloni, M. R. (2016). The increasing trend in caesarean section rates: Global, regional and national estimates: 1990–2014. *PloS One, 11*(2), e0148343.

Bruce, S. G., Blanchard, A. K., Gurav, K., Roy, A., Jayanna, K., Mohan, H. L., ... & Avery, L. (2015). Preferences for infant delivery site among pregnant women and new mothers in Northern Karnataka, India. *BMC Pregnancy and Childbirth, 15*(1), 49.

Divyamol, N., Raphael, L., & Koshy, N. (2016). Caesarean section rate and its determinants in a rural area of South India. *Int J Community Med Public Health, 3*(10), 2836–2840.

Douangvichit, D., Liabsuetrakul, T., & McNeil, E. (2012). Health care expenditure for hospital-based delivery care in Lao PDR. *BMC Research Notes, 5*(1), 1–7.

Esteves-Pereira, A. P., Deneux-Tharaux, C., Nakamura-Pereira, M., Saucedo, M., Bouvier-Colle, M. H., & Leal, M. D. C. (2016). Caesarean delivery and postpartum maternal mortality: A population-based case control study in Brazil. *PloS One, 11*(4), e0153396.

Ghosh, S., & James, K. S. (2010). Levels and trends in caesarean births: Cause for concern?. *Economic and Political Weekly, 45*(5), 19–22.

Govil, D., Mohanty, S. K., & Narzary, P. K. (2020). Catastrophic household expenditure on caesarean deliveries in India. *Journal of Population Research, 37*(2), 139–159.

Joe, W., Perkins, J. M., Kumar, S., Rajpal, S., & Subramanian, S. V. (2018). Institutional delivery in India, 2004–14: Unravelling the equity-enhancing contributions of the public sector. *Health Policy and Planning, 33*(5), 645–653.

Kim, S. J., Kim, S. J., Han, K. T., & Park, E. C. (2017). Medical costs, Cesarean delivery rates, and length of stay in specialty hospitals vs. non-specialty hospitals in South Korea. *PLoS One, 12*(11), e0188612.

Lavender, T., Hofmeyr, G. J., Neilson, J. P., Kingdon, C., & Gyte, G. M. (2012). Caesarean section for non-medical reasons at term. *Cochrane Database of Systematic Reviews, 3*, 1–12.

Lundgren, I., & Berg, M. (2007). Central concepts in the midwife–woman relationship. *Scandinavian Journal of Caring Sciences, 21*(2), 220–228.

Mackintosh, M., Channon, A., Karan, A., Selvaraj, S., Cavagnero, E., & Zhao, H. (2016). What is the private sector? Understanding private provision in the health systems of low-income and middle-income countries. *The Lancet, 388*(10044), 596–605.

Mishra, S., & Mohanty, S. K. (2019). Out-of-pocket expenditure and distress financing on institutional delivery in India. *International Journal for Equity in Health*, *18*(1), 99.

Mohanty, S. K., Panda, B. K., Khan, P. K., & Behera, P. (2019). Out-of-pocket expenditure and correlates of caesarean births in public and private health centres in India. *Social Science & Medicine*, *224*, 45–57.

Molina, G., Weiser, T. G., Lipsitz, S. R., Esquivel, M. M., Uribe-Leitz, T., Azad, T., ... & Haynes, A. B. (2015). Relationship between cesarean delivery rate and maternal and neonatal mortality. *JAMA*, *314*(21), 2263–2270.

National Health Accounts Estimates for India FY 2016–17, National Health Systems Resource Centre, Ministry of Health and Family Welfare, Government of India, New Delhi.

NSS 75th Round, Key Indicators of Social Consumption in India: Health, Ministry of Statistics and Programme Implementation, National Statistical Office, Government of India, New Delhi.

Ologunde, R., Vogel, J. P., Cherian, M. N., Sbaiti, M., Merialdi, M., & Yeats, J. (2014). Assessment of cesarean delivery availability in 26 low-and middle-income countries: A cross-sectional study. *American Journal of Obstetrics and Gynecology*, *211*(5), 504-e1.

Oweis, A., &Abushaikha, L. (2004). Jordanian pregnant women's expectations of their first childbirth experience. *International Journal of Nursing Practice*, *10*(6), 264–271.

Penna, L., &Arulkumaran, S. (2003). Cesarean section for non-medical reasons. *International Journal of Gynecology& Obstetrics*, *82*(3), 399–409.

Pund, S. B., Kuril, B. M., Doibale, M. K., Ankushe, R. T., Kumar, P., & Siddiqui, N. (2017). Study of the changing trends in place of delivery in rural women in relation to pre and post NRHM period in Paithan, Aurangabad, Maharashtra. *International Journal of Community Medicine and Public Health*, *4*(7), 2356–60.

Qadeer, I. (2011). The challenge of building rural health services. *The Indian Journal of Medical Research*, *134*(5), 591.

Ryding, E. L. (1993). Investigation of 33 women who demanded a cesarean section for personal reasons. *Acta Obstetricia et Gynecologica Scandinavica*, *72*(4), 280–285.

Saini, V., Garcia-Armesto, S., Klemperer, D., Paris, V., Elshaug, A. G., Brownlee, S., ... & Fisher, E. S. (2017). Drivers of poor medical care. *The Lancet*, *390*(10090), 178–190.

Sample Registration System (SRS) 2017–19.

Schieber, G. J., Gottret, P., Fleisher, L. K., & Leive, A. A. (2007). Financing global health: Mission unaccomplished. *Health Affairs*, *26*(4), 921–934.

Selvaraj, S., & Karan, A. K. (2009). Deepening health insecurity in India: Evidence from national sample surveys since 1980s. *Economic and Political Weekly*, *44*(40), 55–60.

Shrime, M. G., Dare, A. J., Alkire, B. C., O'Neill, K., & Meara, J. G. (2015). Catastrophic expenditure to pay for surgery worldwide: A modelling study. *The Lancet Global Health*, *3*(Supplement 2), S38–S44.

Singh, P. K., Hashmi, G., & Swain, P. K. (2018). High prevalence of cesarean section births in private sector health facilities-analysis of district level household survey-4 (DLHS-4) of India. *BMC Public Health*, *18*(1), 613.

Singh, P. K., Kumar, V., & Verma, S. (2016). How affordable is childbearing in India? An evaluation of maternal healthcare expenditures. *Newborn and Infant Nursing Reviews*, 16(4), 175–183.

Singh, P. K., Rai, R. K., & Singh, S. S. L. (2018). Rising caesarean births: A growing concern. *Economic and Political Weekly*, 53, 26–27.

Sobhy, S., Arroyo-Manzano, D., Murugesu, N., Karthikeyan, G., Kumar, V., Kaur, I., ... & Zamora, J. (2019). Maternal and perinatal mortality and complications associated with caesarean section in low-income and middle-income countries: A systematic review and meta-analysis. *The Lancet*, 393(10184), 1973–1982.

Stallworthy, G., Boahene, K., Ohiri, K., Pamba, A., & Knezovich, J. (2014). Roundtable discussion: What is the future role of the private sector in health? *Globalization and Health*, 10(1), 55.

Tung, E., & Bennett, S. (2014). Private sector, for-profit health providers in low and middle income countries: Can they reach the poor at scale? *Globalization and Health*, 10(1), 52.

World Health Organization. (2019). *Trends in Maternal Mortality 2000 to 2017: Estimates by WHO, UNICEF, UNFPA, World Bank Group and the United Nations Population Division*. Geneva: WHO Press, World Health Organization.

WHO (2009). *Monitoring Obstetric Care: A Handbook*. Geneva: WHO Press, World Health Organization.

7 Understanding Maternal Healthcare Deprivation in Bihar

Brajesh Kumar

Introduction

Maternal health care (MHC) is a global issue. The evidence from various studies shows that there is a wide difference in access to MHC in developed and developing countries. MHC is significantly associated with maternal morbidity, maternal mortality, infant morbidity, and infant mortality. A good-quality MHC inexplicably contributes to the reduction of maternal mortality. To meet the targets of the Sustainable Development Goal (SDG) of lowering maternal mortality to 70 per 100,000 live births by 2030, access to quality MHC is significant.

According to the World Health Organization (WHO), maternal health refers to the health of women during pregnancy, childbirth, and the postpartum period. These three phases of maternal health care can be referred to as three dimensions of MHC: antenatal care (ANC), delivery care, and postnatal care (PNC). ANC relates to health care sought by women during pregnancy. WHO recommends there should be at least eight quality ANC contacts and the first contact in the first trimester of pregnancy. Quality ANC means ANC from a skilled health professional like doctors, auxiliary nurse midwives, nurses, and lady health visitors. Protection against neonatal tetanus is also an essential component of ANC. For this, pregnant women are required to get at least two tetanus toxoid injections during pregnancy. Furthermore, pregnant women also need to take iron and folic acid during the pregnancy for at least 100 days.

Quality delivery care involves two critical aspects. First, it should be an institutional delivery, i.e. deliveries in a health facility. Second, each delivery must be assisted by skilled health personnel like doctors, auxiliary nurse midwives, nurses, or lady health visitors. Furthermore, it also involves all women who have delivered in a health facility should receive a postnatal health check within 24 hours after delivery (Paswan et al., 2017). Women's health care within six weeks of childbirth is referred to as PNC. For home births, the first postnatal contact should be as early as possible, within 24 hours of birth (WHO, 2015). Despite India's gradual decrease in maternal mortality ratio, reasonable access to quality ANC, delivery care, and PNC remains a challenge in the province of Bihar.

DOI: 10.4324/9781003430636-10

Major Issues

Various studies have documented that specific segments of the population, often those belonging to better-off socioeconomic classes, utilise material healthcare services more frequently. The structural determinants of MHC including education, social position, and place of residence perhaps are the potent forces that determine access to MHC (Saxena et al., 2013). For universal healthcare access and improved maternal health, there is a need to explore the barriers that prevent access to quality MHC services for the poor and marginalised. Various factors, at different levels, affect the use of ANC, delivery care, and PNC services by a skilled health professional (Jat et al., 2011). Previous studies have reported a significant association between socioeconomic status and antenatal care, skilled attendance at delivery, and postnatal care (Bhatia & Cleland, 1995; Navneetham & Dharmalingam, 2002; Jat et al., 2011). There is a low level of maternal healthcare utilisation in many communities, and this is particularly true within low castes in India (Sabarwal & Sonalkar, 2015; Patel et al., 2018). Socio-demographic factors like caste and women's literacy were significantly associated with utilisation of maternal healthcare services (Saroha et al., 2008).

Access to antenatal care by skilled health professionals is fundamental to ensure optimal maternal and child health outcomes (Petrou et al., 2003). A study on the use of ANC services in Madhya Pradesh recorded a significant association between the use of ANC and factors such as women's education, household's standard of living, caste, and religion (Pallikadavath et al., 2004; Jat et al., 2011). Better-educated women are more aware of their health, know more about the availability of maternal healthcare services, and use this awareness and information in accessing healthcare services (Fosu, 1994; Costello et al., 1996; Ragupathy, 1996; Navneetham & Dharmalingam, 2002; Jat et al., 2011). Studies also suggest a significant disparity in delivery care attendance among urban and rural women. Besides, demographic factors like children ever born found statistically significant in influencing maternal health care (Kenea & Jisha, 2017)

WHO recommends that the first PNC must be within 24 hours of childbirth and four and more PNC checks within six weeks of childbirth; however, studies indicate that there is a low level of PNC within 24 hours of delivery (WHO, 2015; Patel et al., 2018). The findings from various studies suggest that the use of ANC had a significant effect on the use of skilled attendance at delivery and the use of both ANC and skilled attendance at birth had a positive influence on the use of PNC (Singh et al., 2012).

While a few studies on MHC focus on the role of ANC, other studies focus on delivery care or PNC, and others on all three dimensions separately. However, none of the studies attempts to use all three dimensions to develop a single index of MHC and this paper attempts to address this gap by taking Bihar as a case as the state is grappling with poor maternal outcomes alongside the low sociocultural context. Furthermore, this study is limited to Bihar as its performance on MHC is the poorest among empowered action group (EAG) states. According to NFHS-4, only 3.3 per cent of pregnant women in Bihar received all recommended types of ANC, which is increased to 23% in 2019–20; however, it remains the lowest among the EAG states in India. Likewise, institutional delivery which was 64 per cent in 2015–16 increased to 84% in 2019–20 but was lower than the national average.

Figure 7.1 compares ANC, delivery care, and PNC among the EAG states and India, and it was observed the MHC utilisation was lower in Bihar among all the EAG states during 2015–16 and the pattern remains the same in 2019–20 (NFHS-5).

According to the special bulletin on maternal mortality in 2018–20, the maternal mortality ratio (MMR) in Bihar is 118 compared to the national figure of 97. Generally, the MMR and maternal morbidity are considered as the best measure of maternal health although such measures do not measure the intended concept and hence are not valid measures of MHC deprivation. Furthermore, the multidimensional nature of maternal health is itself a challenge to address the problem of MHC.

Incorporating the multidimensionality of MHC for creating a single index may be very significant in understanding patterns of MHC utilisation

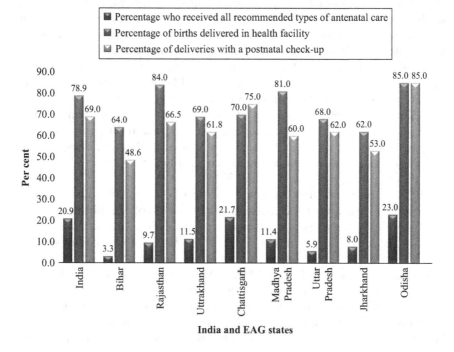

Figure 7.1 Comparison of ANC, Delivery Care, and PNC Among the EAG States and India

Note: Figure constructed from data compiled from 2015–16 NFHS-4

though computing such index is a challenging task. This study aims to put forward a multidimensional index for measuring maternal healthcare deprivation based on the deprivations experienced by women on different dimensions/indicators of maternal health care. The Alkire-Foster method (Alkire et al., 2015) is used to identify women that are multidimensionally deprived of MHC. After that adjusted headcount ratio of MHC deprivation (M) is calculated, which is referred to as an index of MHC deprivation. This method gives a scientific basis for measuring and monitoring maternal morbidity.

Data and Methods

The data for the study have been taken from the 2015–16 National Family Health Survey-4 (NFHS-4). The sample was designed to provide estimates of key indicators at national and state levels. The data on Bihar were collected from 36,772 households which included 45,812 women in the age group of 15–49. Since many cases in the data set have missing values on one or the other variables, the cases were list-wise deleted. Finally, 16,433 women in the age group 15–49 who had at least one birth in the preceding five years of the survey were considered for analysis.

Seven critical variables used in this study correspond to seven indicators in measuring MHC deprivation. These are the first ANC, number of ANCs, iron and folic acid, tetanus toxoid injection, place of delivery, assistance in the delivery, and PNC as described in Table 1. Furthermore, five socio-demographic variables used in this study are caste, religion, level of education, wealth index, and residence. Caste is divided into five categories: General, Other Backward Class (OBC), Scheduled Caste (SC), Scheduled Tribe (ST), and others. Religion takes two values: Hindu and Muslim. The level of education takes four values: no education, primary education, secondary education, and higher education. The wealth index shows the economic status and carries five categories: poorest, poor, middle, rich, and richest. Finally, the residence takes on two values: rural and urban.

The Alkire-Foster Methodology

The Alkire-Foster methodology is a promising approach to measure poverty. Nevertheless, it has the potential to measure many other kinds of deprivations as well. This study uses the Alkire-Foster methodology to develop an index of MHC deprivation. The multidimensional healthcare deprivation index identifies deprivations in three dimensions: ANC, delivery care, and PNC. These dimensions further consist of several indicators. There are four indicators for ANC, two for delivery care, and one for PNC. In all, there are seven indicators in three dimensions.

Each respondent is assigned zero or one score in each of the seven indicators based on the deprivation cut-off. Deprived women are given a score of one and non-deprived were scored zero. Each dimension is equally weighted, i.e. 1/3. Furthermore, nested weight is used, i.e. weight of each dimension is similarly divided equally into the indicators constituting that dimension. The ANC has four indicators, so each is weighted as 1/12. Delivery care has two indicators, each weighted 1/6, and PNC consists of only one indicator and is weighted 1/3. In this way, the total weights of all the seven indicators are equal to one i.e. $\sum_{j=1}^{7} wj = 1$. Dimensions, indicators, weights, and deprivation cut-off are given in Table 7.1.

The total of each woman's weighted score on all indicators/ dimensions represents their deprivation score. Since each dimension is equally weighted, any respondent's maximum possible deprivation score can be one and minimum zero. A zero deprivation score means the women are not deprived in any of the indicators/dimensions, and a deprivation score of one means the respondent is deprived in all the indicators/dimensions. Here, deprivation cut-off is applied to identify multidimensionally deprived (MD) women. In this study, a deprivation cut-off of 0.33 is applied. Accordingly, a woman has multidimensionally deprived of MHC if her score is greater than or equal to 0.33. Those women whose score is less than 0.33 are censored; i.e., they are not considered multidimensionally deprived of MHC. After that, this study focuses on only those women who are multidimensionally deprived of MHC.

The headcount ratio, *H*, is the proportion of multidimensionally deprived women in the population. If *q* is the number of women who are

Table 7.1 Dimensions, Indicators, Weight, and Deprivation Cut-Off

Dimensions	Indicators	Weight (w_j)	Deprivation cut-off
Antenatal care	First ANC	1/12	First ANC by skilled health personnel in the first trimester of pregnancy
	Number of ANCs	1/12	At least eight ANCs by skilled health personnel during pregnancy
	Iron and folic acid	1/12	Iron and folic acid are taken for at least 100 days during pregnancy
	Tetanus toxoid injection	1/12	At least two tetanus toxoid injections are given during pregnancy
Delivery care	Place of delivery	1/6	Delivery at a health facility (institutional delivery)
	Assistance in delivery	1/6	Delivery assisted by skilled health personnel
Postnatal care	Postnatal care	1/3	Received first postnatal care by skilled health personnel within 24 hours of delivery

multidimensionally poor and n is the total population, then multidimensional headcount ratio or incidence H is given as:

$$H = \frac{q}{n}$$

However, this measure of incidence violates *dimensional monotonicity* (Alkire & Foster, 2011a). Dimensional monotonicity requires that a multidimensionally deprived woman who is not deprived in all indicators becomes deprived in an additional indicator; then, MHC deprivation should increase. This means that the headcount ratio *(H)* is not a good measure of MHC deprivation because the increase in deprivation in an additional indicator does not change H. To overcome this limitation, another measure, intensity *(A)*, is used, which takes into account the deprived women in multiple dimensions/indicators. After that, *adjusted headcount ratio (M)* is measured. MHC deprivation intensity *(A)* is the weighted average deprivation among multidimensionally deprived women. To calculate A, deprivation scores of multidimensionally deprived women are summed and divided by the total number of multidimensionally deprived women and given as:

$$A = \frac{\sum_{i}^{q} ci}{q}$$

where c_i is the deprivation score of the ith multidimensionally deprived woman.

The deprivation score c_i of the ith multidimensionally deprived woman can be expressed as the sum of the weights associated with each indicator j ($j = 1, 2 \ldots 7$) in which woman i is deprived, $^{c}i = {^{c}i_1} + {^{c}i_2} + \cdots + {^{c}i_7}$.

The adjusted multidimensional MHC deprivation *(M)* value is the product of two measures, the incidence *(H)* and the intensity *(A)*, and given as:

$$M = H \cdot A = \frac{\sum_{i}^{n} ci}{n}$$

M refers to the proportion of maternal deprivations that multidimensionally deprived women in a society experience as a share of the deprivations that would be experienced if all women were deprived in all dimensions.

Subgroup decomposition of M is used for analysing MHC deprivation by caste, religion, level of education, wealth index, and residence. Population subgroup decomposability allows understanding and monitoring of adjusted headcount ratio of the subgroup and comparing them with the aggregate M. So if there are m subgroups, then

$$M = \sum_{i=1}^{m} \left(\frac{ni}{n} \right) (Mi)$$

where M_i is the adjusted headcount ratio of the ith subgroup (S_i). Furthermore, the contribution of an ith subgroup to the overall adjusted headcount ratio is given as follows:

$$S_i = \left(\frac{ni}{n}\right)\left(\frac{Mi}{M}\right)$$

The adjusted MHC deprivation also satisfies the dimensional breakdown. It hence can be used to analyse the dimensional composition of M. So, the contribution of dimension j (D_j) to the overall adjusted headcount ratio is given as follows:

$$D_j = w_j \frac{hj}{M}$$

where w_j is the relative weight attached to the jth indicator and h_j is the censored headcount ratio of the jth indicator.

As mentioned above, a woman is identified as multidimensionally deprived of MHC if the weighted sum of deprivation is below a certain measure, and here, this measure is 0.33. The selection of this cut-off lies somewhere between the union and intersection approach. The union approach identifies that the ith woman is multidimensionally deprived if she is deprived in any indicator, i.e. if $c_i > 0$. On the contrary, the intersection approach identifies a woman as multidimensionally deprived only if she is deprived in all seven indicators, i.e. if $c_i = 1$. Between these two approaches is the dual-cut-off method. Both these approaches give a disquieting figure. Thus, for this paper, a cut-off of 0.33 is selected.

Results

Table 7.2 shows that the number of multidimensionally deprived women depends on the weighted deprivation cut-off level selection. We can see that if the union definition is adopted, 99.5 per cent of women are multidimensionally deprived of MHC. If an intersection approach is used, 0.51 per cent of women are multidimensionally deprived.

Table 7.2 Maternal Healthcare Deprivation for Different Cut-Offs

Multidimensional deprivation cut-off ()	Incidence (H)	Intensity (A)	Adjusted headcount ratio (M)
Union approach ($c_i > 0$)	0.995	0.539	0.536
Midway ($c_i \geq 0.33$)	0.660	0.709	0.468
Intersection approach ($c_i = 1$)	0.051	0.051	0.051

For a cut-off of 0.33, we find that:

$H = 0.66$, $A = 0.709$, and $M = 0.468$.

The estimates show that the incidence of MHC deprivation is 66 per cent. In other words, about 66 per cent of women in Bihar are multidimensionally deprived of MHC. The intensity or the average MHC deprivation score among the deprived women is 0.709. Furthermore, the adjusted headcount ratio of MHC is 0.468, i.e. the proportion of MHC deprivations that deprived women in Bihar experience as a share of the deprivations that would be experienced if all women were deprived in all indicators. Disaggregating the adjusted headcount ratio down by dimensions/indicators reveals the underlying structure of deprivations in MHC.

Table 7.3 indicates the dimension/indicator-wise composition of MHC deprivation. It is observed that ANC contributes 34.5 per cent to MHC deprivation, delivery care contributes 22.6 per cent, and PNC contributes 42.9 per cent. This suggests the most considerable contribution to MHC deprivation is PNC. The results provide important policy insights. As PNC deprivation contributes substantially to overall MHC deprivation, policies and strategies should be formulated and implemented with the aim of reducing PNC deprivation among women. This will control the MHC deprivation to a large extent.

Table 7.3 Dimension/Indicator-Wise Composition of MHC Deprivation

Dimensions/Indicators	Censored headcount ratio	Per cent contribution
Antenatal care		
First antenatal care	0.043	9.1
Number of antenatal cares	0.054	11.5
Iron and folic acid	0.051	11.0
Tetanus toxoid injection	0.014	2.9
Total	**0.162**	34.5
Delivery care		
Place of delivery	0.057	12.1
Assistance in delivery	0.049	10.5
Total	0.106	22.6
Postnatal care	0.021	42.9
Total	0.201	42.9
M	0.468	
H	0.660	
A	0.709	

Subgroup Decomposition

This section analyses how the subgroup decomposition property of the Alkire-Foster methodology allows an understanding of the contribution of subgroups to overall MHC deprivations. A review of previous work indicates wide variation in MHC according to critical variables. By considering some critical socioeconomic variables like residence, caste, religion, age, birth order, level of education, and wealth index, an attempt is made to identify the contribution of such variables to MHC deprivation. All these variables are categorical and allow for subgroup decomposition of MHC deprivation. Table 7.4 gives the subgroup decomposition of MHC deprivation on some key socioeconomic variables.

The adjusted headcount ratio of MHC deprivation by caste group shows that general caste women perform better, followed by OBC and SC women. ST women have the highest adjusted headcount ratio of MHC deprivation. Similar is the trend for the headcount ratio as well. However, it is interesting to note that OBC women contribute the highest (57.7 per cent) to the overall adjusted headcount ratio and ST women contribute only 4.7 per cent. This is because of the largest share (59.3 per cent) of the population of OBC women

Table 7.4 Subgroup Decomposition of MHC Deprivation

Group/subgroup	Population share in per cent	H	Per cent contribution to H	M	Per cent contribution to M
Caste					
General	14.1	0.590	12.6	0.406	12.2
OBC	59.3	0.647	58.1	0.456	57.7
SC	21.9	0.704	23.3	0.516	24.1
ST	3.7	0.833	4.7	0.591	4.7
Other	1.1	0.831	1.4	0.576	1.3
Religion					
Hindu	82.2	0.645	80.3	0.451	79.1
Muslim	17.8	0.731	19.7	0.549	20.9
Level of education					
No education	55.3	0.726	60.3	0.539	63.7
Primary education	12.3	0.665	12.4	0.469	12.4
Secondary education	27.7	0.576	24.2	0.370	21.9
Higher education	4.6	0.372	2.6	0.206	2.0
Wealth index					
Poorest	22.5	0.765	26.0	0.582	27.9
Poorer	22.2	0.715	24.0	0.523	24.8
Middle	20.7	0.658	20.6	0.462	20.5
Rich	18.9	0.617	17.6	0.415	16.7
Richest	15.7	0.490	11.6	0.302	10.1
Residence					
Urban	10.7	0.541	8.8	0.360	8.2
Rural	89.3	0.675	91.2	0.481	91.8

and the low share (3.7 per cent) of the ST population. The MHC deprivation pattern will be more evident if we compare the population share in per cent of each caste group with their per cent contribution to the adjusted head-count ratio of MHC deprivation (M).

The per cent contribution to M for General (12.2) and OBC (57.7) is less than their population share in 14.1 and 59.3 per cent, respectively. However, per cent contribution to M by SC (24.1) and ST (4.7) is more than their population share in per cent. Also, the actual proportion of MHC deprivation among ST is maximum (0.591), and the proportion of MHC deprivation among the General caste is minimum (0.406).

A similar pattern of MHC deprivation according to religion, level of education, wealth index, and residence has been observed. For religion, Muslims have 17.8 per cent of the population share but contribute more (20.9) per cent to M. The MHC contribution by wealth quintile reveals the contribution of MHC is linearly associated with the economic class. The contribution to MHC deprivation is highest among the poor (27.9) followed by the poorest (24.8) and so on. Similarly, women having no education belong to the poorest and poorer wealth quintile and women from rural areas in Bihar have more contribution to M than their population share.

Dimensional/Indicator-Wise Breakdown

Dimension/indicator-wise breakdown of MHC deprivation also gives exciting information to guide policy formulation and implementation. From Table 7.5, it is clear that PNC deprivation is the maximum for all subgroups. Let us consider caste for instance. The values presented in the table show that the measure M for the General caste is 0.406 and it is clear that General caste women perform better on the first indicator, i.e. most of them take first ANC by a trained health professional within the first trimester. They also perform relatively better on other indicators of MHC deprivation except for PNC. However, it is interesting to note that they perform worst in PNC. These figures need to be explained thoroughly.

Among the seven indicators of MHC deprivation, the contribution of PNC to adjusted MHC deprivation is maximum for the General caste. This is also true for all other castes. However, the General caste's contribution of PNC to the adjusted headcount ratio of MHC deprivation is 44.8 per cent. This figure is 43.1 per cent for OBC, 43.2 per cent for ST, and the lowest at 41.3 per cent for SC. Among seven indicators, the contribution of PNC is maximum for the General caste and least for the SC. The first six indicators share lower MHC deprivation in the case of the General caste compared to SC and other caste groups. However, more MHC deprivation is shared by the first six indicators in the case of SC women, and they are left with relatively more minor to contribute to PNC deprivation.

Table 7.5 Dimensional Decomposition of MHC Deprivation as Evident from NFHS-4

Group/subgroup	Antenatal care				Delivery care		Postnatal care	M
	H_1	H_2	H_3	H_4	H_5	H_6	H_7	
Caste								
General	0.034	0.047	0.045	0.011	0.048	0.040	0.182	0.406
Per cent contribution	8.3	11.6	11.1	2.8	11.7	9.7	44.8	100.0
OBC	0.042	0.053	0.050	0.013	0.054	0.047	0.196	0.456
Per cent contribution	9.1	11.6	11.0	2.8	11.9	10.4	43.1	100.0
SC	0.049	0.058	0.056	0.015	0.067	0.059	0.213	0.516
Per cent contribution	9.4	11.2	10.8	2.9	12.9	11.4	41.3	100.0
ST	0.054	0.068	0.065	0.019	0.071	0.059	0.255	0.591
Per cent contribution	9.2	11.4	11.1	3.2	12.0	9.9	43.2	100.0
Other	0.057	0.068	0.064	0.021	0.057	0.045	0.264	0.576
Per cent contribution	9.9	11.8	11.1	3.6	9.9	7.8	45.9	100.0
Religion								
Hindu	0.042	0.053	0.051	0.013	0.052	0.045	0.196	0.451
Per cent contribution	9.2	11.7	11.1	2.9	11.5	10.0	43.5	100.0
Muslim	0.048	0.060	0.058	0.016	0.078	0.067	0.223	0.549
Per cent contribution	8.7	10.9	10.5	2.9	14.2	12.2	40.6	100.0
Level of education								
No education	0.050	0.060	0.058	0.016	0.071	0.063	0.221	0.539
Per cent contribution	9.4	11.1	10.7	3.0	13.2	11.7	41.0	100.0
Primary education	0.043	0.054	0.052	0.013	0.057	0.048	0.202	0.469
Per cent contribution	9.2	11.6	11.2	2.7	12.1	10.3	43.0	100.0
Secondary education	0.032	0.047	0.043	0.010	0.035	0.029	0.175	0.370
Per cent contribution	8.5	12.6	11.6	2.8	9.3	7.7	47.4	100.0
Higher education	0.013	0.027	0.025	0.005	0.013	0.010	0.112	0.206
Per cent contribution	6.6	12.9	12.3	2.5	6.3	5.0	54.4	100.0

(*Continued*)

Table 7.5 Continued

Group/subgroup	Antenatal care				Delivery care		Postnatal care	M
	H_1	H_2	H_3	H_4	H_5	H_6	H_7	
Wealth index								
Poorest	0.054	0.063	0.061	0.018	0.080	0.072	0.234	0.582
Per cent contribution	9.4	10.9	10.5	3.1	13.7	12.3	40.1	100.0
Poorer	0.049	0.059	0.057	0.015	0.067	0.058	0.218	0.523
Per cent contribution	9.4	11.3	10.8	2.9	12.8	11.1	41.1	100.0
Middle	0.043	0.054	0.052	0.014	0.055	0.047	0.197	0.462
Per cent contribution	9.4	11.6	11.1	3.1	12.0	10.2	42.6	100.0
Richer	0.036	0.050	0.047	0.011	0.044	0.038	0.189	0.415
Per cent contribution	8.7	12.2	14.4	2.5	10.6	9.2	45.5	100.0
Richest	0.023	0.039	0.035	0.007	0.026	0.021	0.150	0.302
Per cent contribution	7.8	12.8	11.7	2.4	8.7	6.8	49.8	100.0
Residence								
Urban	0.029	0.044	0.042	0.008	0.038	0.033	0.166	0.360
Per cent contribution	8.1	12.2	17.7	2.2	10.6	9.1	46.1	100.0
Rural	0.044	0.055	0.053	0.014	0.059	0.051	0.205	0.481
Per cent contribution	9.2	11.5	10.9	3.0	12.2	10.6	42.6	100.0

Similarly, the dimensional composition of MHC deprivation can be explained by religion level of education, wealth index, and residence. Per cent contribution of PNC for Hindus (43.5) is more than that of Muslims (40.6); for women with higher education (54.4) is more than women with no education (41.0); for women in the richest wealth index (49.8) is more than women in poorest wealth index (40.1); and for women in an urban area (46.1) is more than women in a rural area (42.6).

It is clear from the above analysis that PNC is the most neglected indicator among all women. The government must develop a precise and targeted approach to emphasise PNC and thereby reduce MHC deprivation.

Conclusion

The construction of a single index for measuring MHC deprivation using the Alkire-Foster methodology helps understand the patterns and structure of MHC deprivation. This study is perhaps the first to construct a composite index for measuring MHC deprivation using seven indicators related to three dimensions of MHC: ANC, delivery care, and PNC for the state Bihar. Many studies reveal that structural features like caste, religion, education, wealth, and residence are significantly associated with access to MHC (Saxena et al., 2013; Saroha et al., 2008). There is significant variation in MHC deprivation according to these structural features, which have been observed. Several studies find that PNC contribute most significantly to MHC deprivation (Singh et al., 2012; Bhatia & Cleland, 1995). The findings of this study also support the findings and reveal the significant contribution of postnatal care to MHC deprivation. However, the dimensional breakdown of MHC deprivation reveals striking results. PNC seems to be the most neglected and the most significant contributor to MHC deprivations and the general caste women perform worse than OBC, SC, and ST women in PNC.

The Alkire-Foster methodology is a promising approach to measure MHC deprivation. It gives the systematic and scientific basis for understanding patterns of MHC deprivation. The results show a high incidence and intensity of maternal healthcare deprivation in Bihar. The study also finds widespread differences in maternal healthcare deprivation according to key socioeconomic variables like caste, religion, level of education, wealth index, and residence. This methodology is also helpful in measuring dimensional/indicator-wise composition and their contribution to MHC deprivation, thereby delineating the underlying structure of MHC deprivation.

The study reveals that the composition of MHC deprivation differs for different subgroups of women. It provides valuable policy visions. The most ignored dimension of maternal health care is PNC, the leading cause of maternal mortality. Overall, maternal healthcare utilisation in Bihar is far from satisfactory. There are several interventions made by the government to improve maternal health care in Bihar over time. Under National Rural Health Mission (NRHM), many innovations have been introduced in the states to deliver maternal healthcare services effectively. Janani Suraksha Yojana offers cash incentives for women of lower socioeconomic status to prefer institutional delivery. Recognising the role of community workers in sensitising women to MHC, one of the core strategies was creating a village-level female social activist designated ASHA (Accredited Social Health Activist) for every village. She is expected to create awareness of maternal and child health and its determinants, mobilise the community, and increase utilisation of the existing health services. Accredited Social Health Activists (ASHA) play a significant role in facilitating access to health services and strengthening public health service delivery. But these interventions did not work to make headway in MHC in Bihar.

Subgroup composition, the dimensional composition of MHC deprivation, and postnatal care may be given particular emphasis in maternal healthcare policies. The findings of the study recommend the strategies to improve maternal health care need to incorporate measures that will improve the utilisation of postnatal care services in Bihar. To enhance PNC care, it is essential to monitor the role of ASHA workers and promote them to sensitise women to receive PNC care.

References

Alkire, S., & Foster, J. (2011). Counting and multidimensional poverty measurement. *Journal of Public Economics, 95*(7–8), 476–487.

Alkire, S., Foster, J., Seth, S., Santos, M. E., Roche, J. M., & Ballon, P. (2015). *Multidimensional Poverty Measurement and Analysis*. Oxford: Oxford University Press.

Bhatia, J. C., & Cleland, J. (1995). Determinants of maternal care in a region of South India. *Health Transition Review, 5*, 127–142.

Costello, M. A., Lleno, L. C., & Jensen, E. R. (1996). *Determinants of Two Major Early Childhood Disease and Their Treatment in the Philippines: Findings from the 1993 National Demographic Survey*. East-West Center.

Fosu, G. B. (1994). Childhood morbidity and health services utilisation: Cross-national comparison of user-related factor from DHS data. *Social Science and Medicine, 38*, 1209–1220.

Jat, T. R., Nawi, N., & Sebastian, M. S. (2011). Factors affecting the use of maternal health services in Madhya Pradesh state of India: A multilevel analysis. *International Journal for Equity in Health, 10*(59), 1–11.

Kenea, D., & Jisha, H. (2017). Urban-rural disparity and determinants of delivery care utilisation in Oromia region, Ethiopia: Community-based cross-sectional study. *International Journal of Nursing Practice, 24*, 1–10.

Navneetham, K., & Dharmalingam, A. (2002). Utilisation of maternal health care services in Southern India. *Social Science and Medicine, 55*, 1849–1869.

Organisation, W. H. (n.d.). Maternal Health. Retrieved March 14, 2019, from World Health Organization: https://www.who.int/maternal-health/en/

Pallikadavath, S., Foss, M., & Stones, R. W. (2004). Antenatal care in rural Madhya Pradesh: Provision and inequality. In A. R. Chaurasia, & R. W. Stones, *Obstetric Care in Central India* (pp. 111–128). Southampton: University of Southampton.

Paswan, B., Singh, S. K., Lhungdim, H., Shekhar, C., Arnold, F., Kishor, S., et al. (2017). *National Family Health Survey (NFHS-4) 2015–16*. Mumbai: International Institute for Population Sciences (IIPS) and ICF.

Patel, P., Das, M., & Das, U. (2018). The perception, health-seeking behaviour and access to scheduled caste women to maternal health services in Bihar. *Reproductive Health Matters*, 26(54), 114–125.

Petrou, S., Kupek, E., Vause, S., &Maresh, M. (2003). Antenatal visits and adverse perinatal outcomes: Results from a British population-based study. *European Journal of Obstetrics Gynecology and Reproductive Biology*, 106(1), 40–49.

Ragupathy, S. (1996). Education and the use of maternal health care in Thailand. *Social Science and Medicine*, 43(4), 459–471.

Sabarwal, S. N., & Sonalkar, W. (2015). Dalit women in India: At the crossroads of gender, class and caste. *Global Justice Theory Practice Rhetoric*, 8(1), 44–73.

Saroha, E., Maja, A., & Sibley, L. M. (2008). Caste and maternal health care service use among rural hindu women in Maitha, Uttar Pradesh, India. *Journal of Midwifery and Women's Health*, 53(5), 41–47.

Saxena, D., Vangani, R., Mavalankar, D. V., & Thomsen, S. (2013). Inequality in maternal health care service utilisation in Gujarat: Analysis of district-level health survey data. *Global Health Action*, 6(1), 19652, DOI: 10.3402/gha.v6i0.19652.

Singh, A., Padmadas, S. S., Mishra, U. S., Pallikadavath, S., Johnson, F. A., & Matthews, Z. (2012). Socioeconomic inequalities in the use of postnatal care in India. *PLoS ONE*, 7(5), 1–9.

WHO (2015). Maternal Health. Retrieved March 14, 2019, from WHO Maternal health: https://www.who.int/maternal-health/en/

Part III
Nutrition and Well-being

8 Nutritional Status of Mothers and Children

Trends and Determinants

Neha Yadav and Krishna Kumar Choudhary

Introduction

Since its independence, India's public health care has been a concern, mainly in rural areas. Poverty, population growth, malnutrition, and high child and maternal mortality have afflicted the country for decades (Zodpey & Negandhi, 2018). While entering the 21st century, the maternal mortality ratio (MMR) estimates stood at 327 maternal deaths per 100,000 live births, and infant mortality rate (IMR) was pegged at 68, well above the global average (SRS, 2000). Almost half of the children (47 per cent) under three years of age were underweight, a similar proportion (45.5 per cent) were stunted, and 15.5 per cent were wasted (Ghosh & Shah, 2004). Overall, 52 per cent of women and 74 per cent of children aged 6–35 months were anaemic. Among the primary states, anaemia among women was most common in Assam, Bihar, Orissa, and West Bengal, where more than six out of 10 women were anaemic (National Family Health Survey, 1998-99).

In health, two important things happened in India in the Year 2000. For the first time, the Indian government announced the National Population Policy (known as NPP 2000), and India became a signatory to commit to MDG (Sharma, 2018). After two years, India announced the National Health Policy (NHP) 2002, which reflects the concerns of the MDGs. The NHP may be considered the forerunner of the National Rural Health Mission (NRHM), which started in 2005 (Yadav, 2018). MDGs 4 and 5 aimed to increase the coverage of essential maternal, newborn and child health interventions, and reduction in the prevalence of underweight children (under five years of age). It has been included as an indicator for one of the targets to eradicate extreme poverty and hunger (Goal 1) (WHO, 2018). NRHM has been viewed as the state-governed holistic mission mode intervention in health. The cornerstone of NRHM was decentralized planning and enabling the states to address their priorities (Prasad et al., 2013).

Maternal and child health was the principal concern of the NHM and at least 12 of the 17 SDGs comprise indicators pertinent to nutrition. The World Health Assembly recognized an inclusive plan on maternal, infant, and young child nutrition targets to be achieved by 2025. To catalyse the progress, the GoI launched the National Nutrition Mission in 2015. Despite

DOI: 10.4324/9781003430636-12

India's commitment to improving the health of its people and improvements made in economic development, agricultural production, and child survival, the nation lags behind the world and its neighbours on the nutritional status of children. According to the India Health Report on Nutrition 2015, in children under-five age group, stunting accounts for 38.7 per cent and wasting for 15.1 per cent (Raykar et al., 2015).

India has succeeded in halving poverty rates from the 1990 levels but failed to address the prevalence of hunger. As per the Census 2011 report, around 89 million children in the age group 0–3 were malnourished, with 35.6 million underweight. India lags in checking maternal mortality and child mortality to expected levels (Venkat, 2015). Attainment of the low IMR target set by the MDGs cannot be seen as an achievement in the presence of high under-nutrition rates. Children's nutritional deficiency outcome in India (stunting, wasting, and underweight) has considerably declined, especially during the last decade (2005-15) and further in 2019–21, but still exceeds levels observed in other countries at similar income levels.

Considering early detection and management will reverse wasting and prevent stunting in children, SDGs have advocated using stunting and wasting rates to assess undernutrition. Goal 2 of the SDGs drives to end hunger, achieve food security and improved nutrition, and promote sustainable agriculture; however, at least 12 of the 17 goals contain highly relevant indicators of nutrition (Ritchie et al., 2018).

The study aims to provide a general overview of national trends and state-level variability in nutrition status, determinants, and intervention coverage and investigate the impact of nutritional status on maternal and child health outcomes between the EAG states and the rest of India. This study helps to bring together data to support policy decisions for nutrition at the national level and especially for the EAG states.

The Interrelationship between Maternal Nutrition and Child Health

A mother's nutrition status and health have substantial effects on the outcome of her pregnancy. The foetal growth, birthweight, perinatal development rate, and survival probabilities determine nutritional status before and during pregnancy (maternal nutrition). Low birthweight (LBW) increases the risk of early mortality and morbidity at a later age (Osrin, 2000). Women in the reproductive age group and young children are most susceptible to malnutrition owing to low dietary intakes (both quantity and quality), inequitable distribution of food within the household (between female and male), inadequate food storage and preparation, dietary restrictions, poor hygiene, infectious diseases, and lack of care (Woldemariam & Timotiows, 2002). Predominantly for women, the high nutritional costs of pregnancy and lactation contribute considerably to the poor nutritional status.

Malnutrition in infancy and childhood negatively impacts the cognitive, motor-skill, physical, social, and emotional development of the afflicted child and reduces labour productivity in adulthood (UNICEF, 1998). The occurrence of an intergenerational link between maternal and child nutrition suggests a small mother will have small offspring who in turn grow to become small mothers. Some outcomes on the relationship between maternal and child nutrition (Genebo, 1999; Loaiza, 1997; Teller et al., 2000)

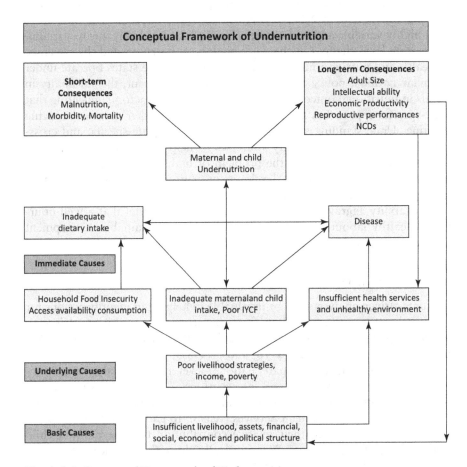

Figure 8.1 Conceptual Framework of Undernutrition

Source: adapted from UNICEF (1990) framework for studying malnutrition and death.

UNICEF. (1990). UNICEF Nutrition Strategy. https://www.unicef-irc.org/files/documents/d-3978-UNICEF%20Nutrition%20Strategy%20Document.pdf

*The black arrows indicate the long-term consequences of the undernutrition can give feedback to the underlying and basic causes of undernutrition, continuing the cycle of undernutrition and inequalities.

exhibited that a high proportion of low birthweight and stunted children were observed among malnourished mothers.

Variability in State-Level Health and Nutrition Outcome

India has made substantial progress in child nutrition outcomes between 2005–06 and 2015–16, and considerable progress was observed in the last five years (NFHS-4 to NFHS-5). However, these improvement rates have been highly variable across the states (Figure 8.2). It is likely due to variability in state-level changes in the determinants of nutrition and the coverage of health and nutrition interventions. Although all the states operate under a similar national policy and programmatic environment, the variability in trends in nutritional outcomes points to state-specific factors, indicating that state-specific approaches are necessary to achieve further gains in reducing stunting. Understanding such factors can facilitate state-specific and cross-state learning and help identify strategies to help India accelerate progress in nutrition. India overlooks the problem of undernutrition and its impact on maternal health and child development at its risk of substantial health, social, and economic consequences for future generations. While inequality and instability aggravate undernutrition, it is also factual that a well-nourished, healthy labour force is a pre-condition for sustainable development (Nguyen et al., 2021).

Material and Methods

The data-driven analysis shall be invaluable in helping to identify actions for accelerating advancement and areas where more investment is precarious to accelerate progress to attain the goals set by SDGs pertinent to nutrition. We used data from NFHS-4, 2015–16, and NFHS-5, 2019–21, national report and state factsheets to compare national-level trends, analyse nutrition-specific status, determinants, and interventions. We also reviewed national policies on maternal and child health and two national programs, NHM and Integrated Child Development Services (ICDS), to gather a list of nutrition-specific interventions for their relative contribution to maternal and child health during the last decade. We specifically chose those indicators that we consider suitable for this study and for which data are available in NFHS-5 and NFHS-4 for national- or state-level trend analysis.

Results

National Trends in Nutrition Status, Determinants, and Intervention Coverage

Nutritional Status

In the last five years, India has made substantial progress on several maternal and child nutritional status indicators (2015–16 to 2019–21). The incidence

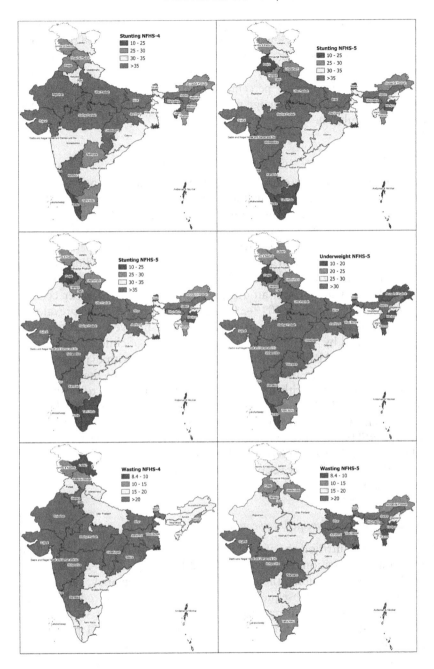

Figure 8.2 Prevalence of Malnutrition (%), Across the State, NFHS-4 and NFHS-5
Source: Authors' creation from the NFHS-4 and NFHS-5 India factsheets
NFHS 4 INDIA FACT SHEET R 10 FINAL.indd (rchiips.org)
NFHS 5 India.pdf (rchiips.org)

of stunting among children below five years has decreased by ~3 percentage points, and underweight declined by ~4 percentage points, while the decline in the wasting prevalence was 1.7 percentage points. The proportion of low birthweight children declined by ~3 percentage points, whereas exclusive breastfeeding increased by ~9 percentage points. Anaemia among pregnant women increased by ~2 percentage points, and it declined by ~9 percentage points among children.

Immediate Determinants

For the past five years, there have been modest and mixed improvements in the immediate determinants of nutrition. The percentage of women with low body mass index (BMI) declined from 22.9 per cent to 18.7 per cent, suggesting an improvement in the nutritional status of women. Early breastfeeding initiation remains unchanged (from 41.6 percent to 41.8 percent), and only 11 and 12.7 per cent of breastfeeding and non-breastfeeding children received an adequate diet, respectively. However, per cent of non-breastfeeding children who received an adequate diet declined (14.3 per cent in 2015–16 to 11.1 per cent in 2019–21), which could increase the prevalence of malnutrition. The proportion of children under five years infected with diarrhoea declined by ~2 points, while the percentage of children with acute respiratory disease (ARI) remains unchanged. Children with diarrhoea were taken to health facilities have increased by one point percentage. Around 69 per cent of children with fever (due to ARI) were taken to hospital in 2019–21, whereas 73.2 per cent of children with the same illness took treatment from a hospital in 2015–16. The lower level of receiving health service during the NFHS-5 by the children who had a fever with ARI symptoms was due to COVID-19. It advocates that more efforts to prevent illness are indispensable, primarily because low national levels could hide high illness burdens in some states and districts.

Coverage of Nutrition-Specific Interventions

The coverage of nutrition-specific interventions, which affect the immediate determinants of nutrition, improved during 2015–16 to 2019–21. The coverage of these interventions, the first 1,000 days of pregnancy, the first six months of life, and the subsequent early childhood period have been examined. For interventions, during pregnancy, the proportion of women who had at least four antenatal care (ANC) visits increased from 51 per cent to 58 per cent. The consumption of iron–folic acid (IFA) supplements during pregnancy, institutional deliveries, and birth assisted by skilled birth attendants, and birth registration also shows improvement. For childhood interventions, attention is given to immunization and vitamin A supplementation enhanced remarkably in the last five years (2016 to 2021). The percentage of children getting an oral rehydration solution (ORS) during diarrhoea has also intensified.

These improvements in the coverage of interventions followed a considerable change in India's policy and programmatic environments, primarily for the two nationwide programs—the ICDS and NHM. The ICDS and health programs increase coverage and reach by providing funds and guidance for the states to act on nutrition. Regardless of these changes, though, average national-level coverage did not extend 90 per cent for any interventions.

State Trends in Nutrition Status, Determinants, and Intervention Coverage

In India, during the last two consecutive NFHS rounds, although stunting in children under the age of five declined, the rate of stunting reduction varied significantly across the states. Some states experienced a very high percentage of decrease of around 7–10 percentage points (Madhya Pradesh 9.8, Rajasthan 9.1, and Uttar Pradesh 7.4), while Nagaland, Kerala, Telangana, Jammu and Kashmir, Assam, Tripura, Himachal Pradesh, and West Bengal showing improvement in stunting). State-level disparities in stunting prevalence are considerable, and in 2019–21, stunting occurrence persisted high in several states. Meghalaya had the highest level (46.5 per cent) followed by Bihar (42.9 per cent), Uttar Pradesh (39.7 per cent), and Jharkhand (39.6 per cent), while Puducherry had the lowest level of stunting (20 per cent). The transformation in wasting also varied extensively among states and union territories. Twelve states had substantial wasting reduction; in contrast, wasting increased in 22 states. In 2019–21, Maharashtra documented the highest levels of wasting (25.6 per cent), followed by Gujarat (25.1 per cent) and Bihar (22.9 per cent), while Chandigarh showed the lowest wasting levels (8.4 per cent). The overall prevalence of underweight among children under five years declined by around four points in the last five years, but the magnitude varied across the states. In 2019–21, Bihar had the highest proportion of underweight children (41 per cent), trailed by Gujarat (39.7 per cent) and Jharkhand (39.4 per cent), whereas Mizoram had the lowest (12.7 per cent).

In between the NFHS-4 and NFHS-5, LBW rates fell across the country except for Kerala, increasing by 0.2 per cent. In 2019–21, Rajasthan had the highest low birthweight rate (22.4 per cent), closely trailed by Madhya Pradesh (22.1 per cent), and Uttar Pradesh (20.5 per cent). At the state level, maximum states noticed an increase in exclusive breast feeding, with the exclusions of Uttar Pradesh, West Bengal, Chhattisgarh, Karnataka, Arunachal Pradesh, and Kerala.

Nationwide, anaemia among women of reproductive age increased slightly by four percentage points. The rate of anaemia reduction is diverse by state and union territories (UTs). UTs like Lakshadweep (10 percentage points), Chandigarh (10 percentage points), and Daman and Diu (10 percentage points), whereas states like Assam, Jammu Kashmir, Chhattisgarh, Odisha, Tripura, Gujarat, and Mizoram saw an increase of more than 10 percentage

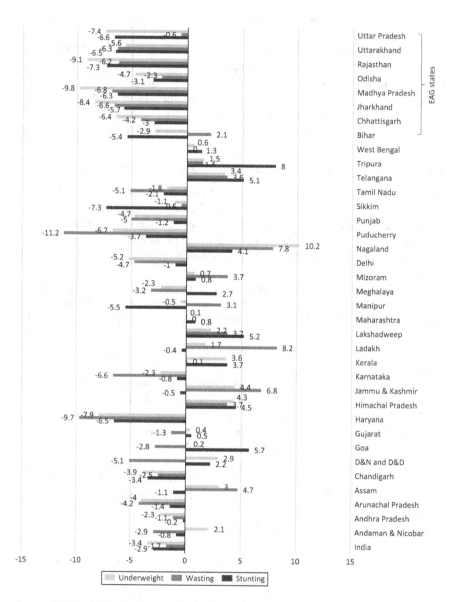

Figure 8.3 Declining Percentage Point Prevalence of Malnutrition Among Children from NFHS-4 to NFHS-5

Source: NFHS-4 and NFHS-5 India factsheet

NFHS 4 India report 60263_National_Report_Full File 05-07-2018 WEB.pdf (rchiips .org)

NFHS 5 India report FR375.pdf (dhsprogram.com)

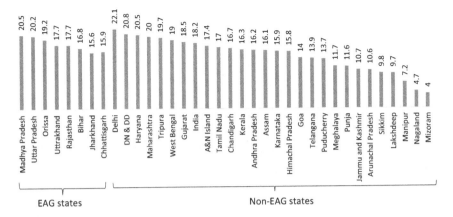

Figure 8.4 Prevalence of Lower Birthweight (>2.5kg) Babies, NFHS-5, 2019–21

Source: National Family Health Survey - 5

FR375.pdf (dhsprogram.com)

points (annexure Table 1). Anaemia among pregnant women increased by 1.8 percentage points from 2015–16 to 2019–21. More than half of the states show an increase in anaemia among pregnant women. Anaemia among children showed significant variability among states; the highest reduction was in Chandigarh, where Assam showed a 32.7 percentage point increase in anaemia prevalence among children, followed by Mizoram (27 percentage points) and Chhattisgarh (25.6 percentage points).

Trends in Immediate Determinants

The NFHS-5 India report indicates a steady decrease in the percentage of women with a body mass index (BMI) below the normal threshold, defined as 18.5 kilograms per meter of height. In 2015-16, the rate stood at 22.9 per cent, which fell to 18.7 per cent in 2019-21. In 2021, the states of Jharkhand, Bihar, Gujarat, Madhya Pradesh, Maharashtra, and Odisha saw the highest rates of underweight women, with percentages exceeding 20 per cent. Specifically, Jharkhand registered a rate of 26.2 per cent, Bihar 25.6 per cent, Gujarat 25.2 per cent, Madhya Pradesh 23 per cent, Maharashtra 20.8 per cent, and Odisha 20.8 per cent. Conversely, the lowest prevalence of underweight women was observed in Ladakh (4.4%), Jammu and Kashmir (5.2%), Mizoram (5.3%), Arunachal Pradesh (5.7%), and Sikkim (5.8%).

The percentage of Early Initiation of Breast Feeding (who started breastfeeding within 1 hour of birth) rates remained unchanged in the last two rounds of NFHS. In 2019–21, Jharkhand and Uttar Pradesh had the lowest

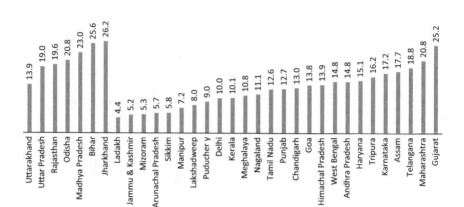

Figure 8.5 Prevalence of Malnutrition (BMI > 18.5kg/m²) Among Women, NFHS-5
National Family and Health Survey -4 India Report 60263_National_Report_Full
File 05-07-2018 WEB.pdf (rchiips.org)

Early Initiation of Breast Feeding (>30 per cent). Meghalaya, Lakshadweep, and Kerala reported the highest level of (>=70) Early Initiation of Breast Feeding. The fraction of young children (6–8 months) who were fed complementary foods declined in India during the last two rounds.

Trends in Coverage of Nutrition-Specific Interventions

The section examines the state-level trends in antenatal care (ANC) among pregnant women and nutrition-specific interventions among the mothers and children impacting the continuum of care. There has been an increase in the proportion of women who get ANC during the first trimester, the states including Nagaland (50 per cent), Bihar (52.9 per cent), Arunachal Pradesh (53.1 per cent), and Meghalaya (53.9 per cent), where coverage was lowest. At the same time, Kerala (93.6 per cent), Telangana (88.5 per cent), and Lakshadweep (99.6 per cent) had the highest ANC coverage in the first trimester. In 2019–21, the proportion of women who received four or more ANC visits showed that half of the states had made more than 70 per cent coverage. In contrast, five states had fewer than 50 per cent coverage; Nagaland and Bihar showed the lowest coverage at 21 and 25 per cent, respectively. Janani Suraksha Yojana's (JSY) coverage was better in the EAG states than in other states. Thus, there has been a remarkable rise in skilled attendants' coverage at birth. Substantial improvements are seen in institutional deliveries in states with low coverage in 2016, and the EAG states have far more scope for improvement. Although the percentage of pregnant women consuming iron and folic acid (IFA) supplements for at least 100 days continued to be low, only 20 states had more than 50 per cent.

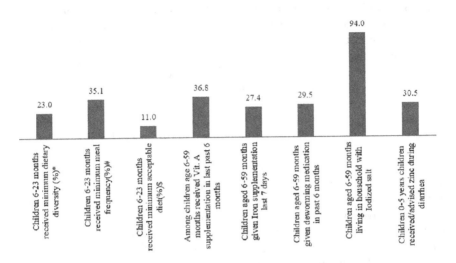

Figure 8.6 Prevalence of Nutrition-Specific Intervention Indicators, NFHS-5, 2019–21*

National Family and Health Survey -5 India Report. FR375.pdf (dhsprogram.com)

* Children receive foods from 5 or more of the following food groups: a. infant formula, milk other than breast milk, cheese or yoghurt, or other milk products; b. foods made from grains or roots, including porridge or gruel, fortified baby food; c. vitamin A-rich fruits and vegetables; d. other fruits and vegetables; e. eggs; f. meat, poultry, fish, shellfish, or organ meats; g. beans, peas, lentils, or nuts.

Children are fed the minimum recommended number of times per day according to their age and breastfeeding status: For breastfed children, the minimum meal frequency is receiving solid or semi-solid food at least twice a day for infants 6–8 months and at least three times a day for children 9–23 months; for non-breastfed children age 6–23 months, minimum meal frequency is receiving solid or semi-solid food or milk feeds at least four times a day. At least one of the feeds must be solid or semi-solid food.

$ Children aged 6–23 months are considered to be fed a minimum acceptable diet if they receive breast milk, other milk, or milk products (breastfeeding, or not breastfeeding and receiving two or more feedings of commercial infant formula, fresh, tinned, and powdered animal milk, and yoghurt), are fed the minimum dietary diversity (children receive foods from 5 or more of the following food groups: a. infant formula, milk other than breast milk, cheese or yoghurt, or other milk products; b. foods made from grains or roots, including porridge or gruel, fortified baby food; c. vitamin A-rich fruits and vegetables; d. other fruits and vegetables; e. eggs; f. meat, poultry, fish, shellfish, or organ meats; g. beans, peas, lentils, or nuts), and are fed the minimum recommended number of times per day according to their age and breastfeeding status: For breastfed children, the minimum meal frequency is receiving solid or semi-solid food at least twice a day for infants 6–8 months and at least three times a day for children 9–23 months; for non-breastfed children age 6–23 months, minimum meal frequency is receiving solid or semi-solid food or milk feeds at least four times a day. At least one of the feeds must be solid or semi-solid food.

Infants and young children are sensitive to undernutrition, including stunting and micronutrient deficits, as well as increased morbidity and mortality. To support proper growth and development, infants and young children require a minimum acceptable diet (MAD). Twenty-three per cent of all children (breastfed + non-breastfed) had an adequately diverse diet since they had been given foods from the appropriate number of food groups, while 35.1 per cent had been fed the minimum number of times appropriate for their age. According to the IYCF indicators for the minimum acceptable diet for all children aged 6 to 23, the minimal appropriate diet was served to 11 per cent of all children.

As children are weaned, vitamin A and iron-rich foods intake increases. Iron supplements were given to 27.4 per cent of children aged 6–59 months in the seven days preceding the study. 36.8 per cent of children aged 6–59 months received vitamin A supplements in the six months preceding the study, and 29.5 percent received deworming medicine. Iodized salt is used in the homes of 94 per cent of children aged 6 to 59 months. This is comparable to NFHS-4 when 93 per cent of households used iodized salt. Iodized salt is used the least in Andhra Pradesh (83 per cent), Dadra and Nagar Haveli, and Daman and Diu (89 per cent), and Meghalaya (91 per cent).

Discussion and Conclusion

As can be seen from the changes in nutritional status, India improved in some areas of undernutrition between 2015–16 and 2019–20, while others remained relatively unchanged. Almost 35.5 per cent of children in India under the age of five are stunted, and 19.3 per cent are wasted, making it one of the world's leading contributors to the worldwide burden of undernutrition. When India signed up for the 2030 Agenda for Sustainable Development in 2015, it included nutrition as a priority. The World Health Assembly approved a strategy for improving the nutrition of mothers and young children in 2012. By 2025, the program optimisms to have reduced the prevalence of stunting, wasting, and low birthweight, increased the prevalence of exclusive breastfeeding, and decreased the prevalence of anaemia in women of reproductive age by half (WHO, 2014). The GoI announced the National Nutrition Mission, popularly known as the POSHAN Abhiyaan, in December 2017 with the goal of lowering undernutrition to 20.7 per cent by 2022. Outcomes seen over the past decade (2005–06, 2015–16, and 2019–21) suggest that despite strong constitutional and legislative policies, dedicated plans, and program commitments towards improving maternal and child health, there are significant inter-state variations in the coverage of nutrition-specific interventions and nutrition status determinants. Together, wasting (at over 20%) and anaemia (affecting more than 50% of women of reproductive age) remain serious public health issues for India (Global Nutrition Report: The state of global nutrition, 2021). For many indicators, results are poor in the EAG states compared with the non-EAG states. In the last decade (2005-15), there has been a significant decline in child under-nutrition. However, declines have not been unvarying across the states of India, while furthermore, some states showed a decrease, and some showed improvement from 2015–16 to 2019–21. Even though all states function under a comparable broad national policy and programmatic environment, regional variability in the results opinions to state-specific factors affecting improvement. At the state level, careful examination of severe stunting, wasting, and anaemia in specific regional pockets will be desirable to identify the extent and level of intervention needed to tackle the issues. It is likely that in some parts, the severe wasting is seasonal or limited to sub-populations that necessitate immediate consideration, whereas, in others, it could imitate broader deprivation. What is important is that states emphasize action on those determinants of nutrition where gaps are prevalent. Understanding such influences can enable cross-state learning and identify state-specific areas for strategic investments to improve nutrition outcomes and help India accelerate improvements in nutrition. There is a critical need to bring together data to sustain policy decisions for nutrition at the national level and across the states. A state-by-state analysis of districts' trends, changes, and internal variability is crucial to identify factors affecting progress. It is essential to recognize areas of advancement and areas where more investment is critical to accelerating overall progress. It will necessitate state-level analyses to expose the diversity, both among and within the states, to develop strategies for geographically specific actions to achieve the SDG targets.

References

David Osrin, Anthony M.de L Costello. (2000). Maternal nutrition and fetal growth: practical issues in international health. *Seminarsin Neonatology*, 209–219.

Genebo, T., Girma, W., Hadir, J., and Demmissie, Y. (1999). The association of children's nutritional status to maternal education in Ziggbaboto, Guragie Zone South Ethiopia." *Ethiopian Journal of Health Development*, 13, 55–61.

Global Nutrition Report. (2021). *Global Nutrition Report: The State of Global Nutrition*. Bristol: Development Initiatives Poverty Research Ltd. Retrieved May 31, 2022, from 2021 Global Nutrition Report | The state of global nutrition - Global Nutrition Report.

Ghosh, S., & Shah, D. (2004). Nutritional problems in urban slum children. *Indian Paediatrics*, 41(7), 682–696.

Loaiza, E., Status, E. M. N., & Studies, D. C. (1997). No. 24, Macro International. Calverton, MD.

National Family Health Survey (2000). *National Family Health Survey (1998–99)*. Mumbai: International Institute for Population Sciences.

National Family Health Survey (2005–06). *National Family Health Survey (NFHS-3)*. Mumbai: International Institute for Population Sciences. National Family Health Survey (rchiips.org).

National Family Health Survey (2015–16). *National Family Health Survey (NFHS-4)*. Mumbai: International Institute for Population Sciences. National Family Health Survey (rchiips.org).

National Family Health Survey (2019–21). *National Family Health Survey (NFHS-5)*. Mumbai: International Institute for Population Sciences. National Family Health Survey (NFHS-5) (rchiips.org).

Nguyen, P. H., Scott, S., Headey, D., Singh, N., Tran, L. M., Menon, P., & Ruel, M. T. (2021). The double burden of malnutrition in India: Trends and inequalities (2006–2016). *Plos One, 16*(2), e0247856.

Office of Registrar General, India (2011). *Annual Health Survey (AHS) in 8 EAG States and Assam: Release of AHS Bulletin: 2010–11*. New Delhi: Ministry of Home Affairs, Government of India.

Prasad, A. M., Chakraborty, G., Yadav, S. S., & Bhatia, S. (2013). Addressing the social determinants of health through health system strengthening and intersectoral convergence: The case of the Indian National Rural Health Mission. *Global Health Action, 6*(1), 20135.

Raykar, N., Majumder, M., Laxminarayan, R., & Menon, P. (2015). *India Health Report: Nutrition 2015*. New Delhi, India: Public Health Foundation of India.

Ritchie, H., Reay, D., & Higgins, P. (2018). Sustainable food security in India—Domestic production and macronutrient availability. *PloS One, 13*(3), e0193766.

Sharma, A. K. (2018). Sociological critique of the national rural health mission: Issues and priorities. AK Sharma, Professor, HSS Department, IIT Kanpur, Kanpur–208016. Paper on NRHM.pdf (iitk.ac.in).

SRS (2000). *Sample Registration System Bulletin*. Government of India, New Delhi: Registrar General, India.

Teller, C. H., & Yimer, G. (2000). Levels and determinants of malnutrition in adolescent and adult women in southern Ethiopia. *Ethiopian Journal of Health Development, 14*(1), 57–66.

UNICEF (1998). *The State of the World's Children*. New York: Oxford University Press.

Venkat, V. (2015). India yet to achieve UN Millennium Development Goals. *The Hindu*. September 15. Accessed March 11, 2022. https://www.thehindu.com/news/national/india-yet-to-achieve-un-millennium- development-goals/article7654764 .ece.

WHO (2014). *Global Nutrition Targets 2025: Policy Brief Series*. World Health Organization. Retrieved from https://www.who.int/publications/i/item/WHO-NMH-NHD-14.2

WHO (2018, February 19). *Progress Report on the Health-related MDGs*. Retrieved May 31, 2022, from World Health Organization: https://www.who.int/news-room/fact- sheets/detail/millennium-development-goals-(mdgs)

Woldemariam Girma, & Timotiows Genebo. (2002). *Determinants of Nutritional Status of Women and Children in Ethiopia*. Calverton, MD: ORC Macro.

Yadav, N. (2018). The Shift in India's Health policy Paradigm and their Implication on Healthcare Needs. *International Journal of Research in Social Sciences, 8*(3), 557–570.

Zodpey, S. P., & Negandhi, P. H. (2018). Tracking India's progress in health sector after 70 years of independence. *Indian Journal of Public Health, 62*(1), 1.

Annexure

Table 8A1 Prevalence of Anaemia Among Women (15–49 Years) and Children (0–59 Months) Across States

States	Reproductive Age group[1]		Pregnant women[2]		Children[2]	
	NFHS-4	NFHS-5	NFHS-4	NFHS-5	NFHS-4	NFHS-5
India	**53.1**	**57**	**50.4**	**52.2**	**58.5**	**67.1**
Non-EAG states						
Andaman and Nicobar	65.7	57.5	61.4	53.7	49	40
Andhra Pradesh	60	58.8	52.9	53.7	58.6	63.2
Arunachal Pradesh	43.2	40.3	37.7	27.9	54.2	56.6
Assam	46	65.9	44.9	54.2	35.7	68.4
Chandigarh	75.9	60.3	76.8	0	73.1	54.6
Dadra and Nagar Havel and Daman and Diu	72.9	62.5	62.3	60.7	82	75.8
Delhi	54.3	49.9	46.3	42.2	59.7	69.2
Goa	31.3	39	26.8	41	48.3	53.2
Gujarat	54.9	65	51.2	62.6	62.6	79.7
Haryana	62.7	60.4	55	56.5	71.7	70.4
Himachal Pradesh	53.5	53	50.4	42.2	53.7	55.4
Jammu and Kashmir	49.4	65.9	47.4	44.1	54.5	72.7
Karnataka	44.8	47.8	45.4	45.7	60.9	65.5
Kerala	34.3	36.3	22.6	31.4	35.7	39.4
Lakshadweep	46	25.8	39	20.9	53.6	43.1
Maharashtra	48	54.2	49.3	45.7	53.8	68.9
Manipur	26.4	29.4	26	32.4	23.9	42.8
Meghalaya	56.2	53.8	53.2	45	48	45.1
Mizoram	24.8	34.8	27.2	34	19.3	46.4
Nagaland	27.9	28.9	32.6	22.2	26.4	42.7
Puducherry	52.4	55.1	25.9	42.5	44.9	64
Punjab	53.5	58.7	42	51.7	56.6	71.1
Sikkim	34.9	42.1	23.6	40.7	55.1	56.4
Tamil Nadu	55	53.4	44.4	48.3	50.7	57.4
Telangana	56	57.6	48.6	53.2	60.7	70
Tripura	54.5	67.2	54.4	61.5	48.3	64.3
West Bengal	62.5	71.4	53.5	62.3	54.2	69
EAG states						
Bihar	60.3	63.5	58.3	63.1	63.5	69.4
Chhattisgarh	47	60.8	41.5	51.8	41.6	67.2
Jharkhand	65.2	65.3	62.6	56.8	69.9	67.5
Madhya Pradesh	52.5	54.7	54.6	52.9	68.9	72.7
Odisha	51	64.3	47.6	61.8	44.6	64.2
Rajasthan	46.8	54.4	46.7	46.3	60.3	71.5
Uttar Pradesh	52.4	50.4	51	45.9	63.2	66.4
Uttarakhand	45.2	42.6	46.5	46.4	59.8	58.8

Source: Author's calculations from NFHS-4, 2015–16; [1]Anaemia level for women is <12.0 g/dl; [2] For pregnant women and children, the value is <11.0 g/dl.

Table 8A2 Trends in Nutritional Status of Children NFHS-4 and NFHS-5 Across States

136 Neha Yadav and Krishna Kumar Choudhary

State	NFHS-4			NFHS-5			Changes in nutritional status		
	Stunting	Wasting	Underweight	Stunting	Wasting	Underweight	Stunting	Wasting	Underweight
India	**38.4**	**21**	**35.5**	**35.5**	**19.3**	**32.1**	**-2.9**	**-1.7**	**-3.4**
Non-EAG states									
Andaman and Nicobar	23.3	18.9	21.6	22.5	16	23.7	-0.8	-2.9	2.1
Andhra Pradesh	31.4	17.2	31.9	31.2	16.1	29.6	-0.2	-1.1	-2.3
Arunachal Pradesh	29.4	17.3	19.4	28	13.1	15.4	-1.4	-4.2	-4
Assam	36.4	17	29.8	35.3	21.7	32.8	-1.1	4.7	3
Chandigarh	28.7	10.9	24.5	25.3	8.4	20.6	-3.4	-2.5	-3.9
Dadra and Nagar Haveli and Daman and Diu	37.2	26.7	35.8	39.4	21.6	38.7	2.2	-5.1	2.9
Goa	20.1	21.9	23.8	25.8	19.1	24	5.7	-2.8	0.2
Gujarat	38.5	26.4	39.3	39	25.1	39.7	0.5	-1.3	0.4
Haryana	34	21.2	29.4	27.5	11.5	21.5	-6.5	-9.7	-7.9
Himachal Pradesh	26.3	13.7	21.2	30.8	17.4	25.5	4.5	3.7	4.3
Jammu and Kashmir	27.4	12.2	16.6	26.9	19	21	-0.5	6.8	4.4
Karnataka	36.2	26.1	35.2	35.4	19.5	32.9	-0.8	-6.6	-2.3
Kerala	19.7	15.7	16.1	23.4	15.8	19.7	3.7	0.1	3.6
Ladakh	30.9	9.3	18.7	30.5	17.5	20.4	-0.4	8.2	1.7
Lakshadweep	26.8	13.7	23.6	32	17.4	25.8	5.2	3.7	2.2
Maharashtra	34.4	25.6	36	35.2	25.6	36.1	0.8	0	0.1
Manipur	28.9	6.8	13.8	23.4	9.9	13.3	-5.5	3.1	-0.5
Meghalaya	43.8	15.3	28.9	46.5	12.1	26.6	2.7	-3.2	-2.3
Mizoram	28.1	6.1	12	28.9	9.8	12.7	0.8	3.7	0.7
Delhi	31.9	15.9	27	30.9	11.2	21.8	-1	-4.7	-5.2
Nagaland	28.6	11.3	16.7	32.7	19.1	26.9	4.1	7.8	10.2
Puducherry	23.7	23.6	22	20	12.4	15.3	-3.7	-11.2	-6.7
Punjab	25.7	15.6	21.6	24.5	10.6	16.9	-1.2	-5	-4.7

(Continued)

Table 8A2 Continued

State	NFHS-4			NFHS-5			Changes in nutritional status		
	Stunting	Wasting	Underweight	Stunting	Wasting	Underweight	Stunting	Wasting	Underweight
Sikkim	29.6	14.2	14.2	22.3	13.7	13.1	-7.3	-0.5	-1.1
Tamil Nadu	27.1	19.7	23.8	25	14.6	22	-2.1	-5.1	-1.8
Telangana	28	18.1	28.4	33.1	21.7	31.8	5.1	3.6	3.4
Tripura	24.3	16.8	24.1	32.3	18.2	25.6	8	1.4	1.5
West Bengal	32.5	20.3	31.6	33.8	20.3	32.2	1.3	0	0.6
EAG states									
Bihar	48.3	20.8	43.9	42.9	22.9	41	-5.4	2.1	-2.9
Chhattisgarh	37.6	23.1	37.7	34.6	18.9	31.3	-3	-4.2	-6.4
Jharkhand	45.3	29	47.8	39.6	22.4	39.4	-5.7	-6.6	-8.4
Madhya Pradesh	42	25.8	42.8	35.7	19	33	-6.3	-6.8	-9.8
Odisha	34.1	20.4	34.4	31	18.1	29.7	-3.1	-2.3	-4.7
Rajasthan	39.1	23	36.7	31.8	16.8	27.6	-7.3	-6.2	-9.1
Uttarakhand	33.5	19.5	26.6	27	13.2	21	-6.5	-6.3	-5.6
Uttar Pradesh	46.3	17.9	39.5	39.7	17.3	32.1	-6.6	-0.6	-7.4

9 Association between Parental Migration and Undernutrition Among the Children Left Behind in Rural Empowered Action Group (EAG) States, India

Monalisha Chakraborty and Subrata Mukherjee

Introduction

Migration is an intricate episode that brings up a range of economic, social and security aspects which affects the daily lives of people in an increasingly interconnected world (International Organization for Migration, 2018). Identifying a migrant is often conceptually complicated because of the subject's dynamic, temporal and spatial nature. The United Nations (1998) defines an international migrant as 'any person who changes his or her country of usual residence'. The Indian Census defines migration as the change of residence from one civil division to another, and the volume of migration to a considerable degree is a function of the size of the areas chosen for compilation (Census of India, 2001). The National Sample Survey in its 64th Round survey (2007–08) considered migrants as those individuals who had changed their usual place of residence within or outside the state (NSSO, 2010).

In the majority of cases, migration is considered the only strategy for survival and an available way for enhancing livelihood conditions (McDowell and de Haan, 1997; Islam et al., 2019). Internal migration in Asia, particularly South-East Asia is high and showing a rise over the period (Deshingkar, 2015; Srivastava et al., 2017). India too has experienced a huge wave of internal migration, particularly from its rural to urban areas (Bhagat, 2017). Historically, the volume of migration in the Indian subcontinent was comparatively low predominantly due to the prevalence of caste system, language and cultural diversity, educational backwardness, joint family system, traditional values and preponderance of agriculture (Davis, 1951). However, in the last few decades, transposition of the Indian economy, expansion of transport and communication facilities, and advancement in education pledged momentum for people to migrate (Bhagat, 2017). Since the 1990s, the volume of migration in India registered a significant increase. Moreover, urbanisation and industrialisation have fuelled employment-related migration in India. Over time the number of internal migrants increased from 33 million in 2001 to 51 million in 2011 (Census of India, 2001; 2011). Though

DOI: 10.4324/9781003430636-13

no recent Census data are available, it is quite expected that in the last 10 years, these figures have inflated substantially. Census 2011 data show that in India about 62 per cent of the internal migrants are short-distance and intra-district migrants. Long-distance and inter-state migrants account for 12 per cent of total internal migrants, which is quite low compared to other developing countries like Brazil and China (Rajan et al., 2020).

The inter-state migration from backward states and both inter-state and intra-state migration from backward regions of states have experienced a huge increase during the post-reform period. Many underdeveloped districts have experienced losing their adult male population of productive age group to developed and industrialised/more urbanised districts through migration (Bhattacharjee, 2020). At the state level, migration flow has remained persistent towards the richer states (in terms of per capita income), namely, Maharashtra, Punjab, Haryana, Gujarat, Kerala, Tamil Nadu and Karnataka (Bhagat, 2017). The states such as Bihar, Orissa, Uttar Pradesh, Assam, Madhya Pradesh and Rajasthan have remained net out-migrating with Bihar, and Uttar Pradesh topped the list since Census 2011 data were released.

The EAG states are socio-economically backward states and lag other states in Human Development Index values (Pandey et al., 2007) as well. These states together account for about 46 per cent of India's population (Census of India, 2011) and are characterised by a higher prevalence of child undernutrition and higher infant mortality rates (Arokiasamy and Gautam, 2008; Kumar et al., 2020; Kumar and Paswan, 2021). Though the Sustainable Development Goals (SDGs) have targeted to end all forms of malnutrition by 2030, the average decline in undernutrition has been slow in India, especially in the EAG states that are characterised by large economic disparities and higher share of poor children in the country (Pathak and Singh, 2011; Gupta et al., 2016). Out-migration from these states is mostly led by underdevelopment and poverty, where people migrate for employment opportunities and to secure a better earning (Rahaman et al., 2021). As a result, a substantial fraction of children from these states is confronting parental migration during the course of their childhood. Table 9.1 shows out-migration among the working-age population (15–64 years) for all eight EAG states to the five dominant destination states and Delhi (union territories) in India.

Parental Migration and Child Nutrition

Migration is found to have a multifaceted effect on individuals, families, societies, economies and cultures, both in the place of origin of the migrants and their destinations (Shen et al., 2009). Parental migration may cause children's health and education to suffer due to the disruption created to their lives (Konseiga et al., 2009). The children who are left behind by their migrant parents (single or both parents) in the countryside are usually taken care of by single parents, or other extended family members, such as grandparents, relatives and even non-relatives. Studies have found that parental migration

Table 9.1 Inter-State Out-Migration Among Working Age Population (15–64 Years) from the EAG States to Five Major States and Delhi

Source (EAG) States	Top five destination states [a]							EAG states [b]	Other states/ Union Territories
	Maharashtra	Gujarat	Delhi	Haryana	West Bengal	Punjab	Karnataka		
Bihar	10.29	8.06	16.90	6.86	9.43	5.42	2.11	33.37	7.56
Chhattisgarh	24.91	2.90	2.10	2.71	1.03	1.66	1.81	52.85	10.03
Jharkhand	9.19	5.44	5.46	1.91	20.83	1.46	2.58	45.60	7.53
Madhya Pradesh	27.27	11.49	4.71	2.78	0.45	1.16	1.35	46.98	3.81
Orissa	11.54	18.35	3.62	1.66	7.24	0.85	8.90	27.45	20.39
Rajasthan	15.81	22.44	7.35	15.33	1.04	4.99	5.09	20.72	7.23
Uttar Pradesh	22.95	10.49	20.27	9.56	1.18	5.63	1.32	23.56	5.04
Uttarakhand	5.49	1.56	26.84	8.34	0.40	5.67	1.01	42.47	8.22

Source: Census of India, 2011
Note: [a] It includes five dominant destination states and the union capital territory of Delhi receiving migrants from the EAG states, [b] EAG states other than the source state of out-migration is included.

affects the physical, mental and emotional health of the children left behind both positively and negatively since the day-to-day supervision provided to children when one or both parents are absent likely to be not the same when both parents are present (McKenzie, 2005; Pescaru, 2015; Davis and Brazil, 2016; Mazzucato and Cebotari, 2017). On the one hand, migration could enhance the well-being of families left behind (Yang, 2008; De Brauw and Rozelle, 2008; Mu and De Brauw, 2015) as remittances received from migration could support the family by minimising economic risk (Stark and Taylor, 1991; Massey et al., 1993) and allow the household to spend more on children's nutrition and education (Islam et al., 2019). There is evidence in the literature from Mexico (McKenzie, 2005), Pakistan (Mansuri, 2006) and New Zealand (Stillman et al., 2012) that left-behind children have better health than the children of non-migrant households. On the other hand, literature also shows the negative consequences of parental migration on the physical health of left-behind children (Konseiga et al., 2009; Shen et al., 2009). As family composition and roles change due to migration, older children are more required to take care of their younger siblings, perform more household responsibilities and play additional roles in supporting the household (Hanson and Woodruff, 2003). Parental absence also reduces the time allocated to child care within households, causes caregiver rearrangement and changes feeding practices, especially when both parents migrate (Choudhary and Parthasarathy, 2009; Coffey, 2013; Xu and Xie, 2015). A stream of literature has found that left-behind children are more likely to be stunted, underweight and wasted when compared with other children (Ning and Chang, 2013; Tian et al., 2017; Lei et al., 2017).

Despite its importance, the effect of migration and remittances on the left behind children is notably understudied in Indian context. Moreover, studies focusing on the health of left-behind children in rural EAG states where parental out-migration is high are also glaring. This chapter makes an attempt to assess undernutrition among children based on their parent's migration status in the EAG states of India.

Data and Methods

The study utilises the second wave of India Human Development Survey (IHDS, 2011-12) Data pertaining to eight EAG states. The analysis considers the bottom 40 per cent of the population as per economic status proxied by per capita household expenditure, as an approximately similar percentage of the population in those states taken together live below the poverty line (Planning Commission, 2013) (Table 9.2). By confining our analysis to the bottom 40 per cent of the population, we are able to restrict our analysis to a more-or-less homogeneous population sub-group in terms of economic conditions which may have a bearing on their decision to migrate for work and child's nutritional health status.

Table 9.2 Percentage of Population Below Poverty Line in the EAG States, 2011–12 (Tendulkar Methodology)

EAG states	Rural	Urban	Total
Bihar	34.06	31.23	33.74
Madhya Pradesh	35.74	21.00	31.65
Chhattisgarh	44.61	24.75	39.93
Uttar Pradesh	30.40	26.06	29.43
Rajasthan	16.05	10.69	14.71
Jharkhand	40.84	24.83	36.96
Odisha	35.69	17.29	32.59
Uttarakhand	11.62	10.48	11.26

Source: Press note on Poverty Estimates, 2011–12, Planning Commission, 2013

IHDS-II considered migrants as those individuals who had stayed outside their home districts for at least six months in the last year. The variable parent's migration status in the study is constructed using the following information: First, in the household questionnaire, the respondent was asked if any woman/man in the household had a husband/wife who lived outside the household. If a husband/wife were away at the time of the survey, we have considered him/her as a current migrant in our analysis. In addition, the survey asked whether any household members had left home to find seasonal/short-term work for at least one month during the past five years and returned back. We have considered them as returned migrants. The survey also collected information on the number of months the household members had stayed outside the home district in the last year. Based on parental migration status, we categorise the children into three mutually exclusive groups: (1) children of non-migrant parent(s) (C-NM); (2) left-behind children of returned migrant parents (LBC-RM); and (3) left-behind children of currently migrant parents (LBC-CM). Our analysis has considered only rural to urban migration and children belonging to the age group 0–14 years.

Outcome Variables

The study uses the data on anthropometric measurements (i.e., height and weight) for analysing the impact of parental migration on children's nutritional health status. The three most commonly used indices for nutritional health status are weight-for-age, height-for-age and body mass index (BMI), which allow us to compare a child's health with a reference population (Mansuri, 2006). We use height-for-age and BMI for analysing a child's nutritional health status. BMI is an indirect measure of body fatness, which can be used to detect thinness. Height-for-age is used to identify children who suffer from stunting. These variables are converted into z-scores using WHO's age- and gender-specific international reference standards, which are based on a sample of children from developed and developing countries and provide a suitable reference for standardising our sample of children (WHO Multicentre Growth Reference Study Group, 2006). The deviation function is

$$Z_{it}^* = \frac{y_i - M_t}{StDev(t)} \tag{1}$$

where y_i is the ith child's measured height or weight and M_t and $StDev(t)$ are the mean and standard deviation of height or weight of reference age-sex group t, respectively.

The BMI z-score (BMIZ) is categorised as underweight and normal/over-weight. Studies evidenced obesity in children appeared to be predominantly a problem of non-poor or well-off households in low- and middle-income countries (Dinsa et al., 2012). As our study focuses on children belonging to households of low-income groups, we consider underweight among children as one category and clubbed together normal and overweight to form the other category.

Control Variables

Based on the review of the literature, a number of predictors for outcome variables are considered for the analysis. These predictors or independent variables are found to influence children's nutritional health in different contexts (Table 3). The predicting variables fall under the following broad categories: (a) Spatial and demographic variables: parental migration status (children of non-migrant parents/left-behind children of returned migrant parents/left-behind children of current migrant parents); child age group (0–5 years/6–10 years/11–14 years); child sex (boy/girl), (b) variables capturing socio-economic status: caste (ST/SC/OBC/Others); religion (Hindu/Muslim/others); mother's education (illiterate/primary/secondary/above secondary); mother's occupation (non-working/self-employed in agriculture/self-employed in non-agriculture/agricultural waged labour/non-agricultural waged labour/salaried and others); mother's exposure to mass media (never/sometimes or irregular/regular or often) – we have taken women's exposure to mass media as a proxy of mother's exposure to mass media; per capita household expenditure (low/medium/high), (c) sanitation and hygiene related variables: sanitation facility (no facility/public or shared toilet/traditional pit toilet in household/semi-flush or flush toilet in household).

Analysis

To explore the relationship between a child's nutritional status and his/her parental migration status, a logistic regression model is estimated. A logistic regression model is useful in this case since our outcome variables can be considered as binary variables which are influenced by a number of independent variables. The logistic model is specified as (Wooldridge, 2019)

$$Y_i = ln\left(\frac{P_i}{1-P_i}\right) = \beta_0 + \beta_1 D_i + \beta_2 S_i + \beta_3 H_i + \beta_4 I_i + u_i \qquad (2)$$

where Y_i is the value of outcome variable of ith child; $\left(\frac{P_i}{1-P_i}\right)$ is the odds ratio; outcome variables are underweight and stunting taking binary values (underweight/stunted=1;0 otherwise); β_j $(j = 0,....,4)$ is the vector of coefficients; D_i is the spatial and demographic variables, S_i is the socio-economic variables, H_i is the health and hygiene variables, I_i is an interaction term between parental migration status and child's sex variables, and u_i is the error term. Analyses are carried out using Stata 14. In models, adjusted odds ratios (OR[a]) with 95% confidence intervals (CI) are reported for variables.

Results

Sample Characteristics

Select summary statistics of the sample is presented in Table 9.3. It is observed that almost three-fourth of the study population/children (74.8 per cent) live in less-developed villages[1] with children left behind by the current migrant parents showing the highest share (78.6 per cent) compared to other two groups (viz. children of non-migrant parents and left behind children of returned migrant parents). Almost half of the children belong to Other Backward Class (48.6 per cent) with children left behind by current migrant parents showing the highest share (60.7 per cent). Among the mothers, 69.0 per cent are found to be illiterate. Majority of the children (87.3 per cent) live in households with no sanitation facility, with left-behind children of returned migrant parents showing the highest share (91.2 per cent).

Parental Migration and Child Undernutrition

The percentage of underweight and stunted children by parental migration status is shown in Figure 9.1. It is evident that parents' migration status portrays a remarkable variation in the prevalence of undernutrition among children. Children of non-migrant parents are more likely to be underweight (19.5 per cent) when compared with the other groups of children. It is worth noticing that underweight is found less among the left-behind children of currently migrant parents (15.5 per cent). Stunting is higher among the left-behind children of returned migrant parents (48.1 per cent) compared to other groups children.

Table 9.3 Select Summary Statistics

Background characteristics	Children of non-migrant parent(s) (n = 6481)	Left-behind children of returned migrant parent(s) (n = 754)	Left-behind children of current migrant parent(s) (n = 591)	Total (n = 7826)
Living in less developed villages (%)	74.6	72.8	78.6	74.8
Child age group				
0–5 years (%)	34.0	44.2	50.5	36.5
6–10 years (%)	37.9	36.4	36.4	37.6
11–14 years (%)	28.1	19.5	13.1	25.8
Female (%)	50.3	47.3	52.3	50.2
Caste				
ST (%)	12.8	15.0	3.3	12.1
SC (%)	26.6	30.2	22.4	26.5
OBC (%)	47.6	44.7	60.7	48.6
Others (%)	13.0	10.2	13.6	12.8
Religion				
Hindu (%)	87.5	91.7	76.1	83.6
Muslim (%)	11.5	8.2	23.0	12.3
Others (%)	1.0	0.0	0.9	0.9
Mother's education				
Illiterate (%)	69.2	68.8	67.1	69.0
Primary (%)	14.3	16.8	15.0	14.6
Secondary (%)	14.6	13.4	16.3	14.6
Higher secondary and above (%)	1.9	1.0	1.7	1.8
Mother's occupation				
Non-working (%)	81.9	78.7	79.7	81.4
Self-employed in agriculture (%)	5.4	5.9	3.9	5.3
Self-employed in non-agriculture (%)	1.1	0.1	0.5	1.0
Agricultural waged labour (%)	5.0	8.2	12.1	6.1
Non-agricultural waged labour (%)	5.3	7.0	3.0	5.2
Salaried/others (%)	1.3	0.1	0.9	1.1
Mother's exposure to mass media				
Never (%)	47.5	41.6	47.8	47.0
Irregular/sometimes (%)	38.6	48.1	41.8	39.8
Regular/ often (%)	13.9	10.2	10.4	13.2
Per capita household expenditure				
Low (≤ Rs. 11725) (%)	68.7	64.1	68.3	68.2
Moderate (Rs. 11729–Rs. 19498) (%)	24.1	30.1	22.4	24.5
High (> Rs. 19510) (%)	7.2	5.5	9.3	7.3

(Continued)

Table 9.3 Continued

Background characteristics	Children of non-migrant parent(s) (n = 6481)	Left-behind children of returned migrant parent(s) (n = 754)	Left-behind children of current migrant parent(s) (n = 591)	Total (n = 7826)
Sanitation facility				
No facility/open defecation (%)	87.0	91.2	86.2	87.3
Shared/public (%)	1.9	1.3	0.4	1.7
Traditional pit toilet in household (%)	5.8	5.6	5.8	5.8
Semi-flush/flush toilet in household (%)	5.3	1.9	7.6	5.3

Source: Authors' estimation from IHDS-II (2011–12) unit-record data
Note: ST – Scheduled Tribe; SC – Scheduled Caste; OBC – Other Backward Class

Econometric Analysis

Table 9.4 presents the results of the logit regression model which examined the effects of parental migration on children's nutritional health status after controlling for all other relevant covariates. Though parental migration is not found to have any significant effect on underweight among children, it has a positive effect on children being stunted. Left-behind children of returned migrant parents are found 1.43 times (95% CI 1.05–1.93) more likely to be stunted than children of non-migrants. No relation is found between remittances received by the household and underweight among children. However, children of

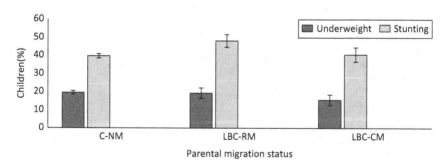

Figure 9.1 Undernutrition Among Children by Parent's Migration Status

Source: Authors' estimation from IHDS-II (2011–12) unit-record data

Note: C-NM – children of non-migrant parent(s), LBC-RM – left-behind children of returned migrant parent(s), LBC-CM – left-behind children of currently migrant parent(s).

Table 9.4 Logistic Regression Model Results for Undernutrition Among Children (0–14 Years)

Covariates	Underweight		Stunting	
	OR[a]	CI (95%)	OR[a]	CI (95%)
Parent's migration status (Ref: *Children of non-migrant parents*)				
Left-behind children of returned migrant parents	0.87	0.63–1.20	1.43**	1.05–1.93
Left-behind children of current migrant parents	0.67	0.41–1.10	1.37	0.94–2.02
Remittances received by household (Ref: *No*)				
Yes	1.25	0.99–1.69	0.69***	0.54–0.88
Place of residence (Ref: *More developed villages*)				
Less developed villages	1.13	0.94–1.36	0.95	0.82–1.11
Age (Ref: *0–5*)				
6–10	1.37***	1.13–1.66	0.68***	0.58–0.79
11–14	1.74***	1.41–2.15	0.79***	0.67–0.94
Sex (Ref: *Boy*)				
Girl	0.84*	0.71–1.00	1.11	0.96–1.29
Caste (Ref: *ST*)				
SC	0.70***	0.54–0.90	1.40***	1.13–1.74
OBC	0.70***	0.56–0.88	1.10	0.90–1.35
Others	0.63***	0.46–0.87	1.10	0.84–1.46
Religion (Ref: *Hindu*)				
Muslim	0.85	0.64–1.12	1.28**	1.02–1.58
Others	0.58	0.25–1.37	0.64	0.31–1.33
Mother's education (Ref: *Illiterate*)				
Primary	0.95	0.77–1.18	0.64***	0.53–0.78
Secondary	0.92	0.72–1.18	0.73***	0.59–0.90
Above secondary	0.43**	0.21–0.88	0.75	0.42–1.32
Mother's occupation (Ref: *Non-working*)				
Self-employed in agriculture	1.03	0.71–1.48	1.62***	1.23–2.14
Self-employed in non-agriculture	1.22	0.61–2.44	1.04	0.58–1.89
Agricultural waged labour	0.75*	0.54–1.05	0.93	0.72–1.21
Non-agricultural waged labour	1.13	0.81–1.59	1.02	0.76–1.38
Salaried work/ others	0.89	0.41–1.93	0.99	0.53–1.85
Mother's exposure to mass media (Ref: *Never*)				
Sometimes/irregular	0.89	0.75–1.07	0.99	0.85–1.14
Regular/often	1.23**	1.00–1.56	0.65***	0.53–0.80
Per capita household expenditure (Ref: *Low*)				
Medium	0.99	0.80–1.17	0.84*	0.72–0.99
High	0.86	0.65–1.14	0.46***	0.36–0.60
Sanitation facility (Ref: *No facility/ open defecation*)				
Shared/public	1.56	0.81–3.02	0.90	0.50–1.63

(*Continued*)

Table 9.4 Continued

Covariates	Underweight		Stunting	
	OR[a]	CI (95%)	OR[a]	CI (95%)
Traditional pit toilet in household	1.31	0.96–1.79	0.80	0.60–1.05
Semi-flush/flush toilet in household	0.93	0.68–1.26	0.82	0.62–1.09
Parent's migration status # child sex				
Left-behind children with returned migrant parents#girl	1.52*	0.95–2.42	0.97	0.64–1.47
Left-behind children with current migrant parents#girl	1.28	0.69–2.39	0.95	0.59–1.51

Source: Authors' estimation from IHDS-II (2011–12) unit-record data
Note: OR[a] shows the adjusted odd ratios; ***, ** and * – significant at 1%, 5% and 10% level. ST – Scheduled Tribe; SC – Scheduled Caste; OBC – Other Backward Class; CHC – Community Health Centre

remittance-recipient households are found 0.69 times (95% CI 0.54–0.88) less likely to be stunted than children of remittance non-recipient households.

Among the other covariates, compared to children of 0–5 years of age group, the likelihood of being underweight is found 1.37 times (95% CI 1.13–1.66) and 1.74 times (95% CI 1.41–2.15) higher among the children of 6–10 years and 11–14 years of age groups, but children of the same age groups are found 0.68 (95% CI 0.58–0.79) and 0.79 times (95% CI 0.67–0.94) less likely to be stunted than children of 0–5 years of age group. The girls are found 0.84 times (95% CI 0.71–1.00) less likely to be underweight than the boys. It is observed that the likelihood of being both underweight and stunted decreases with increasing years of education of the mother. Children whose mothers are self-employed in agriculture are found more likely to be stunted (OR[a] 1.62, 95% CI 1.23–2.14) than children of non-working mothers. The children whose mothers are engaged as agricultural wage labourers are found 0.75 times (95% CI 0.54–1.05) less likely to be underweight than the children of non-working mothers. The children of the mothers, who are regularly exposed to mass media, are less likely to be stunted (OR[a] 0.65, 95% CI 0.53–0.80) than the children of mothers who are never exposed to mass media. It is striking to find that mothers' regular exposure to mass media increases the likelihood of 'being underweight' among the children by 1.23 times (95% CI 1.00–1.56). Controlling for all other factors, the likelihood of being stunted is found to be monotonically lower among the children belonging to medium- and high-expenditure class households compared to the children belonging to low-expenditure class households. The results do not show any significant effect of sanitation facilities on undernutrition among children. The estimated coefficients of the interaction terms between parental migration status and sex of the child indicate that left-behind girl children of returned migrant parents are 1.52 times (95% CI 0.95–2.42) more likely to be underweight than children of non-migrants and boys.

Discussion

Migration has a multifaceted effect on individuals, families, societies, economies and cultures, both in the places of origin and destination (Shen et al., 2009). In India, migration for economic reasons by adult men is a common livelihood strategy adopted by families. In most cases, migrants leave their wives and children in their places of origin because initial low incomes, uncertainty about work, subsistence living arrangement, lack of social support and expected high cost of living with family at the destination places do not allow them migrate with families (Bhattacharjee, 2020). Labour migration is high from the EAG states, mostly from rural areas, due to underdevelopment and poverty (Rahaman et al., 2021). As a result, a substantial proportion of children in rural areas of the EAG states are living separately either from one or both parents due to parental out-migration. The relationship between parental migration and the health outcomes of children left behind has taken a central place in migration and health discourse. In particular, the remittances that migrants send to their left-behind families highlight the possibility of migration to serve as a key pathway to development in resource-constrained settings (De Brauw and Rozelle, 2008; Mu and De Brauw, 2015). One of the focal questions here is whether adult migration enhances the well-being of left-behind children, as the absence of single/both parents could also affect a child's health negatively. The present study attempted to analyse the effect of parental out-migration on the nutritional health status of children.

Our study finds that left-behind children of returned migrant parents are more likely to be stunted. This could be because of the reason that households with migrant parent(s) may have fewer family members and less time available to take care of a child, and also to provide the latter with nutritious home-cooked meals (De Brauw and Mu, 2011; Mu and De Brauw, 2015). Chen and Liu (2012) in their study found that grandparents often fail to understand the health risks of their grandchildren and channel inadequate resources towards their nutritional and health betterment. Although our study did not find any relation between remittances received by the household and underweight among children, children of remittances recipient households are found less likely to be stunted. Studies found that remittances sent home by migrant parents are generally used by left-behind families in improving children's health and nutrition through increased investment in more nutritious food (McKenzie 2005; Yang, 2008; De Brauw and Rozelle, 2008; Mu and De Brauw, 2015). However, it is to be noted that height-for-age is a typical measure of chronic malnutrition and the varied period of migration of parents with its transitory nature might not be long enough to capture the long-term effect on child health.

Our study finds that girls are less likely to be underweight than boys, which suggests that the nutrient intake of boys may be lower than that of girls and also boys spend more time playing outdoors which potentially causes them to be underweight (Syahrul et al., 2016; Deren et al., 2018). This finding challenges the commonly held presumption in the context of nutritional gender difference that girls are more likely to be affected by undernutrition in poor families because of gender-based discrimination. However, there are studies that corroborate our finding. A study by NCD Risk Factor Collaboration (NCD-RisC) (2017) found that underweight is more among boys of 5–19 years of age group compared to the girls of the same age group (30.7 per cent as against 22.7 per cent). As per Urban HUNGaMA Report (2014), survey conducted in 10 big cities of India found that boys are more malnourished than girls in India. The coefficients of the interaction term in our estimated logit model indicated that left-behind girls of returned migrant parents were more likely to be underweight.

Our analysis also identified major risk factors such as age, caste, religion, mother's education, mother's occupation, mother's exposure to mass media and household economic status associated with underweight and stunting among children. One of the important points to discuss is that our study finds that children whose mothers are engaged as agricultural wage labours are less likely to be underweight than children of non-working mothers. This may be because mother's who are engaged in income earning activities are able to spend more on their children's nutrition and education. Studies have found that mother's income plays a vital role in alleviating undernutrition among children (Rathnayake and Weerahewa, 2003; Malapit et al., 2015). Although our study has found that incidence of stunting is lower among children whose mothers are regularly exposed to mass media, it has found positive effect on underweight among children. Studies have found that mothers who are exposed to mass media are more aware about their children's health and nutrition risk (Kim et al., 2018). However, our study highlights an unclear impact of mother's exposure to mass media on undernutrition among children.

Conclusion

The paper has highlighted how parental migration and different social and economic attributes of a child influence and interact with each other and shape his/her nutritional health status. The results indicate existing inequalities in child nutrition across different population sub-groups, even within poor rural. We found that left-behind children of returned migrant parents are more likely to be stunted. Also, left-behind girls of returned migrant parents are more likely to be underweight than their peers. This empirical evidence may be crucial for sharpening our policy focus. Scholars have argued that nutritional policies for children must focus on groups that have systematically worse outcomes; and those who are disadvantaged in several dimensions would require greater policy attention. The potential interventions should aim at raising awareness of the mothers of the children through local health workers about health and nutritional risks faced by their children.

To the best of our knowledge, hardly any study is based on large-scale household data, which has explored the connection between parental out-migration and nutritional health status of their children in the EAG states. More studies should be conducted among children in these states before making generalisation.

Note

1 IHDS identifies urban and rural areas based on Census (2001 and 2011) data. It divides villages into two approximately equal groups according to an index of infrastructural development. The more developed villages generally appear closer to urban areas on most human development outcomes (Desai et al., 2009).

References

Arokiasamy, P., & Gautam, A. (2008). Neonatal mortality in the empowered action group states of India: Trends and determinants. *Journal of Biosocial Science*, *40*(2), 183–201.

Bhagat, R. B. (2017). Internal migration in India: Are the underclass more mobile? In *Irudaya Rajan "India Migration Reader"*. London: Routledge.

Bhattacharjee, M. R. (2020). Development and internal outmigration in India in post-economic reform era. *Asia-Pacific Journal of Regional Science*, *4*(3), 713–735. Doi: 10.1007/s41685-020-00156-6

Census of India (2001). Migration Data: Abstract on data highlights. Retrieved from http://censusindia.gov.in/Data_Products/Data_Highlights/Data_Highlights_link/data_highlights_D1D2D3.pdf

Census of India (2011). Migration. Retrieved from http://censusindia.gov.in/Ad_Campaign/drop_in_articles/08-Migration.pdf

Chen, F., & Liu, G. (2012). The health implications of grandparents caring for grandchildren in China. *J. Gerontol. B Psychol. Sci. Soc. Sci.*, *67B*, 99–112. Doi: 10.1093/geronb/gbr132.

Choudhary, N., & D. Parthasarathy. (2009). Is migration status a determinant of urban nutrition insecurity? Empirical evidence from Mumbai City. *Journal of Biosocial Science*, *41*, 583–605.

Coffey, D. (2013). Children's welfare and short-term migration from rural India. *J Dev Stud.*, *49*(8), 1101–1117.

Davis, J., & Brazil, N. (2016). Migration, remittances and nutrition outcomes of left behind children: A national-level quantitative assessment of Guatemala. *PloS One*, *11*(3), e0152089. Doi:10.1371/journal.pone.0152089.

Davis, K. (1951). *The Population of India and Pakistan*. Princeton: Princeton University Press.

De Brauw, A., & Mu, R. (2011). Migration and the overweight and underweight status of children in rural China. *Food Policy*, *36* (1), 88–100.

Dereń, K., Nyankovskyy, S., Nyankovska, O., Łuszczki, E., Wyszyńska, J., Sobolewski, M., & Mazur, A. (2018). The prevalence of underweight, overweight and obesity in children and adolescents from Ukraine. *Scientific Reports*, *8*(1), 3625. Doi:10.1038/s41598-018-21773-4.

Desai, S., Dubey, A., Joshi, B. L., Sen, M., Shariff, A., & Vanneman. R. (2009). India Human Development Survey: Design and Data Quality. IHDS Technical Paper 1.

Deshingkar, P., & Zeitlyn, B. (2015). South-South Migration for Domestic Work and Poverty. *Geography Compass*, 9(4), 169–179. Doi:10.1111/gec3.12200

Dinsa, G. D., Goryakin, Y., Fumagalli, E., & Suhrcke, M. (2012). Obesity and socioeconomic status in developing countries: A systematic review. *Obes Rev.*, 13(11), 1067–1079. Doi:10.1111/j.1467-789X.2012.01017.x.

Gupta, A. K., Ladusingh, L., & Borkotoky, K. (2016). Spatial clustering and risk factors of infant mortality: District-level assessment of high-focus states in India. *Genus*, 72, 2. Doi: 10.1186/s41118-016-0008-9

Hanson, G. H., & Woodruff, C. (2003). Emigration and educational attainment in Mexico. Mimeo: University of California at San Diego. Retrieved from http://citeseerx.ist.psu.edu/viewdoc/download?doi=10.1.1.716.5969&rep=rep1&type=pdf.

International Institute for Population Sciences (IIPS) and Macro International (2007). *National Family Health Survey (NFHS-3), 2005–06, India.* Mumbai.

International Institute for Population Sciences (IIPS) (2016). *National Family Health Survey (NFHS-3), 2016, India.* Mumbai.

International Organisation for Migration (2018). *World Migration Report 2018.* The UN Migration Agency. Retrieved from https://www.iom.int/sites/g/files/tmzbdl486/files/country/docs/china/r5_world_migration_report_2018_en.pdf.

Islam, M., Kashem, S., Morshed, S., Rahman, M. M., & Das, A. (2019). Dynamics of Seasonal Migration of Rural Livelihood, *Advanced Journal of Social Science*, 5(1), 81–92. Doi:10.21467/ajss.5.1.81-92

Ji, M., Zhang Y., Zou J., Yuan T., Tang A., Deng J., Yang L., Li M., Chen J., Qin H., et al. (2017). Study on the Status of Health Service Utilization among Caregivers of Left-Behind Children in Poor Rural Areas of Hunan Province: A Baseline Survey. *International Journal of Environmental Research and Public Health*, 14. Doi: 10.3390/ijerph14080910.

Kim, S. S., Roopnaraine, T., Nguyen, P. H., Saha, K. K., Bhuiyan, M. I., & Menon, P. (2018). Factors influencing the uptake of a mass media intervention to improve child feeding in Bangladesh. *Maternal and Child Nutrition*, 14(3), e12603. Doi: 10.1111/mcn.12603.

Konseiga, A., Zulu, M. E., Bocquier, P., Muindi, K., Beguy, D., & Ye, Y. (2009). Assessing the effect of mother's migration on childhood mortality in the informal settlements of Nairobi. In Collinson, M., Adazu, K., W. M, & F. S. (Eds.), *The Dynamics of Migration, Health and Livelihoods: INDEPTH Network Perspectives* (pp. 123–138). England.

Kumar, R., & Paswan, B. (2021). Changes in socio-economic inequality in nutritional status among children in EAG states, India. *Public Health Nutrition*, 24(6), 1304–1317. Doi:10.1017/S1368980021000343

Kumar, S., Sahu, D., Mehto, A., & Sharma, R. K. (2020). Health inequalities in under-five mortality: An assessment of empowered action group (EAG) states of India. *JHEOR*, 7(2), 189–196. Doi:10.36469/jheor.2020.18224

Lei, L., Liu, F., & Hill, E. (2017). Labour Migration and Health of Left-Behind Children in China. *The Journal of Development Studies*, 54, 1–18. Doi:10.1080/00220388.2017.1283015.

Lusome, R., & Bhagat, R. B. (2006). Trends and patterns of internal migration in India, 1971–2001. In Annual Conference for the Study of Population (IASP), Thiruvananthapuram.

Malapit, H. J. L., Kadiyala, S., Quisumbing, A.R., Cunningham, K., & Tyagi, P. (2015). Women's empowerment mitigates the negative effects of low production diversity on maternal and child nutrition in Nepal. *Journal of Development Studies*, 51, 1097–123.

Mansuri, G. (2006). *Migration, Sex Bias, and Child Growth in Rural Pakistan*. World Bank Policy Research Working Paper Series 3946.

Massey, D. S., Arango, J., Hugo, G., Kouaouci, A., Pellegrino, A., & Taylor, J. E. (1993). Theories of international migration: A review and appraisal. *Population and Development Review*, 19(3), 431–466.

Mazzucato, V., & Cebotari, V. (2017). Psychological well-being of Ghanaian children in transnational families. *Population Space and Place*, 23(3). Doi:10.1002/psp.2004.

McDowell, C., & de Haan, A. (1997). Migration and Sustainable Livelihoods: A Critical Review of the Literature, IDS Working Paper 65, Brighton: IDS.

McKenzie, D. (2005). Beyond remittances: The effects of migration on Mexican households. In Ozden, C., & Schiff, M. (Eds.), *International Migration, Remittances and the Brain Drain* (pp 123–147). Washington, DC: McMillan and Palgrave.

Mishra, S. V. (2014). Understanding needs and Ascribed Quality of life – through maternal factors: Infant mortality dialectic. *Asian Geographer*, 32(1), 19–36. Doi :10.1080/10225706.2014.962551

Meng, X., & Yamauchi, C. (2015). Children of Migrants: The Impact of Parental Migration on Their Children's Education and Health Outcomes. *IZA Discussion Papers 9165*, Bonn: Institute for the Study of Labour (IZA).

Mu, R., & De Brauw, A. (2015). Migration and young child nutrition: Evidence from rural China. *Journal of Population Economics*, 28(3), 631–657. Doi:10.1007/s0 0148-015-0550-3.

NCD Risk Factor Collaboration (NCD-RisC) (2017). Worldwide trends in body-mass index, underweight, overweight, and obesity from 1975 to 2016: A pooled analysis of 2416 population-based measurement studies in 128·9 million children, adolescents, and adults. *Lancet*, 390, 2627–42. Doi: 10.1016/ S0140-6736(17)32129-3.

NSSO (2010). Migration in India, 2007–08. Ministry of Statistics and Programme Implementation, Government of India (June, 2020). Retrieved from http://mospi .nic.in/sites/default/files/publication_reports/533_final.

Ning, M., & Chang, H. (2013). Migration decisions of parents and the nutrition intakes of children left at home in rural China. *Agricultural Economics/ ZemedelskaEkonomika*, 59(10), 467–477.

Pandey, R. P., & Astone, N. M. (2007). Explaining son preference in Rural India: The independent role of structural versus individual factors. *Population Research and Policy Review*, 26(1), 1–29. Retrieved from http://www.jstor.org/stable/40230884

Pathak, P. K., & Singh, A. (2011). Trends in malnutrition among children in India: Growing inequalities across different economic groups. *Social Science and Medicine*, 73(4), 576–585. Doi: 10.1016/j.socscimed.2011.06.024.

Pescaru, M. (2015). Consequences of parents' migration on children rearing and education. *Procedia-Social and Behavioral Sciences*, 180, 674–681. Doi: 10.1016/j. sbspro.2015.02.177.

Planning Commission (2013). *Poverty Estimates*, 2011-12. Government of India, PRS. Retrieved from https://www.prsindia.org/tags/planning- commission

Rahaman, M., Hossain, B., Kundu, S., & Ajmer, S. (2021). Duration of father out-migration and its impact on nutritional status of left-behind children: A cross-sectional study in rural EAG states in India. *Indian Journal of Public Health Research & Development*, 12(3), 389–395. Doi: 10.37506/ijphrd.v12i3.16090

Rajan, S. I., Sivakumar, P., & Srinivasan, A. (2020). The COVID-19 pandemic and internal labour migration in India: A 'crisis of mobility'. *Indian Journal of Labour Economics*, 63, 1021–1039. Doi: 10.1007/s41027-020-00293-8.

Rathnayake, I., & Weerahewa, J. (2003). Intra-household allocation of calories among low income households in Sri Lanka: impact of female sources of income. Globalisation and Distribution in SriLanka. Retrieved from https://www.pep -net.org/sites/pep- net.org/files/typo3doc/pdf/files_events/1st_PMMA- MPIA/ Rathnayake.pdf

Rathnayake, I. M., & Weerahewa, J. (2005). Maternal employment and income affect dietary calorie adequacy in households in Sri Lanka. *Food and Nutrition Bulletin*, 26(2), 222–229. Doi:10.1177/156482650502600206

Shen, M., Yang, S., Han, J., Shi, J., Yang, R., Du, Y., et al. (2009). Non-fatal injury rates among the "left-behind children" of rural China. *Injury Prevention*, 15(4), 244–247.

Srivastava, R. (2020). Labour Migration, Vulnerability, and Development Policy: The Pandemic as Inflexion Point?. *Indian Journal of Labour Economics* 63, 859–883. https://doi.org/10.1007/s41027-020-00301-x

Stark, O., & Taylor, J. E. (1991). Migration incentives, migration types: The role of relative deprivation. *The Economic Journal*, 101(408), 1163–1178.

Stillman, S., Gibson, J., & Mckenzie, D. (2012). The impact of immigration on child health: Experimental evidence from a migration lottery program. *Economic Inquiry*, 50(1), 62–81. Doi:10.1111/J.1465-7295.2009.00284.X

Syahrul, S., Kimura, R., Tsuda, A., Susanto, T., Saito, R., & Ahmad, F. (2016). Prevalence of underweight and overweight among school-aged children and it's association with children's socio demographic and lifestyle in Indonesia. *International Journal of Nursing Sciences*, 3(2), 169–177.

Tian, X., Ding, C., Shen, C., & Wang, H. (2017). Does parental migration have negative impact on the growth of left-behind children?: New evidence from longitudinal data in rural China. *International Journal of Environmental Research and Public Health*, 14(11), 1308. Doi:10.3390/ijerph14111308

United Nations (1998). *Recommendations on Statistics of International Migration, Revision-1*. Department of Economics and Social Affairs Statistics Division. Retrieved from https://unstats.un.org/unsd/publication/seriesm/seriesm_58rev1e .pdf

Urban HUNGaMA Report (2014). *Nutrition and the City*. Naandi Foundation. Retrieved from https://www.naandi.org/images/3b29cd5d8d8dfbac30c6275 c916862ac.pdf.

Vlassoff, C. (2013). The importance of sons in Indian culture. In *Gender Equality and Inequality in Rural India*. New York: Palgrave Macmillan. Doi:10.1057/9781137373922_1

WHO Multicentre Growth Reference Study Group (2006). WHO child growth standards based on length/height, weight and age. *Acta Pædiatrica*, 2006(Suppl

450), 76/85. Retrieved from https://www.who.int/childgrowth/standards/Growth_standard.pdf

Wooldridge, J. M. (2019). *Introductory Econometrics A Modern Approach.* 5th Edition, Cengage Press.

Xu, H., & Xie, Y. (2015). The causal effects of rural-to-urban migration on children's wellbeing in China. *European Sociological Review, 31*(4), 502e519. Doi:10.1093/esr/jcv009.

Yang, D. (2008). International migration, remittances, and household investment: Evidence from Philippine migrants' exchange rate shocks. *The Economic Journal, 118*(5), 591–630.

10 Utilisation of Integrated Child Development Services (ICDS) and Nutritional Outcomes in Empowered Action Group (EAG) States of India

Evidence from Two National Surveys

Rudra Narayan Mishra

Introduction

India remains one of the leading countries in the world in terms of under-nourished population. The recent Global Hunger Index (GHI) has once again highlighted the issue of high prevalence of undernutrition in the country. Compared to GHI 2021, in the year 2022 the country slips by six positions from 101 to 107 among the 122 countries and also ranks below the poorer neighbouring countries. The report highlights the task of achieving 'zero hunger', i.e. Goal 2 of the Sustainable Development Goals (SDG) adopted by all United Nations member countries in 2015, for the country a difficult proposition given the pace of improvement. With an overall score of 29.1 in the composite score for GHI, India is in the category of 'serious' in hunger related matters. Despite impressive economic growth after reforms in 1990s which coincide with the first national-level reliable data base for nutritional information of reproductive age women and children in India (National Family Health Surveys-NFHS) shows the hypothesis for direct relation between 'higher economic growth leading to better nutritional outcome', is somewhat truncated in Indian context (Rai et al; 2014).

National Family Health Survey (NFHS) started in the early 1990s is one of the prominent sources for understanding the prevalence of undernutrition in India in terms of anthropometric and clinical indicators. As per the latest survey (2019-21), among children of age below five years, 36% are reportedly stunted (short height for their age), 32% are underweight (less weight for their given age), and 19% were wasted (thin for their given height). In the prevalence of wasting, the country occupied the top position among the 122 countries that were evaluated for GHI 2022. Among children of age 6–59 months, 67% were having mild-to-severe anaemia. Among reproductive age women and adult men, the prevalence of low body mass index (low BMI), 19% of adult female and 16% of adult male were thin or undernourished. In terms of the prevalence of anaemia, 57% of adult women and 25% of adult men were reportedly anaemic.

DOI: 10.4324/9781003430636-14

Compared to 2015–16, when the data for NFHS-4 round were released, the decline in child stunting and underweight was 2% and 4%, respectively, whereas wasting increased by 2.0 percentage points. In the case of child anaemia, there is a 7 percentage points increase at all India levels in 2019–21 over 2015–16. For both adult women and men, the prevalence of low BMI has declined by 4 percentage points from 2015–16 to 2019–21. Despite these reductions in overall prevalence, the country remains one of the largest repositories of undernourished population in the world. Given the size of its population, India's measures to address the issue of hunger and malnutrition are crucial at the global stage to remove the 'Hunger' as per SDG goals. Under recently launched POSHAN Abhiyaan, India aims to reduce prevalence of stunting and underweight among pre-school children and low birthweight by 2% each per annum and the prevalence of anaemia among pre-school children, women and adolescent girls by 3% per annum. However, given the rate of decline in these indicators between 2015–16 and 2020–21, the goals look hard to be realised any time soon.

Undernutrition in the context of India though declining for most of the anthropometric indicators, in terms of number counts in millions it has been increasing (Oxford Poverty and Human Development Initiative , 2019, 2021). The prevalence of undernutrition among children and women is one of the major factors towards multidimensional poverty around the globe (ibid). Studies show that adults who face undernutrition in their childhood could earn 20% less compared to adults who did not face any deficiency regarding their nutrition in childhood (*Comprehensive National Nutrition Survey (CNNS)*, 2019). With an increase in 1 CM height in the case of a male child, he is likely to earn 4 times more in adulthood, while the same for girl children is a recorded 6% increase in wages in case she did not face any undernutrition (ibid). A recent study predicts, because of loss of livelihood and disruption in social welfare schemes due to COVID-19 pandemic, especially among socio-economically poorer households the prevalence of underweight children below six years of age and lower BMI among reproductive-age women could go up by 5% (Joe et al; 2020).

In India, the incidence of monetary poverty, ill health and undernutrition is more prevalent among certain social groups than others. For example, among scheduled tribes (STs), the prevalence of multidimensional poverty which includes monetary poverty, ill health and undernutrition shows despite they constitute less than 10% of the total population, over 50% of them face multidimensional poverty. Among the scheduled caste (SC) population, the same is found to be 33.3%. Not only prevalence but also the incidence of deprivation in multidimensional poverty index was found to be higher for these two social groups than others (Oxford Poverty and Human Development Initiative, 2021). Five out of six households reporting multidimensional poverty in India belongs to a SC/ST/OBC (other backwards caste) households (ibid). Over the years the socio-economic inequality in undernutrition has increased in EAG states (Kumar and Paswan, 2021).

Since independence, one of the major welfare interventions for India was to achieve zero hunger and nutritional well-being. The largest subsidised food programme in terms of public distribution system through fair price shops (PDS), mid-day meal (MDM) for school going children and ICDS scheme for pre-school children, girl children not going to school and expecting and lactating mothers was launched in the 60s and 70s to address the issue of hunger and undernutrition among the masses (Mishra, 2020, Kumar et al, 2020). Over the years, different programmes to reduce the prevalence of undernutrition have been initiated through these institutions. But it is observed the lion's share of the budget allocated to nutritional programmes like ICDS goes towards salaries, honorariums and infrastructure, and only a little goes towards supplementary food being provided (Kapur et al; 2021). In this paper, we will look at the utilisation of ICDS at the household level, specifically among the EAG states.

Nonetheless the ICDS interventions for young mother and children need to be complemented by interventions from other sectors like poverty alleviation schemes through convergence for vulnerable households like Scheduled Caste and Scheduled Tribes (Rajpal et al; 2020a, 2020b), households belonging to minorities (Kumar et al, 2021), occupationally vulnerable households whose livelihood depends upon agricultural labour and fishing (Smita et al, 2021), empowering women through imparting skill and education (Kumar and Lakhtakia, 2021) and strengthening the health infrastructure in rural areas (Kumar and Singh, 2016, Jose et al; 2020). Nonetheless the social, economic, cultural and service related barriers (both from demand and supply side) need multipronged strategy to improve the health outcomes for women and children in India (Mahapatro, 2022) and ICDS is crucial to address them. The economic growth and distribution of economic gain are important to finance the mission to improve the women and Child health in India (Panda et al, 2021). It is also essential to address inherent inequality within various population groups while measuring progress in health-related indicators vis-à-vis population averages to design interventions addressing the specific needs of each sub group (Mishra, 2016).

Empowered Action Group States: Why They Hold the Key to Improve India's Nutritional Scenario

EAG states refer to eight socio-economically backward states in India, viz. Bihar, Chhattisgarh, Jharkhand, Madhya Pradesh, Odisha, Rajasthan, Uttarakhand and Uttar Pradesh. These states were characterised by poor health outcomes among women and children and at the same time low utilisation of maternal and child health services (Arokiyasami and Gautam; 2008, Mishra et al; 2015). These eight states have 46% of the total population in

India as per the 2011 census and 61% of the below poverty line population as per the 2011 household consumer survey by NSSO (Kumar et al., 2016). These eight states together also constitute a major share of the burden of disease among the Indian population and the accessibility to basic health care is still not available to a majority of the people in these states (ibid). These EAG states also show higher socio-economic inequalities for prevalence of undernutrition among pre-school children in different anthropometric indicators (Kumar and Paswan, 2021). The EAG states like Bihar and Uttar Pradesh reportedly account for higher burden of child anaemia among Indian states due to early marriages of girls, higher number of births and short birth intervals (Rana et al, 2019). In 2013, the Government of India (GOI) introduced the concept of 'high priority districts (HPD)', to improve maternal and child health outcomes under National Rural Health Mission (NRHM) and identified 184 districts out of 718 total districts in India for improving the reproductive, maternal, newborn, child and adolescent health (referred to as RMNCH+A). The initiative has resulted in marked improvement in service delivery for the EAG states vis-à-vis non-EAG states but the improvement for respective HPD within a given EAG states vis-à-vis the non-HPD districts are found to be not much different (Ramesh et al; 2020). The study identified mother's education level as one of the major factors towards service utilisation (ibid). In the EAG states, it is also observed that the poor maternal health of the mothers determines the outcome for nutritional health of children and the result is statistically significant (Prasad et al, 2015). Studies found that in the EAG states where migration is a continuous phenomenon, the children in those households have higher risk of various forms of undernourishment than households without migration (Margubur et al., 2021). Another study shows despite the increase the health spending, especially on primary health, remained inadequate in the EAG states which contribute towards higher incidence of undernutrition in these states (Salve, 2022, Dash, 2016).

The women in the EAG states were found to have higher unmet needs, one of the major factors being their poor economic condition, which is affecting the health and nutritional outcomes of the women in these states (Malik and Akhtar, 2021). It is also observed the improvement in healthcare access and utilisation is lagging in rural areas compared to their urban counterparts leading to higher prevalence of poor nutrition status in rural and remote areas of these states (Roy, 2021). The supply-side issues in health care in rural India, viz. availability of physical infrastructure and manpower in the case of primary health care, are reflected in poor nutritional health outcomes among women and children in the EAG states (Bhatia et al; 2021). The improvement in supply-side challenges will lead to a reduction in inequality in nutritional outcomes between poor and rich households in these states (ibid). According to NITI Ayog's recent observation, all the EAG states, except Chhattisgarh, were in the bottom half in terms of overall performance in the Health Index for 2019–20, despite having improvement over 2018–19 (page 25). Therefore, any study on the EAG states will add insights to the policy making for better provision of various social safety nets in general and preventive/curative health care in particular. A recent study shows there is a decline in the number of Supplementary Nutrition Programme (SNP) beneficiaries during the COVID-19 lockdown between June 2019 and June 2020 in four out of eight EAG states; Madhya Pradesh (50%), Jharkhand (37%), Odisha (11%) and Uttar Pradesh (6%) though in Bihar and Chhattisgarh the number of beneficiaries increased by 31% and 26%, respectively, followed by 6% in Uttar Pradesh and 4% in Rajasthan (Kapur et al; 2021). The same study also shows that the budgetary allocation towards SNP fell short of the estimated required cost for most of the states in India including EAG states in 2020–21, which could have resulted in the denial of SNP to millions of children and women beneficiaries (ibid, page 5). Among the EAG states, the highest shortfall was 71 per cent for Rajasthan, followed by Bihar (66%), Uttar Pradesh (53%), Jharkhand (49%), Madhya Pradesh (46%), Chhattisgarh (29%) and Odisha (19%) in COVID-19 pandemic year. As per the above study, over the years the proportion of ICDS allocations out of projected demand has declined from 80% in 2017–18 to 70% during 2020–21 financial years (revised estimates). Without adequate financial support, the nutritional intervention will not achieve the desired result in the planned time period. Out of the total budget allocated towards nutritional programmes in any given financial year, over 95 per cent goes towards implementation of ICDS (ibid, page 3) which justifies the purpose of this paper to look at its utilisation across the EAG states.

Objective

The present study has a very specific objective to look at the utilisation of ICDS. The reason being in the Indian context the ICDS is the institutional multipurpose vehicle which takes care of access to both food inadequacy and health care, the immediate causes of undernutrition in various forms among pre-school children and young mothers (UNICEF, 2020). Since the EAG states as the evidence above shows face higher incidence of poverty and lack adequate health facilities to take care of the burden of disease due to poor living condition, it is the anganwadis of the ICDS which address the hunger due to poverty through supplementary nutrition programme and health care through regular health check-ups for mothers and children below age 6 years, immunisation, micronutrient supplementation and nutrition education. Therefore, the present chapter will look into the service delivery aspect at anganwadis through ICDS programme for households who belong to rural areas, marginalised sections like SC/ST/OBCs and poorer households (Figure 10.1).

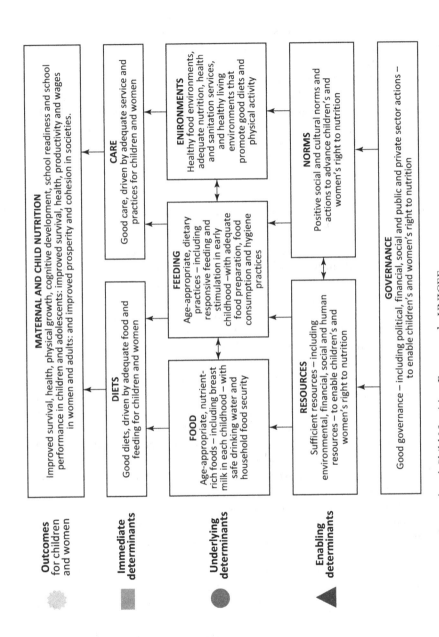

Outcomes for children and women

Immediate determinants

Underlying determinants

Enabling determinants

MATERNAL AND CHILD NUTRITION
Improved survival, health, physical growth, cognitive development, school readiness and school performance in children and adolescents: improved survival, health, productivity and wages in women and adults: and improved prosperity and cohesion in societies.

CARE
Good care, driven by adequate service and practices for children and women

ENVIRONMENTS
Healthy food environments, adequate nutrition, health and sanitation services, and healthy living environments that promote good diets and physical activity

FEEDING
Age-appropriate, dietary practices – including responsive feeding and stimulation in early childhood – with adequate food preparation, food consumption and hygiene practices

NORMS
Positive social and cultural norms and actions to advance children's and women's right to nutrition

DIETS
Good diets, driven by adequate food and feeding for children and women

FOOD
Age-appropriate, nutrient-rich foods – including breast milk in each childhood – with safe drinking water and household food security

RESOURCES
Sufficient resources – including environmental, financial, social and human resources – to enable children's and women's right to nutrition

GOVERNANCE
Good governance – including political, financial, social and public and private sector actions – to enable children's and women's right to nutrition

Figure 10.1 Maternal and Child Nutrition Framework: UNICEF

Source: Nutrition For Every Child, UNICEF Nutrition Strategy 2020–2030, UNICEF, New Work, page 32.

Methodology

To achieve the objectives, we have used the child files from both NFHS-4 and NFHS-5 rounds. We have taken into account the utilisation of any ICDS services for pregnant and breastfeeding mothers separately and for children below age six years. Since the protocol for nutritional supplementation, immunisation, health check-up and nutritional education varies among these two groups of mothers, a separate analysis is justified on the account. Recently, under Janani Suraksha Yojana (JSY), the direct monetary benefits were provided to needy mothers from poorer households, which is basically coordinated and supervised at the level of anganwadi centres, we include the analysis of the same in the chapter.

Results and Discussions

Prevalence of Undernutrition Among Women and Children in the EAG States: 2015–16 and 2019–21

The prevalence of undernutrition among children has come down across the EAG states confirming to all India patterns in anthropometric indicators such as stunting, underweight and wasting, the exception being Bihar in the case of wasting. But what is worrying is in most of the EAG states, except for Jharkhand, the prevalence of anaemia among children is rising, the highest being Chhattisgarh followed by Odisha and Rajasthan which is clearly an outcome of inadequate food and frequent infections (UNICEF; 2020). ICDS system in India is designed to take care of these twin immediate factors of child anaemia through supplementary food intake, immunisation and regular health check-up for children below six years of age. All EAG states show at least three out of five children below age six years are still facing anaemia which is definitely a public health challenge to be addressed on a priority basis. If we look at anthropometric measures, then at least two out of every five children are facing stunting and three out of five children are facing underweight across the EAG states. Similarly, one out of five children across all EAG states are having wasting, an extreme form of undernutrition. Though rural parts of the EAG states show a higher decline than their urban counter parts for most of the EAG states, still the prevalence of stunting, underweight and wasting is higher for the former (Table 10.1).

For women of reproductive age, the prevalence of low BMI has come down between 2015–16 and 2019–21. But the prevalence of anaemia has increased, the highest being in Odisha followed by Bihar, Chhattisgarh and Uttar Pradesh (Table 10.2).

Thus, it is important to assess the functioning of ICDS in these EAG states to understand what measures can be taken to address the dilemma of falling undernutrition albeit at a limited rate in the case of anthropometric measures

Table 10.1 Prevalence of Undernutrition Among Children Below Six Years of Age in Selected Anthropometric Indicators and Anaemia

States	Height-for-age (Stunting)			Wasting (weight-for-height)			Underweight (weight-for-age)			Anaemia		
	2015–16	2019–21	% change	2015–16	2019–21	% change	2015–16	2019–21	% change	2015–16	2019–21	% change
Bihar												
Urban	39.8	36.8	-3.0	21.3	21.6	0.3	37.5	35.8	-1.7	58.8	67.9	9.1
Rural	49.3	43.8	-5.5	20.8	23.1	2.3	44.6	41.8	-2.8	64.0	69.7	5.7
Total	48.3	42.9	-5.4	20.8	22.9	2.1	43.9	41.0	-2.9	63.5	69.4	5.9
Chhattisgarh												
Urban	31.6	30.0	-1.6	20.6	18.9	-1.7	30.2	25.8	-4.4	42.9	71.1	28.2
Rural	39.2	35.8	-3.4	23.7	18.9	-4.8	39.6	32.7	-6.9	41.2	66.2	25.0
Total	37.6	37.6	0.0	23.1	18.9	-4.2	47.1	37.7	-9.4	41.6	67.2	25.6
Jharkhand												
Urban	33.7	26.8	-6.9	26.8	23.0	-3.8	39.3	30.0	-9.3	63.2	65.5	2.3
Rural	48.0	42.3	-5.7	29.5	22.3	-7.2	49.8	41.4	-8.4	71.5	67.9	-3.6
Total	45.3	39.6	-5.7	29.0	22.4	-6.6	47.8	39.4	-8.4	69.9	67.4	-2.5
Madhya Pradesh												
Urban	37.4	30.1	-7.3	22.0	19.9	-2.1	36.5	28.6	-7.9	66.2	72.5	6.3
Rural	43.6	37.2	-6.4	27.1	18.7	-8.4	45.0	34.2	-10.8	69.8	72.7	2.9
Total	42.0	35.7	-6.3	25.8	18.9	-6.9	42.8	33.0	-9.8	68.9	72.6	3.7
Odisha												
Urban	27.2	24.9	-2.3	17.0	14.9	-2.1	26.2	21.5	-4.7	38.1	56.2	18.1
Rural	35.3	32.0	-3.3	20.9	18.6	-2.3	35.8	31.0	-4.8	45.7	65.6	19.9
Total	34.1	31.0	-3.1	20.4	18.1	-2.3	34.4	29.7	-4.7	44.3	64.2	19.9

(Continued)

Table 10.1 Continued

States	Height-for-age (Stunting)			Wasting (weight-for-height)			Underweight (weight-for-age)			Anaemia		
	2015–16	2019–21	% change	2015–16	2019–21	% change	2015–16	2019–21	% change	2015–16	2019–21	% change
Rajasthan												
Urban	33.0	28.3	-4.7	21.6	18.3	-3.3	30.7	25.4	-5.3	55.7	68.3	12.6
Rural	40.8	32.6	-8.2	23.4	16.4	-7.0	38.3	28.1	-10.2	61.6	72.3	10.7
Total	39.1	31.8	-7.3	23.0	16.8	-6.2	36.7	27.6	-9.1	60.3	71.5	11.2
Uttar Pradesh												
Urban	37.9	33.0	-4.9	18.0	18.7	0.7	33.7	28.2	-5.5	65.0	65.3	0.3
Rural	48.5	41.3	-7.2	17.8	17.0	-0.8	41.0	33.1	-7.9	62.7	66.7	4.0
Total	46.2	39.7	-6.5	17.9	17.3	-0.6	36.1	32.1	-4.0	63.2	66.4	3.2
Uttarakhand												
Urban	32.5	24.3	-8.2	18.6	17.4	-1.2	25.6	21.0	-4.6	59.3	63.8	4.5
Rural	34.0	28.2	-5.8	19.9	11.3	-8.6	27.1	20.9	-6.2	52.8	56.6	3.8
Total	33.5	27.0	-6.5	19.5	13.2	-6.3	26.6	21.0	-5.6	54.9	58.8	3.9
All India												
Urban	31.0	30.1	-0.9	20.0	18.5	-1.5	29.1	27.3	-1.8	56.0	64.2	8.2
Rural	41.2	37.3	-3.9	21.4	19.5	-1.9	38.3	33.8	-4.5	59.5	68.3	8.8
Total	38.4	35.5	-2.9	21.0	19.3	-1.7	35.7	32.1	-3.6	58.5	67.1	8.6

Source: Author's calculation from NFHS data.

Table 10.2 Prevalence of Undernutrition (BMI and Anaemia) Among Women of Reproductive Age (15–49 Years)

States	Women BMI			Women Anaemia		
	2015–16	2019–21	% change	2015–16	2019–21	% change
Bihar						
Urban	22.2	18.7	-3.5	45.4	65.6	20.2
Rural	31.8	26.9	-4.9	45.8	63.1	17.3
Total	30.5	25.6	-4.9	45.7	60.3	14.6
Chhattisgarh						
Urban	17.6	16.0	-1.6	43.3	56.5	13.2
Rural	29.6	25.3	-4.3	48.2	62.2	14.0
Total	26.7	23.1	-3.6	47.0	60.8	13.8
Jharkhand						
Urban	21.6	17.3	-4.3	59.6	61.1	1.5
Rural	35.4	29.2	-6.2	67.3	66.7	-0.6
Total	31.5	26.2	-5.3	65.2	65.3	0.1
Madhya Pradesh						
Urban	20.6	17.1	-3.5	49.6	51.5	1.9
Rural	31.8	25.2	-6.6	53.8	55.8	2.0
Total	28.3	23.0	-5.3	52.5	54.7	2.2
Odisha						
Urban	15.8	12.6	-3.2	39.2	61.5	22.3
Rural	28.7	22.6	-6.1	40.8	64.9	24.1
Total	26.4	20.8	-5.6	40.5	64.3	23.8

(Continued)

Table 10.2 Continued

States	Women BMI			Women Anaemia		
	2015–16	2019–21	% change	2015–16	2019–21	% change
Rajasthan						
Urban	18.6	14.0	–4.6	40.7	49.9	9.2
Rural	29.9	21.3	–8.6	49.0	55.7	6.7
Total	27.0	19.5	–7.5	46.8	54.4	7.6
Uttar Pradesh						
Urban	17.6	14.0	–3.6	39.3	50.1	10.8
Rural	28.1	21.0	–7.1	38.6	50.5	11.9
Total	25.3	19.0	–6.3	38.8	50.4	11.6
Uttarakhand						
Urban	15.5	11.6	–3.9	42.1	45.8	3.7
Rural	20.0	14.9	–5.1	41.2	41.1	–0.1
Total	18.4	13.9	–4.5	41.5	42.6	1.1
All India						
Urban	15.5	13.3	–2.2	50.8	53.8	3.0
Rural	26.8	21.3	–5.5	54.2	58.5	4.3
Total	22.9	18.7	–4.2	53.1	57.0	3.9

Source: Author's calculation from NFHS data.

and at the same time increase in prevalence of anaemia for younger children and adult women in the EAG states.

Utilisation of any ICDS Services Among Expecting Mothers

It is observed that among EAG states, Odisha has the highest reporting of utilisation of ICDS services by women who were pregnant (90.1%) in urban areas followed by Madhya Pradesh and Uttarakhand during 2019–21. Bihar has the lowest utilisation of services (41.6%) followed by Uttar Pradesh, Jharkhand and Rajasthan, and all these four states reportedly have utilisation below the national average during the same period.

Compared to 2015–16, Uttar Pradesh has increased utilisation by more than two times in 2019–21 followed by Rajasthan (nearly twice) of 2015–16. In Bihar, the utilisation of ICDS services remained lowest among all the EAG states for both the periods. Except for Chhattisgarh and Jharkhand, all other states improved the utilisation of ICDS services by more than 10 percentage points between the two periods. In the case of Chhattisgarh, the utilisation has gone up by only 0.4 percentage points during the same period (Figure 10.2).

In rural India, the utilisation is overall higher than in urban India. In Odisha, the utilisation has gone up to 97% followed by Uttarakhand and Chhattisgarh (90% or above). Uttarakhand has registered highest improvement in utilisation of ICDS services by 32.1 percentage points followed by Uttar Pradesh (28.4 percentage points), Rajasthan (16.6 percentage points),

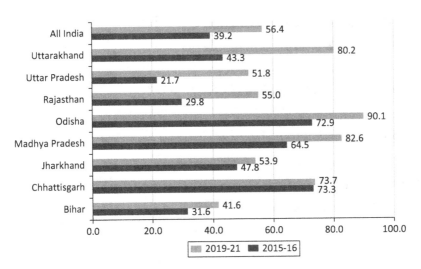

Figure 10.2 Use of Any ICDS Among Pregnant Mothers: EAG States and All India – Urban

Source: Author's calculation from NFHS data.

Madhya Pradesh (14 percentage points) and Bihar (13.9 percentage points). In Chhattisgarh, there is a slight decline in the utilisation of services between the two periods. Except for Bihar and Rajasthan the other EAG states have utilisation of ICDS services for pregnant women more than the national average in 2019–21. This can be attributed towards the effort of the remaining states to improve the ICDS delivery system (Figure 10.3).

By social groups, it is observed that the utilisation of ICDS service for pregnant mothers has increased for all social groups across EAG states except for Chhattisgarh where it has declined for all social groups except for a small increase in the case of 'others'. Odisha is one exception among all the EAG states where the utilisation of ICDS services has been above 96% for marginalised sections like SC, ST and OBCs, highest among all EAG states. Chhattisgarh, Madhya Pradesh and Uttarakhand are the other three states where among SC, ST and OBCs more than 85% of pregnant mothers reported using any ICDS services in 2019–2021. Uttar Pradesh and Uttarakhand have reported more than 25 percentage points increase in utilisation of ICDS services for SC, ST and OBCs between two time periods. Bihar has the lowest utilisation of ICDS services among pregnant women for all EAG states and all of India in both time points (Table 10.3).

By economic status of the households, the utilisation of ICDS by expecting mothers shows an increasing trend for all EAG states except Chhattisgarh. Among all states, Uttarakhand and Uttar Pradesh have registered an increase in ICDS by 25 percentage points to 37 percentage points

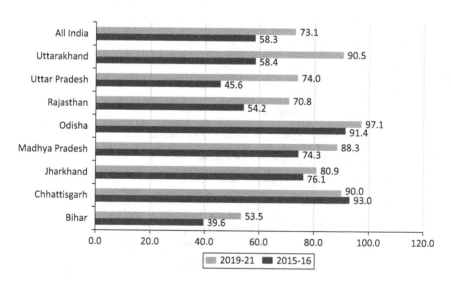

Figure 10.3 Use of Any ICDS Among Pregnant Mothers: EAG States and All India – Rural

Source: Author's calculation from NFHS data.

Table 10.3 Utilisation of Any ICDS for Pregnant Mothers by Social Groups

Caste groups	Time periods	Bihar	Chhattisgarh	Jharkhand	Madhya Pradesh	Odisha	Rajasthan	Uttar Pradesh	Uttarakhand	All India
Scheduled Caste (SC)	2019–21	59.8	86.5	78.1	87.9	96.7	67.3	73.3	85.3	74.1
	2015–16	47.0	90.4	69.4	74.4	90.2	51.6	48.7	58.4	60.1
	% change	*12.8*	*-3.9*	*8.7*	*13.5*	*6.5*	*15.7*	*24.6*	*26.9*	*14.0*
Scheduled Tribe (ST)	2019–21	50.4	90.5	82.9	89.5	97.3	81.0	65.1	94.8	85.8
	2015–16	36.6	92.3	78.7	72.9	91.0	60.6	34.3	68.0	56.8
	% change	*13.8*	*-1.8*	*4.2*	*16.6*	*6.3*	*20.4*	*30.8*	*26.8*	*29.0*
Other Backward Caste (OBC)	2019–21	51.2	86.6	74.8	87.3	96.9	66.6	69.2	89.2	70.9
	2015–16	38.6	89.5	70.6	74.5	90.6	48.7	40.0	46.7	54.3
	% change	*12.6*	*-2.9*	*4.2*	*12.8*	*6.3*	*17.9*	*29.2*	*42.5*	*16.6*
Others	2019–21	40.6	64.2	59.9	81.7	91.6	61.9	64.4	86.5	66.0
	2015–16	28.8	63.8	50.0	58.8	79.5	46.3	32.0	54.3	43.6
	% change	*11.8*	*0.4*	*9.9*	*22.9*	*12.1*	*15.6*	*32.4*	*32.2*	*22.4*

Source: Author's calculation from NFHS data.

for all sections among the EAG states. It is a good sign that among the poorest households in these two states, the utilisation of ICDS has gone up by more than 30 percentage points. Odisha stands out among all the EAG states where across all economic strata the utilisation of services by expecting mothers is above 90 percent except for the richest. Bihar among all EAG states has the lowest utilisation of services by expecting mothers, where among lower economic strata half of the expecting mothers are yet to utilise the services. The high utilisation in certain states for richer sections of Chhattisgarh, Odisha and Uttarakhand is a very good sign for the programme in these states, who despite their affordability to other service providers have chosen state run ICDS programmes. Apart from Bihar, Rajasthan and Uttar Pradesh despite improvement nearly a quarter of expecting mothers were not availing any ICDS according to 2019–21 data (Table 10.4).

Utilisation of any ICDS Among Women Who are Currently Breastfeeding

Among breastfeeding/lactating mothers, the overall utilisation of any ICDS services is found to be less compared to expecting mothers in urban areas. The highest utilisation is reported for Odisha among all EAG states in both the time periods. In Madhya Pradesh and Uttarakhand, more than 75% of lactating women were reportedly using any ICDS. In Chhattisgarh, there is not much change in the utilisation as in both time periods, 70% of lactating women are using any ICDS. All these three EAG states have higher utilisation of ICDS for lactating mothers than the national average in both rounds. Bihar among all the EAG states has lagged behind in both the periods followed by Uttar Pradesh and Rajasthan. In all these three states, less than 50% of lactating mothers use any ICDS. In Jharkhand, little more than 50% of lactating women in urban areas were reportedly using any services as per 2019–21 records. Bihar, Uttar Pradesh, Rajasthan and Jharkhand need to augment their ICDS delivery programmes for women in urban areas (Figure 10.4).

In rural areas, the pattern remains similar to that of urban India for women who were currently lactating/breastfeeding during the survey. Among all EAG states, Odisha reportedly has the highest utilisation in both periods. Uttarakhand, Madhya Pradesh and Chhattisgarh are other three EAG states which reportedly 85.0% or more lactating mothers using any ICDS services as per the survey in 2019–21. Bihar fares worst among all the EAG states in both rounds. As per the survey in 2019–21, less than half of the lactating mothers in rural areas use any services from ICDS in the state. Rajasthan and Uttar Pradesh are the other two EAG states which lagged behind national average for rural areas. However, Uttar Pradesh has improved the utilisation by little more than 33.3 percentage points during the time period. Uttarakhand is closely following Uttar Pradesh in terms of

Table 10.4 Utilisation of Any ICDS for Pregnant Mothers by Wealth Quintiles

Wealth Quintiles	Time periods	Bihar	Chhattisgarh	Jharkhand	Madhya Pradesh	Odisha	Rajasthan	Uttar Pradesh	Uttarakhand	All India
Poorest	2019–21	54.2	89.6	81.5	86.9	96.8	73.0	72.1	88.4	74.0
	2015–16	41.5	92.6	75.6	71.2	90.7	49.5	41.9	52.3	55.1
	% change	**12.6**	**-3.0**	**6.0**	**15.7**	**6.1**	**23.5**	**30.2**	**36.1**	**18.9**
Poorer	2019–21	54.8	90.5	78.8	89.0	97.7	71.9	73.1	90.5	75.3
	2015–16	41.1	94.5	77.2	76.6	91.1	55.6	46.8	60.7	60.6
	% change	**13.7**	**-3.9**	**1.6**	**12.4**	**6.6**	**16.3**	**26.3**	**29.8**	**14.7**
Middle	2019–21	51.1	89.4	76.1	89.8	97.4	70.8	72.6	88.8	75.7
	2015–16	32.3	92.5	71.2	77.5	92.0	52.9	44.0	57.2	59.5
	% change	**18.8**	**-3.1**	**4.9**	**12.3**	**5.4**	**17.9**	**28.7**	**31.6**	**16.2**
Richer	2019–21	42.4	86.5	61.3	88.5	95.7	66.4	66.3	91.2	71.4
	2015–16	23.9	87.4	51.6	74.7	83.0	47.9	37.0	54.3	51.8
	% change	**18.5**	**-1.0**	**9.7**	**13.8**	**12.7**	**18.5**	**29.4**	**36.9**	**19.6**
Richest	2019–21	20.1	63.6	35.9	78.4	84.7	56.2	57.3	80.8	61.2
	2015–16	15.1	62.3	26.8	54.0	58.1	34.2	24.0	43.5	35.3
	% change	**5.0**	**1.3**	**9.1**	**24.4**	**26.6**	**22.0**	**33.3**	**37.3**	**25.9**

Source: Author's calculation from NFHS data.

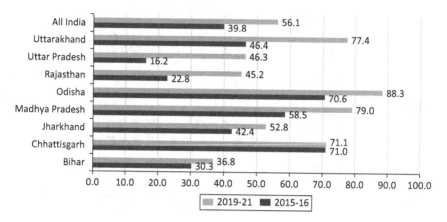

Figure 10.4 Use of Any ICDS Among Breastfeeding Mothers: EAG States and All India – Urban

Source: Author's calculation from NFHS data.

increasing utilisation of ICDS by 26.1 percentage points. Chhattisgarh on the other hand has reported a decline in utilisation though by a small 3 percentage points approximately during the same period. Overall, it is a positive sign that utilisation of ICDS among lactating mothers, except for three states, in the remaining five EAG states is higher than the national average. Still, there is scope to further strengthen the delivery mechanism to cater the needs of breastfeeding mothers under ICDS (Figure 10.5).

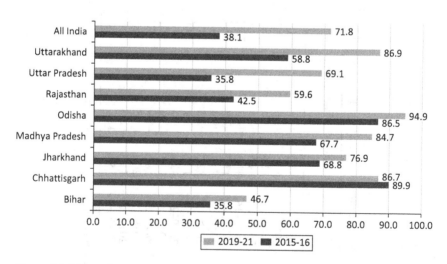

Figure 10.5 Use of Any ICDS Among Breastfeeding Mothers: EAG States and All India – Rural

Source: Author's calculation from NFHS data.

Utilisation of ICDS among breastfeeding mothers according to their social group shows Odisha has the highest utilisation (90%) across all social groups. Among all social groups, SC mothers have the highest utilisation in any given EAG states in both rounds followed by ST women. Uttar Pradesh has registered highest increase in service utilisation for lactating mothers among all the EAG states for SC and ST mothers in 2019–21 over 2015–16 (30.0 percentage points or more) followed by Uttarakhand (17.0 percentage points to 23 percentage points). For OBC mothers, Uttarakhand has registered 39.1 percentage points increase followed by Uttar Pradesh (33.0 percentage points). Chhattisgarh is the only exception among EAG states which has registered negative growth though by a small margin in ICDS service utilisation by lactating mothers for SC, ST and OBC social groups. However, overall utilisation by these three groups in the state remained above 80.0% in both time periods. For Jharkhand, Odisha and Bihar, the improvement in service utilisation by social groups varied between 7.0 and 11.0 percentage points, but these three states are at different levels. Where in Odisha service utilisation is already above 90.0% in both periods, in Bihar for all social groups half of the lactating women were not using any services, Jharkhand is somewhere in the middle where at least one-third of lactating women were reported not using any services (Table 10.5).

Odisha, Chhattisgarh and Uttarakhand, the three EAG states, show more than 85% or more lactating women among any economic strata access some services from ICDS in both time periods. Odisha performed the best among all EAG states. Despite a decline in utilisation, Chhattisgarh comes next. Uttarakhand is close to Chhattisgarh in terms of utilisation in 2019–21. Uttar Pradesh has improved service utilisation by more than 30 percentage points for all economic groups, poorest to richest between two time periods followed by Uttarakhand. Rajasthan and Madhya Pradesh also show improvement by 14–24 percentage points across the five economic groups. Jharkhand has made single digit improvement in lactating mothers' utilisation of ICDS for SC, ST and OBC. Uttar Pradesh, Uttarakhand, Odisha, Madhya Pradesh and Rajasthan made impressive improvements in utilisation of ICDS services among lactating mothers in the richest category which shows the service delivery must have improved in quality to attract the households who otherwise could have availed services from elsewhere, especially from private providers. In Bihar, the utilisation remained lowest for the richest category where less than one-fifth of the lactating mothers were reportedly using ICDS in both periods. In Jharkhand, less than one-third of the lactating mothers reportedly used any ICDS in both periods. The service delivery of ICDS for lactating mothers in the states of Bihar, Jharkhand, Uttar Pradesh and Rajasthan, despite the varying current utilisation status, needs urgent attention to improve the utilisation of services (Table 10.6).

Table 10.5 Utilisation of Any ICDS for Breastfeeding Mothers by Social Groups

Caste groups	Time periods	Bihar	Chhattisgarh	Jharkhand	Madhya Pradesh	Odisha	Rajasthan	Uttar Pradesh	Uttarakhand	All India
Scheduled Caste (SC)	2019–21	51.1	81.7	74.1	83.7	93.4	53.3	67.6	78.0	70.5
	2015–16	42.7	87.4	62.4	67.8	87.1	39.8	38.2	60.1	59.1
	% change	8.4	-5.7	11.7	15.9	6.3	13.5	29.4	17.9	11.4
Scheduled Tribe (ST)	2019–21	45.1	87.8	79.6	86.6	95.9	73.1	59.2	90.5	75.4
	2015–16	32.1	88.3	70.9	66.2	86.5	48.8	27.0	67.1	63.8
	% change	13.0	-0.5	8.7	20.4	9.4	24.3	32.2	23.4	11.6
Other Backward Caste (OBC)	2019–21	45.5	83.3	70.9	84.2	94.9	56.3	64.4	87	67.4
	2015–16	35.1	87.2	63.6	67.4	84	37.7	31.4	47.9	52.1
	% change	10.4	-3.9	7.3	16.8	10.9	18.6	33.0	39.1	15.3
Others	2019–21	34.6	63.6	58.2	76.6	88.9	50.4	59.6	84.5	61.6
	2015–16	26.4	62.4	46.2	54.2	77.9	28.4	24.1	55.1	47
	% change	8.2	1.2	12.0	22.4	11.0	22.0	35.5	29.4	14.6

Source: Author's calculation from NFHS data.

Table 10.6 Utilisation of Any ICDS for Breastfeeding/Lactating Mothers by Wealth Quintiles

Wealth Quintiles	Time periods	Bihar	Chhattisgarh	Jharkhand	Madhya Pradesh	Odisha	Rajasthan	Uttar Pradesh	Uttarakhand	All India
Poorest	2019–21	47.2	87.1	76.8	83.3	94.5	63.3	67.1	84.5	68.8
	2015–16	37.5	88.8	67.9	64.9	85.5	38.6	32.9	50.2	55.1
	% change	9.7	-1.7	8.9	18.4	9.0	24.7	34.2	34.3	13.7
Poorer	2019–21	47.6	86.0	74.9	85.9	95.1	59.8	68.6	87.6	69.8
	2015–16	36.8	91.1	70.2	68.6	86.8	43.8	35.5	59.6	60.6
	% change	10.8	-5.1	4.7	17.3	8.3	16.0	33.1	28.0	9.2
Middle	2019–21	44.8	86.6	74.1	85.9	96.6	59.5	67.1	84.0	70.2
	2015–16	31.0	90.7	64.4	71.6	87.7	40.8	34.8	57.9	59.5
	% change	13.8	-4.1	9.7	14.3	8.9	18.7	32.3	26.1	10.7
Richer	2019–21	38.7	83.4	61.6	84.2	92.7	55.7	61.8	87.5	66.4
	2015–16	22.5	85.1	46.3	69.0	79.4	37.4	28.5	57.1	51.8
	% change	16.2	-1.7	15.3	15.2	13.3	18.3	33.3	30.4	14.6
Richest	2019–21	19.9	61.2	35.0	74.9	82.1	45.6	52.0	78.7	56.1
	2015–16	13.9	60.6	24.3	48.4	55.4	27.1	19.5	46.4	35.3
	% change	6.0	0.6	10.7	26.5	26.7	18.5	32.5	32.3	20.8

Source: Author's calculation from NFHS data.

Utilisation of Health Care in Preceding 12 Months of the Survey for Children below the Age Six

The utilisation of ICDS by children below the age six of age for urban areas shows an increasing trend for all EAG states, the highest utilisation being reported from Odisha (85.7%), followed closely by Madhya Pradesh (85.0%) and Chhattisgarh (84.1%). All EAG states show higher utilisation than all India average (56.1%) for 2019–21. Bihar remained lowest among all the EAG states in both periods for utilisation of ICDS by children below six years of age. Uttar Pradesh reported 49.1% points increase in service utilisation for children below six years of age in urban areas, the highest among all EAG states, followed by Rajasthan (40% points) and Jharkhand (36% points). Bihar, Chhattisgarh, Madhya Pradesh, Odisha and Uttarakhand have registered improvement between 15.1 and 24% points during the same period (Figure 10.6).

For rural areas, Chhattisgarh, Odisha and Madhya Pradesh all reported utilisation of ICDS for children below six years of age in rural areas between 82% and 85% for 2019–21. However, both Odisha and Chhattisgarh registered a small decline in service utilisation in 2019–21 compared to 2015–16 along with Uttarakhand. Uttar Pradesh registered 31.1 percentage points increase in service utilisation during the same period highest among all EAG states, followed by Madhya Pradesh and Bihar (14.3 and 12.1 percentage points, respectively). Rajasthan and Jharkhand reported a 6 percentage points increase during the same period. Compared to national average for service utilisation in 2019–21, Uttarakhand, Rajasthan, Jharkhand and Bihar

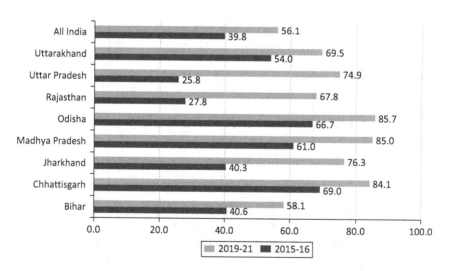

Figure 10.6 Use of Any ICDS Among Children Below Six Years: EAG States and All India – Urban

Source: Author's calculation from NFHS data.

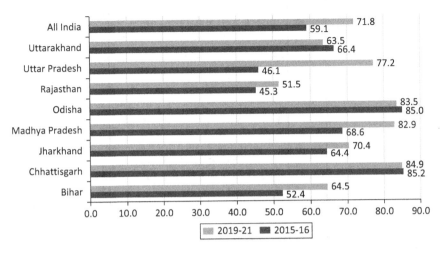

Figure 10.7 Use of Any ICDS Among Children Below Six Years: EAG States and All India – Rural

Source: Author's calculation from NFHS data.

are four EAG states which lag behind in service utilisation for children under age six (Figure 10.7).

By social groups, it is found that children below six years from marginalised sections like SC, ST and OBC improved their service utilisation across EAG states. Odisha clearly stands out among the states where children from all the three vulnerable sections are showing utilisation of some ICDS above 90% followed by Madhya Pradesh and Chhattisgarh (above 80%). Bihar remained lowest in service utilisation among all EAG states for the same in both periods. Both Uttar Pradesh and Rajasthan show 20–29 percentage points improvement in service utilisation for SC, ST and OBC. Despite over 80% utilisation of ICDS, Chhattisgarh reported lowest improvement in service utilisation among SC, ST and OBC children (less than 2 percentage points) among the EAG states (Table 10.7).

By economic status, it is found that children below six years from poorest and poorer households have shown improvement in utilisation of the services. Uttar Pradesh has shown the highest improvement among the poorest and poor households in service utilisation followed by Rajasthan, Uttarakhand and Madhya Pradesh. There is the lowest improvement in service utilisation for Chhattisgarh in all economic strata. Except for Bihar and Rajasthan, all EAG states show service utilisation is higher than national average for respective economic groups. For both periods, Bihar again shows the lowest service utilisation of ICDS for children below age six among all the EAG states (Table 10.8).

Table 10.7 Utilisation of Any ICDS for Children Below Age Six Years by Social Groups

Caste groups	Time periods	Bihar	Chhattisgarh	Jharkhand	Madhya Pradesh	Odisha	Rajasthan	Uttar Pradesh	Uttarakhand	All India
Scheduled Caste (SC)	2019–21	61.2	81.9	73.3	84.1	92.5	62.0	72.3	78.8	70.5
	2015–16	56.9	80.3	61.5	67.9	83.8	42.8	48.6	65.1	59.1
	% change	4.4	1.6	11.8	16.2	8.7	19.3	23.7	13.7	11.4
Scheduled Tribe (ST)	2019–21	60.1	87.5	73.6	87.9	93.5	73.0	63.5	69.9	75.4
	2015–16	47.4	86.4	64.4	69.6	85.9	50.5	34.7	66.8	63.8
	% change	12.7	1.2	9.2	18.3	7.6	22.6	28.8	3.1	11.6
Other Backward Caste (OBC)	2019–21	55.9	82.2	68.5	82.3	93.6	62.1	70.0	78.3	67.4
	2015–16	51.3	81.8	59.4	67.1	82.0	40.9	41.3	59.8	52.1
	% change	4.6	0.4	9.2	15.2	11.6	21.2	28.7	18.5	15.3
Others	2019–21	49.3	65.8	57.7	78.0	87.3	57.4	65.5	75.3	61.6
	2015–16	44.7	62.8	45.4	59.2	74.9	34.0	34.8	62.5	47.0
	% change	4.6	3.0	12.4	18.8	12.4	23.4	30.7	12.8	14.6

Source: Author's calculation from NFHS data.

Table 10.8 Utilisation of Any ICDS for Below Six Years by Wealth Quintiles

Wealth Quintiles	Time periods	Bihar	Chhattisgarh	Jharkhand	Madhya Pradesh	Odisha	Rajasthan	Uttar Pradesh	Uttarakhand	All India
Poorest	2019–21	57.7	86.4	71.5	84.2	93.3	66.4	72.5	76.6	70.0
	2015–16	53.9	85.2	63.8	65.2	85.4	41.6	42.2	58.1	55.1
	% change	**3.8**	**1.2**	**7.7**	**18.9**	**7.8**	**24.8**	**30.2**	**18.5**	**14.9**
Poorer	2019–21	59.0	85.1	71.6	84.7	93.9	65.0	72.7	80.8	72.0
	2015–16	53.2	87.1	64.4	71.0	85.3	46.2	46.7	69.0	60.6
	% change	**5.7**	**–2.0**	**7.2**	**13.7**	**8.7**	**18.8**	**26.0**	**11.8**	**11.4**
Middle	2019–21	58.2	85.2	72.3	84.1	94.1	65.9	71.9	82.3	72.1
	2015–16	46.3	83.2	61.6	71.9	83.4	43.4	45.8	64.5	59.5
	% change	**11.9**	**2.0**	**10.7**	**12.3**	**10.7**	**22.5**	**26.0**	**17.8**	**12.6**
Richer	2019–21	47.4	82.9	63.8	84.1	90.8	61.5	67.3	77.2	66.9
	2015–16	35.8	82.4	42.4	69.9	74.5	42.0	38.8	63.2	51.8
	% change	**11.5**	**0.5**	**21.5**	**14.2**	**16.3**	**19.6**	**28.5**	**14.0**	**15.1**
Richest	2019–21	29.6	62.9	42.9	76.5	78.7	54.2	59.7	69.6	52.9
	2015–16	25.1	59.0	25.8	52.6	53.6	31.4	28.4	55.4	35.3
	% change	**4.5**	**3.9**	**17.2**	**23.8**	**25.2**	**22.7**	**31.3**	**14.2**	**17.6**

Source: Author's calculation from NFHS data.

Financial Assistance Received by Mothers during Childbirth

The data from both rounds show financial assistance received by mothers in urban areas has been around 27% in both periods for all of India. Among EAG states, only Odisha shows some increase by 5.9 percentage points between 2019–21 and 2015–16. All other EAG states show a huge decline in financial assistance extended to mothers for delivery of the child in urban areas, the highest being 14.3% points for Bihar, followed by Chhattisgarh (11.1% points), Uttarakhand and Rajasthan (7.6 and 6.5 percentage points, respectively). Uttar Pradesh and Madhya Pradesh registered a decline of 1.1 and 0.1 percentage points, respectively.

For rural India, there observed a decline in receiving financial assistance. Among EAG states, Chhattisgarh has the highest decline by 17.6% points followed by Uttarakhand (14.1 percentage points), Bihar and Rajasthan (9.7 percentage points each) and Jharkhand (9.4 percentage points). Madhya Pradesh and Uttar Pradesh have registered a decline of 4.7 and 4.5 percentage points, respectively. Odisha has the lowest decline of 0.4 percentage points, but the utilisation remained above 80% in both periods (Figure 10.8).

Except for Chhattisgarh and Madhya Pradesh, all remaining EAG states reported less than 70% for receiving financial assistance towards childbirth, the lowest being Jharkhand at 39.1%. Jharkhand along with Uttarakhand reported less utilisation of financial assistance than the national average among the EAG states for 2019–21 (Figure 10.9).

Across social groups, we found a lesser percent of women received any financial assistance from the state or other sources for childbirth across EAG states except for Odisha and all of India. The highest utilisation for any social groups was found to be highest in Odisha for both time periods. In Odisha, 80% or more women got some financial assistance for childbirth from SC, ST and OBC households in 2019–21. Odisha shows the percent of women

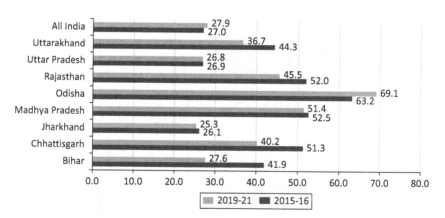

Figure 10.8 Received Any Financial Assistance During Childbirth: EAG States and All India – Urban

Source: Author's calculation from NFHS data

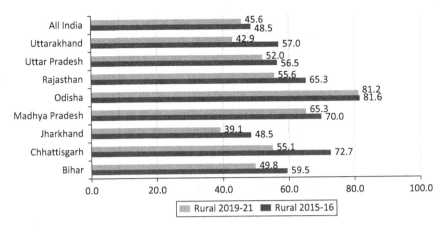

Figure 10.9 Received Any Financial Assistance During Childbirth: EAG States and All India – Rural

Source: Author's calculation from NFHS data.

receiving any financial assistance has even gone up for those women who belong to 'other' households by 10.5 percentage points between the two periods. Jharkhand was found to have the lowest utilisation of any financial assistance for childbirth among all EAG states for any social groups in 2019–21. Jharkhand and Uttarakhand both among EAG states have lower than the national average for receiving any financial assistance by women for childbirth during 2019–21. The decline in receiving assistance for childbirth for SC women (Jharkhand and Uttarakhand), ST and OBC women in Jharkhand is more than 10 percentage points. The causes behind such decline, especially among weaker sections, need deeper investigation (Table 10.9).

Across wealth quintiles, except for Odisha all other EAG states show decline in receiving any financial assistance for childbirth in 2019–21 over 2015–16. Again Odisha registered 80% and above in receiving financial assistance for childbirth for poorest and poorer households among all EAG states. Jharkhand on the other hand reported the lowest number of recipients of any financial assistance during childbirth among all EAG states for any given social groups, and this is below the national average as well. Except for Odisha, 40 to 50% of households among poorer and poorest sections in remaining EAG states not receiving any financial assistance for child delivery raises serious questions on the implementation of such programmes.

Though we look at specific assistance reported by women who got some financial assistance for childbirth, 90% or above received them under Janani Suraksha Yojana (JSY) for all the three background variables, viz. place of residence, social group and household economic status for any given EAG states. So, we are not presenting those figures. It can be concluded the implementation of JSY needs deeper investigation to improve its reach to women, especially those living in rural areas, from marginalised socio-economic groups (Table 10.10).

Table 10.9 Received Any Financial Assistance During Childbirth by Social Groups: EAG States and All India

Caste groups	Time periods	Bihar	Chhattisgarh	Jharkhand	Madhya Pradesh	Odisha	Rajasthan	Uttar Pradesh	Uttarakhand	All India
Scheduled Caste (SC)	2019–21	54.1	51.3	36.8	63.2	82.3	57.5	52.1	44.1	44.4
	2015–16	63.2	65.5	41.5	67.2	77.0	60.3	59.2	56.3	47.3
	% change	*-9.1*	*-14.2*	*-4.7*	*-4.0*	*5.3*	*-2.8*	*-7.1*	*-12.3*	*-2.9*
Scheduled Tribe (ST)	2019–21	43.5	58.2	42.5	68.5	80.8	61.2	55.1	47.7	44.8
	2015–16	50.1	76.1	50.8	65.3	77.8	63.3	53.4	55.3	47.9
	% change	*-6.7*	*-17.9*	*-8.4*	*3.2*	*3.0*	*-2.1*	*1.6*	*-7.6*	*-3.1*
Other Backward Caste (OBC)	2019–21	46.6	50.2	34.3	61.4	79.9	52.2	46.6	35.1	41.2
	2015–16	55.3	64.6	41.3	62.3	72.4	55.1	49.0	43.9	42.6
	% change	*-8.7*	*-14.4*	*-7.0*	*-0.9*	*7.5*	*-2.9*	*-2.4*	*-8.8*	*-1.4*
Others	2019–21	34.9	30.1	29.8	53.3	72.7	44.3	37.6	43.5	31.6
	2015–16	38.4	43.7	26.2	46.4	62.2	48.5	35.4	49.0	30.1
	% change	*-3.5*	*-13.5*	*3.7*	*7.0*	*10.5*	*-4.2*	*2.1*	*-5.5*	*1.5*

Source: Author's calculation from NFHS data.

Table 10.10 Received Any Financial Assistance During Childbirth by Wealth Quintiles: EAG States and All India

Wealth Quintiles	Time periods	Bihar	Chhattisgarh	Jharkhand	Madhya Pradesh	Odisha	Rajasthan	Uttar Pradesh	Uttarakhand	All India
Poorest	2019–21	54.8	58.6	40.6	66.8	80.8	59.5	58.9	54.5	53.6
	2015–16	62.9	77.3	51.0	70.2	77.6	60.9	64.4	56.5	61.5
	% change	*-8.2*	*-18.6*	*-10.4*	*-3.4*	*3.2*	*-1.4*	*-5.5*	*-2.0*	*-7.9*
Poorer	2019–21	49.7	54.1	38.3	69.0	83.3	57.2	54.5	57.5	48.4
	2015–16	54.8	77.2	48.4	68.6	77.7	63.6	60.1	66.7	53.9
	% change	*-5.1*	*-23.1*	*-10.1*	*0.3*	*5.5*	*-6.4*	*-5.6*	*-9.2*	*-5.5*
Middle	2019–21	38.7	53.2	36.4	62.6	82.7	58.2	49.4	46.5	42.0
	2015–16	43.8	69.5	37.7	64.8	75.8	61.0	48.4	62.0	43.0
	% change	*-5.1*	*-16.3*	*-1.4*	*-2.2*	*6.9*	*-2.8*	*1.0*	*-15.6*	*-1.0*
Richer	2019–21	29.6	49.8	27.4	56.3	75.1	50.1	39.1	41.8	34.4
	2015–16	29.9	58.8	25.9	58.1	62.0	55.0	38.2	51.4	32.0
	% change	*-0.2*	*-9.0*	*1.4*	*-1.8*	*13.1*	*-4.9*	*0.9*	*-9.6*	*2.4*
Richest	2019–21	13.2	31.6	14.7	45.1	60.0	44.3	22.5	29.1	23.4
	2015–16	19.1	37.5	11.2	36.3	34.9	39.7	18.1	32.2	19.8
	% change	*-5.9*	*-5.9*	*3.5*	*8.8*	*25.1*	*4.6*	*4.4*	*-3.1*	*3.6*

Source: Author's calculation from NFHS data.

Summary and Policy Prescription

The findings above clearly show there is a lot of scope for improving the functioning of ICDS along with nutrition monitoring in EAG states. Nutritional awareness programmes need to be strengthened through ICT measures to sensitise people about nutritional health of women and children. The recently launched Saksham Anganwadi and POSHAN 2.0, combining several nutritional schemes including ICDS, POSHAN (Prime Minister's Scheme for Holistic Nutrition) Abhiyaan, the Scheme for Adolescent Girls, and the National Crèche Scheme may help to address all three level of factors affecting undernutrition; immediate, household and community level. At the current rate of decline, the commitment to achieve SDG goals looks impossible. Therefore, the implementation of various nutritional schemes and their effective monitoring for course correction needs to be made effective. The adequate grievance redressal mechanism and feedback of the beneficiary mothers and the community through ICT-based technology platforms may go a long way to address shortcomings in the present implementation. The integrated approach is the need of the hour to free India from undernutrition when we are observing the 75 years of independence as 'Azadi ka Amrit Mahotasav'. Over the years, it is observed that the issue of undernutrition is hardly raised in public discourses, especially during electoral exercises. The discourse on nutritional health needs to be included in such public discourses. At the same time, the focus should be on improving awareness and widening the coverage of public programmes related to hygiene, safe drinking water, and use of toilets and safe disposal of human waste at the household level to reduce the morbidity burden. Programmes like Millet Mission can help poorer and other households to get alternative sources of calories and protein other than rice and wheat which are also rich in various micronutrients. At present, we have hardly any large-scale data on the nutritional health of children between 6 and 14 years and of the elderly population which may be suppressing the larger picture about the nutritional scenario prevailing in the country. These two population groups must be included in future surveys like NFHS to help policymakers to devise better targeted programmes and schemes.

References

Ahmad, M. M., & Akhtar, S. N. (2021). medRxiv. Inequalities and policy gaps in maternal health among Empowered Action Group (EAG) States in India: Evidence from Demographic Health Survey. medRxiv 2021.01.15.21249872. https://doi .org/10.1101/2021.01.15.21249872

Arokiasamy, P., & Gautam, A. (2008 Mar). Neonatal mortality in the empowered action group states of India: Trends and determinants. *Journal of Biosocial Science*, 40(2), 183–201. doi: 10.1017/S0021932007002623. Epub 2007 Dec 20. PMID: 18093346.

Bahadur, P. J., Kumar, M., & Singh, M. (2015). Status of maternal nutrition and its association with nutritional status of under-three children in EAG-States and

Assam, India. *International Journal of Humanities and Social Science Invention*, 4(1), 30–38.

Bhatia, M., Dwivedi, L. K., Banerjee, K., Bansal, A., Ranjan, M., & Dixit, P. (2021). Pro-poor policies and improvements in maternal health outcomes in India. Bhatia et al. *BMC Pregnancy and Childbirth*, 21, 389.

Dash, A. (Dec. 2016). Trends and pattern of healthcare outcomes: A study of empowered action group states. *Madhya Pradesh Journal of Social Sciences*, 21(2), 75–105.

International Institute for Population Sciences (IIPS) and ICF (2017). *National Family Health Survey (NFHS-5), India, 2015–16: (Bihar, Chhattisgarh, Jharkhand, Madhya Pradesh, Odisha, Rajasthan, Uttar Pradesh, Uttarakhand and All India Reports)*. Mumbai: IIPS.

International Institute for Population Sciences (IIPS) and ICF (2021). *National Family Health Survey (NFHS-5), India, 2019–21: (Bihar, Chhattisgarh, Jharkhand, Madhya Pradesh, Odisha, Rajasthan, Uttar Pradesh, Uttarakhand and All India Reports)*. Mumbai: IIPS.

Joe William, A., Kumar, R., Rajpal, S., & Subramanian, S. V. (2020). In India: Epidemic growth and impact on maternal and child health. Chapter 4 in *Fighting: Assessments and Reflections* (pp. 34–44). New Delhi: Institute of Economic Growth (IEG).

Jose, S., Gulati, A., & Kurana, K. (2020). Achieving Nutritional Security in India: Vision 2030. NABARD Research Study-9. NABARD and ICRIER. ISBN 978-81-937769-4-0

Kapur, A., Shukla, R., & Pandey, S. (2021). Integrated child development services (ICDS) GoI, 2021–22. *Budget Briefs*, 13(3), 1–12. Available at https://accountabilityindia.in/wp-content/uploads/2021/01/ICDS_2021_22.pdf

Kumar, R., & Lakhtakia, S. (2021). Women's Empowrment and Child Stunting in India. *Journal of Population and Social Studies*, 29, 47–66. http://doi.org/10.25133/JPSSv292021.004

Kumar, R., & Paswan, B. (2021). Changes in socio-economic inequality in nutritional status among children in EAG states, India. *Public Health Nutrition*, 24(6), 1304–1317. doi:10.1017/S1368980021000343

Kumar, R. R., Kumar, S., Sekher, M., Pritchard, B., & Rammohan, A. (2014). A life-cycle approach to food and nutrition security in India. *Public Health Nutrition*, 1–6. doi: 10.1017/S1368980014001037. https://www.researchgate.net/publication/262681004_A_life-_cycle_approach_to_food_and_nutrition_security_in_India/citations#fullTextFileContent

Kumar, S., Sahu, D., Mehto, A., & Kumar Sharma, R. (2020). *Health inequalities in under-five mortality: An assessment of empowered action group (EAG) states of India. Journal of Helath Economics and Outcomes Research (JHEOR)*, 7(2), 189–196. doi:10.36469/jheor.2020.18224

Kumar, V., & Singh, P. (2016). Access to healthcare among the Empowered Action Group (EAG) states of India: Current status and impeding factors. *The National Medical Journal of India (Natl Med J India)*, 29, 267–273.

Mahapatro, S., (2022). Towards Newborn Survival; Challenges and Priorities. Palgrave Macmillan, Singapore. ISBN 978-981-19-3416-2. Pages xi+158.

Margubur, R., Hossain, B., Kundu, S., & Ajmer, S. (2021). Duration of father out-migration and its impact on nutritional status of left-behind children: A cross-sectional study in rural EAG states in India. *Indian Journal of Public Health*

Research & Development, 12(3), 389–395. https://doi.org/10.37506/ijphrd.v12i3 .16090

Ministry of Health and Family Welfare (MoHFW), Government of India, UNICEF, & Population Council. (2019). *Comprehensive National Nutrition Survey (CNNS) National Report*. New Delhi.

Mishra, R. N. (2020). Implications of COVID-19 on India's fight to eliminate undernutrition. https://practiceconnect.azimpremjiuniversity.edu.in/implications -of-covid-19-on-indias-fight-to-eliminate-undernutrition/

Mishra, U.S. (2016). Measuring Progress Towards MDGs in Child Health: Should Base Level Sensitivity and Inequality Matter?. *Evaluation and Programme Planning*, *58*, 70–81.

Mishra, S., Pandey, C. M., Chaubey, Y. P., & Singh, U. (2015). Determinants of Child Malnutrition in Empowered Action Group (EAG) States of India. *Statistics and Applications* {ISSN 2454-7395(online)}, *13*(1&2) 2015 (New Series), 1–9.

NITI Ayog. Health Index Round IV. (2019–20). *Healthy States Progressive India; Report On The Ranks Of States And Union Territories*. https://www.ssca.org.in/ media/1._Determinants_of_Child_Malnutrition_tQ0smd0.pdf

Oxford Poverty and Human Development Initiative (2019). Global Multidimensional Poverty Index 2019; Illuminating Inequalities. https://ophi.org.uk/wp-content/ uploads/G-MPI_Report_2019_PDF.pdf

Oxford Poverty and Human Development Initiative (2021). Global Multidimensional Poverty Index 2021; Unmasking disparities by ethnicity, caste and gender. https:// ophi.org.uk/wp-content/uploads/UNDP_OPHI_GMPI_2021_Report_Unmasking .pdf

Panda, M., Abhishek, K., & William, J. (2021). *Growth Matters; Revisiting the Enigma of Child Undernutrition in India*. IEG working paper no. 418. Institute for Economic Growth, New Delhi.

Prachi, S. (2022). Health check. Despite increased spending, health outcomes remain poor in backward states. https://www.health-check.in/health-finance-governance /despite-increased-spending-health-outcomes-remain-poor-in-backward-states -818519

Rajpal, S., William, J., Rockli, K., Alok, K., & Subramanian, V. (2020a). Child Undernutrition and Convergence of Multisectoral Interventions in India; An Econometric Analysis of National Family Health Survey – 2015-16. *Frontiers in Public Helath*, *8*, 1–10. doi: 10.3389/fpubh.2020.00129

Rajpal, S., Rockli, K., Ranjan, S., Alok, K., William, J., & Subramanian, V. (2020b). Frequently Asked Questions on Child Anthropometric Failures in India. *Economic and Political Weekly*, *LV*(6), 59–64.

Rana, M. J., Gautam, A., Goli, S., Uttamacharya, R. T., Nanda, P., Datta, N., & Verma, R. (2019 Apr). Planning of births and maternal, child health, and nutritional outcomes: Recent evidence from India. *Public Health*, *169*, 14–25. doi: 10.1016/j. puhe.2018.11.019. Epub 2019 Feb 14. PMID: 30772525; PMCID: PMC6483972.

Ramesh, B. M., Dehury, B., Isac, S., Gothalwal, V., Prakash, R., Namasivayam, V., Halli, S., Blanchard, J., & Boerma, T. (2020 Jun). The contribution of district prioritization on maternal and newborn health interventions coverage in rural India. *Journal of Gobal Health* , *10*(1), 010418. doi: 10.7189/jogh.10.010418. PMID: 32373334; PMCID: PMC7182352.

Roy, M. P. (2021). Infant mortality in empowered action group states in India: An analysis of socio-demographic factors. *Journal of Dr. NTR University of Health*

Sciences, 10(6), 21–26. Available at https://www.jdrntruhs.org/text.asp?2021/10 /1/21/316325

Saroj, K., Abhishek, K., Rakesh, K., & William, J. (2021). Social Demographics and Health Achievements An Ecological Analysis of Institutional Delivery and Immunization Coverage in India. IEG working paper no. 427. Institute for Economic Growth, New Delhi.

Smita, S. R., Shiau-Yun, L., & William, J. (2020). Why market orientation matters for agriculture and fishery workers? Unravelling the association between households' occupational background and caloric deprivation in India. *BMC Public Health, 21*(681), 1–13. https://doi.org/10.1186/s12889-021-10644-9

United Nations Children's Fund (UNICEF). (2020). *Nutrition, for Every Child: UNICEF Nutrition Strategy 2020–2030.* New York: UNICEF.

11 Implication of Household Food Security on Child Health

Evidence from Rural Jharkhand

Neha Shri

Introduction

Poverty, food insecurity, and malnutrition are prevalent problems in India. Nationally, thirty-six per cent of children under the age five are stunted (short for their age); 19 per cent are wasted (thin for their height); 32 per cent are underweight (thin for their age) (NFHS-5, 2019-21). There is substantial regional variation in poverty, food insecurity, and malnutrition in the country, and the proportion is substantial in the EAG states. Jharkhand one among the EAG states of India has very high levels of underweight (39%) and wasting (22%) among children aged 0–59 months. The estimated prevalence of stunting in Jharkhand is forty per cent among children under age 5 as compared to the national estimate of thirty-six percent. Jharkhand lies in fourth place in the overall prevalence of stunting in children under age five with the prevalence forty percent (NFHS-5). Jharkhand has made enormous progress in terms of the coverage of its population under National Food Security Act (NFSA) and covers around 87% of its rural population under the state food security act passed in 2015 (state's economic survey 2015–16).

Food security "exists when all people, at all times, have physical and economic access to sufficient, safe and nutritious food to meet their dietary needs and food preferences for an active and healthy life" (FAO, 2012). The three components of food security are availability (having sufficient quantities of appropriate food), accessibility (having adequate income or other resources to access food), and utilization/consumption (having adequate dietary intake and the ability to absorb and use nutrients in the body). India is one of the few countries which have experimented with a broad spectrum of programmes for improving food security. It has already made substantial progress in terms of overcoming transient food insecurity by giving priority to self-sufficiency in food grains and through procurement and public distribution of food grains (i.e. public distribution system), employment programmes, etc. However, despite a significant reduction in the incidence of poverty, chronic food insecurity persists in a large proportion of India's population.

In many studies, the socioeconomic status of the household is identified as a primary risk factor for food insecurity (Abalo, 2009; Dubowitz et al., 2007; Saha et al., 2008). Household food insecurity has been associated with

DOI: 10.4324/9781003430636-15

decreased household food supply, especially of pulses, milk, fruits, and vegetables. Also, food insecurity has been negatively associated with women's food intake (Matheson et al, 2002). Nutrition deficiencies during pregnancy and lactation can contribute to inappropriate growth attainment such as stunting and underweight among young children (Abalo, 2009; Coleman-jensen, 2013). Food insecurity may lead to insufficient dietary intake that can lead to nutrition deficiencies among children (Chaturvedi et al., 2018; Cook et al., 2004; Rahman, 2016).

Malnutrition is the most serious consequence of food insecurity. Adult malnutrition results in lower productivity on farms and in the labour market (Austin et al., 2011). In women, it also results in foetal malnutrition and low birthweights of babies (Ramakrishnan, 2004). Childhood nutritional deficiencies are responsible, in part, for poor school enrolment, absenteeism, early dropout, and poor classroom performance, with consequent losses in productivity during adulthood (Aldernan et al., 2006; Liu & Raine, 2006; Leiva Plaza et al., 2001).

Jharkhand with unacceptable levels of undernutrition, higher the national average, is one of the most vulnerable and high burden states in India. Out of 24 districts in Jharkhand, six districts figure among "200 worst Child Nutritional Districts". As per the India State Hunger Index (ISHI 2008), Jharkhand stands the 16th rank in the state hunger index ranking (second last in the studied 17 states). In context of the food security and child malnutrition scenario, this paper describes the level of household food security in some rural villages of Jharkhand in Bokaro district. It identifies the correlates the household food security and explores the association between food insecurity and malnutrition among children aged 5–9.

Data and Method

To address the objectives, an exploratory study was conducted in selected rural villages of Chandankiyari, Bokaro district of Jharkhand. The villages are selected purposively based on the objectives of the study, and households have been selected using convenience sampling. Since a majority of this area is dominated by tribal population, two villages each with tribal and non-tribal population were selected randomly for the study after listing out all villages in the district. Study areas were villages such as Chamrabad, Karkatta, Sudamdih, and Sabra. These zones are particularly vulnerable from a food and nutritional point of view due to its low level of soil fertility, monsoon dependence for irrigation, and poverty. A cross-sectional domestic survey, including questionnaire and anthropometric measurements, was carried out at household level in order to access the nutritional status, diet diversity, and food security prevailing in the area. The children between 5- and 9-year age group from sampled households were also targeted in order to access the prevalence of malnutrition. The sample size of the study is limited to 85 rural households from different villages of Bokaro district of Jharkhand.

The questions in the survey were asked only to person responsible for food preparation (responsible women in the house).

Based on the questions of household food security, the HDDS indicator was computed. Household food insecurity access was measured using items from the validated Household Food Security (HFS) that was specifically developed for use in developing countries (Frongillo & Nanama, 2006; Knueppel, Demment, & Kaiser, 2009; Maxwell et al., 2003). The HFS consists of nine items specific to an experience of food insecurity occurring within the last month. Each respondent indicated whether they had encountered the following at household level due to lack of food or money to buy food in the last one month: (1) worried about running out of food, (2) lack of preferred food, (3) the respondent or another adult had limited access to a variety of foods due to a lack of resources, (4) forced to eat un preferred food due to lack of resources, (5) eating smaller portions, (6) skipping meals, (7) the household ran out of food, (8) going to sleep hungry, and (9) going 24 hours without food. Endorsed items are then clarified with reported estimates of the frequency of food insecurity (rarely, sometimes, and often). Scores range from 0 to 27 where higher scores reflect more severe food insecurity and lower scores represent less food insecurity.

To determine the status of food insecurity the average Household Food Insecurity Access Scale (HFIAS) score was computed and prevalence of household food insecurity access was calculated (categorized as food secure household, mild food security, moderately food insecurity and severely food insecure) (Castell et al., 2015; Knueppel et al., 2009). Three questions on a household's inability to eat preferred food, inability to eat a variety of food, and inability to eat the food of choice captures the domain of insufficient quality of food. The domain of perception that food is of insufficient quantity is captured by asking whether the respondents had to eat smaller meals or whether they had to eat fewer meals. Three questions on whether the respondents had no food to eat, had to sleep without food, and had to go day and night without food captures the domain of reduction in food intake.

Thus, the HFS indicator categorizes households into four levels of food security: food security, marginal food security, low food security, and very low food security based on the response of the household in nine questions and combining them with specified methods as suggested by the FANTA (Riely et al., 1999). The categorization scheme is designed to ensure that a household's responses can place them in a single, unique category. Households that experience no food insecurity, but rarely experience some anxiety over sufficiency of food are categorized as food secure. Households that worry about not having enough food frequently as well as households that sometimes in last one month could not have their preferred food or have to eat to eat limited variety of food, or food that they really do not want to eat are categorized as mildly food insecure. Households that frequently have to eat food of limited choice and sometimes have to eat lesser quantity of food are categorized as moderately food insecure. Those households that have no food to eat or have to starve day and night are categorized as very low food secure.

For all the questions on food security, a reference period of 12 months prior to survey was used. In order to calculate diet diversity, the reference period used is of last 24 hours, and to calculate the food consumption score, the reference period was of 7 days. The basic measurements taken from children include age, sex, weight, and heights, which are then, compared to the sex-specific National Centre for Health Statistics (NCHS) and WHO guided international reference population as a way to assess the level of under-nutrition. The z-score cut-off point of >+2 SD is used to classify under-nutrition among children. The Standard of Living Index (SLI) was calculated by considering the assets and amenities in the household in order to measure the standard of living as the income may or may not be a reliable indicator because the respondents are daily wage workers and farmers.

Results

The characteristics of surveyed villages are presented in Table 11.1. The majority of the respondents are from age group 36–50, and the next majority group of respondents is from 25- to 36-year age group (Table 11.2). The mean age of the respondents surveyed is 42.10 years. According to the study requirements, the villages were selected with two different ethnicity compositions, i.e. tribal and non-tribal to understand the differentials among tribals and non-tribals. Among the sampled households, 48.24% of the total household surveyed was tribal and 51.76% of households belong to non-tribal community. Around 61.18% of the sample are small or marginal farmers and have less than 2ha of land, and only 3.53% of people are medium and large farmers who have more than two hectares of land. The average land holding size is 0.58 hectares. Around 51.76% of the total population is engaged in agriculture on own land (seasonally) as well as labour in other months.

Table 11.1 Overview of Surveyed Villages

Villages	Chamrabad	Karkatta	Sabra	Sudamdih
Total households	90	100	150	80
Major crop	Rice	Rice	Rice	Rice
Primary occupation	Farmer	Wage worker	Farmer	Farmer
Type of community	Tribal	Non-tribal	Non-tribal	Tribal
Distribution of sample size (HH)	22	21	22	20
Average household size	5.90	5.04	5.72	6.15
Most common source of food	Agriculture	Market	Agriculture	Agriculture
Total no. of eligible children	12	15	17	11

Table 11.2 Demographic Characteristics of Samples

Background characteristics	Frequency	Per cent
Age		
18–25	7	8.24
25–36	29	34.12
36–50	32	37.65
50+	17	20.00
Education		
Illiterate	44	51.76
Upto primary	26	30.59
Higher secondary	12	14.12
Graduate and above	3	3.53
Ethnic group		
Tribal	41	48.24
Non-tribal	44	51.76
Employment		
Agriculture labour	7	8.24
Other labour + self agri.	44	51.76
Self-employed in agriculture	19	22.35
Others	15	17.65
Land holding size		
Landless	30	35.29
Small/marginal (<2ha)	52	61.18
Medium (2–5 Ha)	2	2.35
Large (>5ha)	1	1.18
SLI		
Low SLI	39	45.88
Medium SLI	46	54.12
Household Size		
0–5	52	61.18
5–10	30	35.29
Above 10	3	3.53
PDS availing		
Availing	57	67.06
Not availing	28	32.94
Total	85	100

Only 17.65% of the population is engaged in other types of services and different types of public and government jobs. Out of them 22.35% are engaged only in agriculture. This suggests that they are dependent mainly on agriculture for their income, whereas 8.24% of them are agricultural labour. The majority of the tribal population comes under households having low SLI, i.e. 69.23% of the tribal population have low SLI and only 32.61% of the tribal community have medium SLI, whereas in the non-tribal community people have high standards of living as compared to the tribal population. Around 30.77% of the non-tribal population come under low SLI and the majority of them 67.39% people have medium SLI. The majority of them were having family size <5 people (61.18%) in the household and family size

above 10 were only 3.53%. The average family size is 5.70. Around 67.06% of people are being benefitted from the PDS.

Table 11.3 describes the different dimensions of nutritional security. The three important dimensions of nutritional security are food security, household dietary diversity score, and food consumption score. The three components of food security are child food security, adult food security, and total food security. A positive relationship is observed between household diet diversity and nutritional security. Similarly, a positive relationship occurs between the food consumption score and food security. If a household is adult food security, then it is compulsory that it would be child food security also, but its converse is not true.

Overall, 78.82% of households lie in the very low food security category, 5.88% in high food security, 4.71% in marginal food security, and 10.59% in low food security category. A positive relationship can be observed between the education level and the total food security at the table. As the education level increases, the household is more likely to be

Table 11.3 Household Food Security by Background Characteristics

Background characteristics	Household food security			
	High food security	*Marginal food security*	*Low food security*	*Very low food security*
Education				
Illiterate	2.27	4.55	13.64	79.55
Upto primary	0	0	3.85	96.15
higher secondary	16.67	16.67	16.67	50
graduate and above	66.67	0	0	33.33
Ethnicity				
Tribal	11.90	9.52	14.28	64.28
Non-tribal	0	0	6.97	93.02
Household size				
2–5	3.85	3.85	11.54	80.77
6–10	10.00	6.67	6.67	76.67
Above 10	0.00	0.00	33.33	66.67
Land Holding				
Landless	3.33	0	10	86.67
Small/marginal	5.77	7.69	11.54	75
PDS				
PDS availability	17.86	10.71	7.14	64.29
Non-PDS availability	0	1.75	12.28	85.96
SLI				
Low SLI	5.13	0	12.82	82.05
Medium SLI	6.52	8.7	8.7	76.09
No. of meals				
2	0	0	3.45	96.55
3	8.93	7.14	14.29	69.64
Total	5.88	4.71	10.59	78.82

food secure. Households whose head is illiterate have very low level of food security, i.e. 79.55%. Households whose head received education up to graduation is highly food secure and constitute 66.67% of them. Very low level of food security has been observed in households that are either illiterate or that have received education to primary level. 96.15% of households who have very low level of food security have received education up to primary.

Although the majority of the population comes under the category of very low food security, it is dominated by the non-tribal population. The tribal community is found to be more food secure as compared to the non-tribal community. Around 20% of the tribal community is found to have either high and marginal food security or only 64.28% is under very low food security category. Households with less than five people are found to be more food secure as compared to households with more than five members in the family. Households with more than 10 family members are found to have very low food security. 66.67% of the households with more than 10 members in the family fall in the very low food security category and 33.33% of them are in low food security category. As the PDS is facilitated to the people of low-income level as identified by the government, 17.86% of the households who are not availing of the PDS were highly food secure. Around 85.96% of households that benefit from the PDS scheme have very low levels of total food security. Only 1.75% of households who are availing of PDS have marginal food security. Since, under PDS, households receive mostly grains and not other green vegetables and other varieties of products, this results in PDS secure households having a lower level of food security.

Only 5.88% of households were found to have high food security and 78.82% of them had very low levels of food security. The households that have no land at all are having very low level of food security, whereas the households that have at least some portion of land on which they cultivate are found to be more food secure. This suggests that land is a major livelihood support in the surveyed households. Around 86.67% of households that are landless have very low level of food security. Table 11.3 reveals that 6.52% of households from medium SLI category have high total food security. The household belonging to low SLI was found to have low levels of food security. 76.09% of households that have very low food security belong to the medium SLI category, whereas 82.05% of households are such that they have low SLIs as well very low level of food security. Since households with low SLI have financial hardships, this might restrict them from having a variety of food and impact their eating habits, thus resulting in low level of food security. Although the point worth giving attention is that there are 5.13% of households that are highly food secure despite having low SLI.

Thus, we can interpret that SLI surely has an impact on the total food security of the households. High SLI can lead to higher levels of food security but the converse may or may not be true as seen from Table 11.3.

Table 11.4 shows the per cent of total households lying in different categories of food consumption. The household has been classified according to a predefined set of rules adopted by USAID. Around 14.11% of the total household have poor food consumption scores. Majority of the population lie in "borderline", and they constitute around 77.65% of the total samples surveyed. Only 8.24% of them are at acceptable positions. As evident form the table, households that have dietary diversity index of 6 or more are classified as "high/good dietary diversity". The households with scores lying between 4.5 and 6 are categorized as "medium dietary diversity" and the households having scores less than 4.5 are treated as low dietary diversity. Around 90.59% of households have low dietary diversity and only 7.06% of them have medium dietary diversity. Out of the total samples, only 2.35% have high or good dietary diversity.

Measures of dietary diversity like HDDS have been shown to be associated with nutritional status of children (Table 11.5). However, dietary diversity also tends to increase with income and wealth. This is because the association between dietary diversity and child nutritional status may be confounded by socio-economic conditions. Maximum of the children who have low dietary diversity are stunted (58.82%) and the children who

Table 11.4 Food Consumption Score and Household Dietary Diversity Among Sampled Households

	Freq.	*Percent*
Food consumption score		
Poor	12	14.12
Borderline	66	77.65
Acceptable	7	8.24
Household dietary diversity		
Low dietary diversity	77	90.59
Medium dietary diversity	6	7.06
High dietary diversity	2	2.35
Total	85	100

Table 11.5 Household Dietary Diversity by Different Forms of Malnutrition

	Dietary diversity			
Nutritional status	*Low*	*Medium*	*High*	*Total*
Stunted	58.82	35.29	5.88	100
Not stunted	71.05	23.68	5.26	100
Wasted	68.00	28.00	4.00	100
Not wasted	66.67	26.67	6.67	100
Underweight	58.82	35.29	5.88	10
Not underweight	80.95	14.29	4.76	100

have high dietary diversity are less likely to have stunting, wasting and underweight. This shows a positive association between dietary diversity and prevalence of malnutrition. As the diet becomes more diverse the level of malnutrition decreases. Here, the data show that maximum of the children who do not have any indication of malnutrition are having high and medium diet diversity. Around 68% of the children who are wasted have low dietary diversity.

Figure 11.1 shows different levels of food security as experienced by the children of the households. Majority of the children were measured to have very low food security, and it comprises 55.29% of the total sample. Very few children come under the category of high food security, i.e. 30.59% only and around 14.12% of children come under the category of low food security.

Children from tribal communities are found to be more food secure than children from non-tribal communities. Around half (42.85%) of the children from tribal communities are found to be highly food secure as compared to non-tribal communities (18.6%). Moreover, 45.24% of tribal children fall in the category of very low food secure, whereas 65.12% of children from tribal communities were in the same category.

This may be dependent on various other factors relating to diet diversity, income, and employment level of the household. The prime area of concern is child food security because it is the most important factor of child malnutrition. An interesting thing comes into the picture that children from tribal communities are more food secure as compared to children from non-tribal communities. Dependence on agriculture can be the prime factor for high level of security among children of tribal communities which shows that people from agricultural backgrounds are more food secure.

Figure 11.2 shows the prevalence of different levels of adult food security that is classified as high, marginal, low, and very low food security. Most of

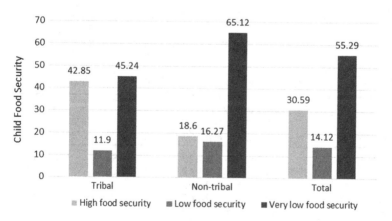

Figure 11.1 Prevalence of Child Food Security by Ethnic Group

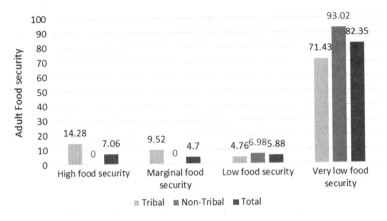

Figure 11.2 Prevalence of Adult Food Security by Ethnic Group

the adult population falls in the category of very low food security. Around 82.35% of the adult are in very low level of food security. A quite alarming situation is seen here that is a very few proportions of total sample; i.e., only 11.76% come under high and marginal food security. A greater portion of very low food secure households is from non-tribal populations. The figure clearly shows that non-tribal households are either very low food security or low food security.

Figure 11.3 shows the prevalence of household food security by ethnic group. As evident from the graph, the majority of the population comes under the category of very low food security and it is dominated by the non-tribal population. Around 78.82% of the household come in very low food security category, 5.88% are in high food security, 4.71% in marginal food secure, and 10.59% in low food security category. The same pattern has also been observed here that the tribal community is found to be more food secure

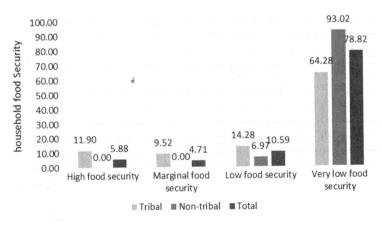

Figure 11.3 Prevalence of Household Food Security by Ethnic Group

as compared to the non-tribal community. Around 20% of the tribal community is found to be either high or marginal food security or only 64.28% if under very low food security category.

Discussion

With more than one-third of the world's undernourished children, India's relatively poor progress in reducing malnutrition is an issue of both national and global concern. Accelerating progress on this front will require a range of nutrition-specific and nutrition-sensitive interventions, including agricultural interventions. The above study reveals that there is a need of attention in nutrition and diet diversity which in turn is dependent on agricultural production. This study furthers our understanding of household food insecurity and child health by considering association between different levels of household food insecurity with health status for a sample of children aged 5–9. Although the economy is mainly agriculture, there is no diversity in the diet. Their diet mainly includes staples such as rice and potato. Their food rarely includes green vegetables and protein-rich foods. So, there is a need of diversification of diet. A large proportion of households are found to be food insecure. So, in order to improve nutrition security, the food security of households needs to improve.

A positive relationship can be observed between the education level and the total food security. Very low level of food security has been observed in households with low levels of education specifically those who are either illiterate or who have received education up to primary. Furthermore, with limited dietary knowledge and power within the households, it is unlikely that women can ensure that their children consumed an adequate diet. The households who have no land at all have very low levels of food security, whereas households who have at least some portion of land on which they cultivate are found to be more food secure. Similar findings were observed in a survey in the Amravati district (Bhagat et al, 2010). Tribal households are more found to be food secure in comparison with non-tribal households. The possible reason behind this can be tribal people's dependency on forest products and their own agricultural products which often includes leafy vegetables which is nutritious in nature thus improving the nutritional status. Jharkhand having low land size and high dependence on agriculture has an urgent need to examine cropping patterns and productivity of land.

It is also found that households belonging to low SLI have low levels of food security. Although the point worth giving attention to is that there are 5.13% of households with low SLI that are highly food secure. High SLI can lead to higher levels of food security but the converse may or may not be true as evident from the study.

Both biological, socio-cultural factors may explain the stronger effects of food insecurity on child health at younger ages. Socio-culturally, younger children's greater dependency on adult household members for food and time spent in the household may increase their vulnerability to the effects of household food insecurity experiences as young children in ages beyond to be breastfed are dependent on their caregivers for nutritionally adequate food (Dewey and Brown 2003). In the sampled households, nutrient-rich foods such as meat, fruits, and vegetables are costlier and thus less consumed than potato and rice, the dietary staples.

A maximum of the children who have low dietary diversity are stunted (58.82%) and the children who have high dietary diversity are less likely to have stunting, wasting, and underweight. This shows a positive association between dietary diversity and prevalence of malnutrition. A maximum of the children who do not have any indicators of malnutrition are having high and medium diet diversity. A negative relationship has been observed in food insecurity levels and nutritional status of children. These findings are consistent with studies in Nepal and Bangladesh (Osei et al., 2010; Saha et al., 2008).

Several limitations need to be considered. First, the data is cross-sectional in nature and is based on a very small geographical location i.e. households with children in Chandankiyari, Bokaro, Jharkhand. Second, seasonal food pattern may also affect the household food insecurity levels. Moreover, the findings are only assumed to be associational and applicable to households in the selected area. Furthermore, these findings can't be generalized unless the study is replicated to other areas.

Conclusion

To conclude, socio-cultural and biological factors may increase the vulnerability to the effects of household food insecurity experiences. The study reveals that tribal households are less food insecure than non-tribal households. Furthermore, limited dietary knowledge and power within the households impacts negatively the consumption of an adequate diet. Households with a maximum of children who do not have any indications of malnutrition are having high and medium diet diversity. A negative relationship has been observed between food insecurity levels and nutritional status of children. Low land size and high dependence on agriculture have an impact on the nutritional status of children and other household members. Thus, there is an urgent need to examine cropping patterns and productivity of the land.

References

Abalo, K. (2009). *Poverty and the Anthropometric Status of Children: A Comparative Analysis of Rural and Urban Households in Togo.* AERC Research Paper 191. African Economic Research Consortium, Nairobi, November 2009. ISBN 9966-778-47-0

Alderman, H., Hoddinott, J., & Kinsey, B. (2006). Long term consequences of early childhood malnutrition. *Oxford economic papers, 58*(3), 450–474.

Austin, O. C., Nwosu, A. C., & Baharuddin, A. H. (2011). Rising food insecurity: Dimensions in farm households. *American Journal of Agricultural and Biological Science. 6*(3), 403–409.

Bhagat, R. B., Unisa, S., Nagdeve, D. A., & Fulpagare, P. (2010). Food security and health status among tribal and non-tribal populations of Amravati district, Maharashtra. IIPS Working paper Number 1, October 2010).

Castell, S., Rodrigo, P., Cruz, D., & Ngo, J. (2015). Household food insecurity access scale (HFIAS). https://doi.org/10.3305/nh.2015.31.sup3.8775

Chaturvedi, A., Patwari, A. K., Soni, D., Pandey, S., Prost, A., Gope, R. K., ... & Tripathy, P. (2018). Progress of children with severe acute malnutrition in the malnutrition treatment centre rehabilitation program : Evidence from a prospective study in Jharkhand, India. *Nutrition journal, 17*(1), 1–9.

Coleman-jensen, A. McFall, W., & Nord, M. (2013). *Food Insecurity in Households With Children Prevalence, Severity, and Household characteristics, 2010-11*, EIB-113, U.S. Department of Agriculture, Economic Research Service, May 2013 (No. 1476-2017-3892).

Cook, J. T., Frank, D. A., Berkowitz, C., Black, M. M., Casey, P. H., Cutts, D. B., ... & Nord, M. (2004). Food insecurity is associated with adverse health outcomes among human infants and toddlers. *Community and International Nutrition* (December 2003), 1432–1438.

Dewey, K. G., & Brown, K. H. (2003). Update on technical issues concerning complementary feeding of young children in developing countries and implications for intervention programs. *Food and nutrition bulletin, 24*(1), 5–28.

Dubowitz, T., Levinson, D., Peterman, J. N., Verma, G., Jacob, S., & Schultink, W. (2007). Intensifying efforts to reduce child malnutrition in India: An evaluation of the Dular program in Jharkhand, India. Food and nutrition bulletin, 28(3), 266–273. doi:10.1177/156482650702800328

FAO. (2012). *The State of Food Insecurity in the World 2012 Key Messages*. FAO.

Frongillo, E. A., & Nanama, S. (2006). Development and validation of an experience-based measure of household food insecurity within and across seasons in Northern Burkina Faso. The Journal of nutrition, 136(5), 1409S–1419S. https://doi.org/10.1093/jn/136.5.1409S.

Knueppel, D., Demment, M., & Kaiser, L. (2009). Validation of the household food insecurity access scale in rural Tanzania. *13*(3), 360–367. https://doi.org/10.1017/S1368980009991121

Leiva Plaza, B., Inzunza Brito, N., Pérez Torrejón, H., Castro Gloor, V., Jansana Medina, JM, Toro Díaz, T., ... & Ivanovic Marincovich, D. (2001). Some considerations on the impact of malnutrition on brain development, intelligence and school performance. *Latin American Nutrition Archives, 51*(1), 64–71.

Liu, J., & Raine, A. (2006). The effect of childhood malnutrition on externalizing behavior. *Current opinion in pediatrics, 18*(5), 565–570.

Matheson, D. M., Varady, J., Varady, A., & Killen, J. D. (2002). Household food security and nutritional status of Hispanic children in the fifth grade. The American journal of clinical nutrition, 76(1), 210–217. https://doi.org/10.1093/ajcn/76.1.210

Maxwell, D., Watkins, B., Wheeler, R., & Collins, G. (2003). The coping strategies index : A tool for rapidly measuring food security and the impact of food aid programmes in emergencies *Nairobi: CARE Eastern and Central Africa Regional Management Unit and the World Food Programme Vulnerability Assessment and Mapping Unit.*

Menon, P., Deolalikar, A., & Bhaska, A. (2008). *India State Hunger Index. Comparisons of Hunger Across States (PDF)*, International Food Policy Research Institute, Welthungerhilfe, University of California, Riverside. Washington, D.C., Bonn, and Riverside.

NFHS-4. (2015). *National Family Health Survey (NFHS-4) India Report.*

Osei, A., Pandey, P., Spiro, D., Nielson, J., Shrestha, R., Talukder, Z., ... & Haselow, N. (2010). Household food insecurity and nutritional status of children aged 6 to 23 months in Kailali District of Nepal. *Food and nutrition bulletin, 31*(4), 483–494.

Rahman, A. (2016). Universal food security program and nutritional intake : Evidence from the hunger prone KBK districts in Odisha. *Food Policy, 63*, 73–86. https://doi.org/10.1016/j.foodpol.2016.07.003

Ramakrishnan, U. (2004). Nutrition and low birth weight: from research to practice. *1–5*(1), 17–21.

Riely, F., Mock, N., Cogill, B., Bailey, L., & Kenefick, E. (1999). *Food Security Indicators and Framework for Use in the Monitoring and Evaluation of Food Aid Programs. Nutrition Technical Assistance Project (FANTA), Washington, DC*

Saha, K. K., Frongillo, E. A., Alam, D. S., Arifeen, S. E., & Lars, A. (2008). Household food security is associated with infant feeding practices in rural Bangladesh. *The Journal of nutrition, 138*(7), 1383–1390.

Saha, K. K., Frongillo, E. A., Alam, D. S., Arifeen, S. E., Persson, L. Å., & Rasmussen, K. M. (2008). Appropriate infant feeding practices result in better growth of infants and young children in rural Bangladesh. *The American journal of clinical nutrition, 87*(6), 1852–1859.

Part IV

Health Governance, Policies and Programmes

12 Factors Affecting Inequity in Institutional Delivery and Choice of Providers

The Role of Janani Suraksha Yojana and Community Health Workers in Bihar

Kakoli Das and Saswata Ghosh

Introduction

To meet the targets to achieve Universal Health Coverage (UHC) as a part of Sustainable Development Goals (SDGs), various initiatives were implemented at the overall country level to reduce maternal and child mortality (Sumner and Melamed, 2010, Requejo et al., 2012). Unlike other developing countries that account for approximately 86% (254,000) of global maternal deaths (WHO, UNICEF, UNFPA, World Bank Group and the United Nations Population Division, 2019), India has shown marked improvements in its maternal and child health (MCH) outcomes at the national level over the past three decades. However, countries with a substantial decline in maternal and child mortality have experienced widening inequities across states and other socio-demographic parameters (Uthman et al., 2012; UNICEF, 2015). India's maternal mortality ratio (MMR) declined from 556 to 103 deaths per 100,000 live births between 1990 and 2019 implies that the country is on track to achieve targets for SDG (70 maternal deaths per 100,000 live-births) (sample registration system (SRS), 2017–19). Despite the progress (103 fatalities during 2017–19), India continues to be responsible for 12% (35,000 deaths; second-highest estimated deaths after Nigeria) of global maternal deaths (WHO, 2019). The nine socio-economically backward states of India, commonly known as empowered action group (EAG) states, are largely responsible for the country's high rates of maternal and infant mortality. In the EAG states, the average MMR is 145 deaths for every 100,000 live births, while southern and other Indian states show only 59 and 79 deaths for every 100,000 live births, respectively. Moreover, mothers from the EAG states have high (0.4%) lifetime mortality risk than mothers from all other Indian states combined (0.15%) (SRS, 2017–19).

Assessment of reproductive health services, as well as the attainment of the UHC, is critical since the MCH outcomes are the complex result of several factors, including socio-economic aspects, spatial-demographic facets, and government interventions (Joshi et al., 2014 and Yamashita et al., 2014). Several empirical researches stated that about 80% of maternal deaths could be avoided by assuring institutional delivery[1] and providing access to quality care (MoHFW, 2005; WHO, 2019; Gupta et al., 2012). According to Baral

DOI: 10.4324/9781003430636-17

et al. (2010), professional birth assistance could reduce maternal fatalities by 13–33% during the antenatal, delivery, and postnatal periods. Hence, institutional delivery[2] and skilled birth attendants (SBAs) have long been considered instrumental in reducing maternal deaths (Yanagisawa, 2014; Wong et al., 2017).

However, demand-side factors such as social tradition, acceptance, and affliction prevent vulnerable communities from accessing maternal care (Ghosh et al., 2015; Jeffery and Jeffery, 2010), even when they have physical access to such facilities. In India, the less-ubiquity of safe delivery and postpartum care among scheduled caste (SC) and scheduled tribes (ST) indicates an embedded disbelief in availing of such services (Saroha et al., 2008; Hazarika, 2011). In this case, cash incentives to protect households from insolvency and indebtedness caused by high out-of-pocket expenditures (OOPE) and catastrophic health spending (CHS) during delivery can act as a pull factor in ensuring optimum health services are delivered (Mohanty and Kastor, 2017). Irrespective of socio-economic and geographic status, greater access and use of MCH services principally depend on the satisfactory antenatal care (ANC), availability and accessibility of health professionals and facilities, quality of transport networks, educational attainment of care-seekers, household economic status, level of women's autonomy, community-level stimuli, and cultural settings of mothers (Ghosh et al. 2015; MoHFW, 2017; Kersterton et al., 2010; Navaneetham and Dharmalingam, 2002).

In addition to the quantitative determinants of institutional delivery, the sufficiency, cost, quality, and continuum of availability of MCH services are found to be important among underserved populations (Ghosh et al., 2015). Owing to such quality issues, OOPE has been increasing as demand for services shifted from public to private sources (Das et al., 2018; Issac et al., 2016; Sharma and Bothra, 2016). These factors, in turn, have critical implications to achieve equitable progress in achieving UHC (Joe et al., 2018). To bridge the gulf, National Rural Health Mission (NRHM; renamed as National Health Mission (NHM) in 2013) was launched in 2005 in India. It aims to improve health security by giving special thrust to susceptible populations, primarily for socio-economically backward states with low MCH indicators and poor health infrastructure.

Under the umbrella of NRHM, the *Janani Suraksha Yojana (JSY)* programme promotes institutional delivery by providing cash incentives (INR 1400) to mothers and has been implemented since 2005 to reduce maternal and child mortality. It also provides cost compensation for transportation and incentives to community health workers (CHWs) or accredited social health activists (ASHAs) to promote enthusiasm for spreading awareness and encouraging mothers to choose (public) institutions as their preferred place for delivery (IIPS, 2017). Joe et al. (2018) confirm that JSY has substantially improved the equity in MCH services, especially in underdeveloped areas. The CHWs/ASHAs are the backbone of the NHRM and are entrusted with enormous responsibilities pertaining to immunization, antenatal and postnatal care, safe abortion, nutrition, and family planning advice, as well as mobilize the community to better utilize healthcare services.

The majority of studies in applied health science have focused on the factors affecting institutional delivery and how $x_{(s)}$ effects y (Das et al., 2018; Navneetham and Dharmalingam, 2002; Tarekegn et al., 2014). However, institutional delivery services and choice of providers are not just an objective outcome of the popular demand-supply nexus; rather, it incorporates a subjective mapping of culture-induced perceptions, previous experiences, cost-quality trade-offs, etc. Moreover, all these aspects are not mutually exclusive and certainly affect availing in-facility delivery services and choice of providers (Lee et al., 2010). For that, one needs to understand the sequential interdependent links involved with institutional delivery and selection of providers. Studies specifically looking at the impact of JSY interventions and the role of CHWs in selecting providers for institutional care are fewer in numbers (Das et al., 2018; Arokiasamy and Pradhan, 2013; Jat et al., 2011; Singh et al., 2012).

Against this backdrop, the present study is a comprehensive assessment of factors that affect inequity in institutional delivery and choice of providers within the context of achieving equitable and universal access to safe delivery care – with a particular focus on the impact of JSY scheme and role of CHWs towards promoting these goals in Bihar, an underdeveloped state in India. Bihar is one of the most disadvantaged states in India, plagued with low MCH indicators since a long, inadequate health infrastructure, and alarmingly low human development indices. In terms of MCH targets, Bihar has had a dismal track record for the past four decades. According to the 75th round of NSS, the percentage of institutional birth in Bihar reached roughly 84% in rural areas and 94% in urban areas. In rural Bihar, approximately one in five mothers use private facilities, compared to three in five mothers in urban Bihar. It is noteworthy to observe that although there is a relatively small percentage of delivery covered by private facilities in rural areas (14.7%, compared to 69.4% delivery in public facilities), the expense gap between public and private facilities is quite large (1:7). In the state, average out-of-pocket medical expenditure (OOPME) for institutional childbirth cases during a stay at a public hospital is 2,466, while in a private hospital, it is 26,234 (at current price) (GoI, 2020). Therefore, studying Bihar could be useful in this regard since it has been a high-priority state for decades and a number of initiatives have been put in place to improve MCH issues, such as the National Health Mission and the Health and Nutrition Strategy under JEEViKA. Yet, the state has a high rate of maternal mortality: 130 deaths for every 100,000 live births, with a high (0.4%) lifetime risk of maternal deaths (SRS, 2017–19). Besides, only 25.2% of women in the state chose to avail themselves of at-least four antenatal visits, and just more than half of the women (57.3%) received postpartum care according to NFHS-5 (IIPS and ICF 2021).

Methods

Data

The present study mainly uses the unit-level data of the Annual Health Survey during 2012–2013 for the study state [AHS, 2013]. It was carried out annually in 284 districts (as per 2001 Census) in eight EAG states (Bihar, Jharkhand, Uttar Pradesh, Uttarakhand, Madhya Pradesh, Chhattisgarh, Odisha, and Rajasthan) and collected information regarding utilization of MCH services, treatment-seeking for pregnancy/delivery/post-delivery complications, awareness of such complications and knowledge of reproductive tract infections (RTI). To understand the reasons behind the lopsided distribution and inaccessibility in the utilization of safe delivery care, this study considered 62,419 women aged between 15 and 49 years in the study state – Bihar by pooling two rounds of AHS.

In addition to AHS, the study used District Census Handbook (2011) of Bihar to explore supply-side variables like: degree of media exposure, the proportion of villages having self-help groups, doctors per 100,000 populations, degree of availability of healthcare providers, and percentage of villages with all-weather roads (RGI, 2011).

Further, unit-level data collected using Schedule 25 of the 60th and 71st rounds of the National Sample Survey (NSS) were used to examine the effect of JSY on institutional delivery in Bihar. In the 60th round, 4,074 households and 23,851 individuals were covered, while 3,167 households and 17,597 individuals were selected in the 71st round for interview in Bihar through a multi-stage stratified sampling design. The number of women pregnant in the 365 days preceding the survey was 567 and 1,020 in the 60th and 71st rounds, respectively (GoI, 2006; GoI, 2016). Data were analysed using Stata SE 16, and appropriate sampling weights were used to ensure the representativeness of the sample.

It may be noted that although unit level data for various demand-side indicators were available in the fourth round of National Family Health Survey (NFHS, 2015–16) data and/or 75th NSS round (GoI, 2017–18), supply-side and contextual factors (as discussed in the earlier section) were missing in this data set. Despite the fact that the data are a decade or more old, the current study had to use AHS data acquired in 2011–12 because of its congruence with Census 2011. To note, Census, 2011 remains the only source of various supply-side and contextual factors which presumably affect MCH uptake. However, for descriptive analyses, data obtained from the last three rounds of NFHS were used.

Variables

Based on the significance of influencing institutional delivery, several predictor variables were considered for the analysis. The main explanatory variable used in the multivariate model is the place of delivery (categorized as home, public, and private facility). The predictor variables used in this study fall under individual-level, household-level, community-level, and contextual/ supply-side variables. At the individual level, the variables are current age of mother (continuous), birth order of children (single child, two children, three children, and three or more children), educational attainment (not-literate, up to primary, middle school, secondary, and higher secondary and above), work status (not working and working), and degree of media exposure (continuous).

Socio-religious category (Hindu, non-Hindu and SC, ST, and others) and household asset index (Bottom, middle, and higher asset quintiles) were taken as the variables operating at the household level. For binary analysis, caste and religion were merged to form a single categorical variable. In the absence of monthly income or expenditure, the household asset index was created by applying principal component analysis (PCA) from various household and economic characteristics namely – the type of house, toilet facility, main fuel for lighting and cooking, main source of drinking water, use of separate room for cooking and ownership of assets such as a house, agricultural land, irrigated land, livestock, and other durable goods.

Variables regarding the functioning of public health providers, percentage of villages having self-help group[3] (SHG), and media exposure were calculated from census 2011. As a proxy to the community-level exposure, proportion of villages having SHG was considered.

Grassroot-level community health providers including the availability of doctors, paramedics, ASHA, ANM (Auxiliary Nurse Midwife) in the village, and maternity financial assistance (JSY, other than JSY, and not availed any scheme) were included as supply-side variables. The variable 'community health workers' was computed by employing PCA. It comprises the number of in-station personal at primary health centres (PHC) per 1,00,000 population, number of in-station para-medical staff at PHCs per 10,000 population, number of in-station para-medical staff at sub-centres per 10,000 population, percentage of villages with ASHAs, and percentage of villages with Anganwadi centres according to Census, 2011. Further, place of residence (rural/ urban) and percentage of villages having all-weathered roads were also controlled in the regression models as contextual variables. PCA was used to compute degree of media exposure. It is a composite index of several variables such as the proportion of households that has transistor/radio, television, computer with Internet facility and mobile with Internet facility.

Analytical Model

The study uses both descriptive and multivariate models. To understand the respondents' background characteristics, binary statistics were used. The present study applied sequential logit (SL) model (Buis, 2007) while studying the net differentials in utilization and choice of institutional delivery services among mothers after controlling for several socio-demographic factors. The model estimates the effect of the explanatory variables on the probabilities of passing through a set of transitions (Buis, 2007; Das and Ghosh 2020). In the present analysis, the first transition refers to respondents' preference regarding safe delivery (institutional delivery vs. home delivery) and model this choice using a conventional logit model. The second transition focuses exclusively on the choice of providers (public vs. private) in institutional delivery using another conventional logit model (Rodrí guez, 2015). Mathematically, suppose there are J alternatives, which are divided into H sub-choice sets, $A_1, A_2, \ldots, A_H$. The decision-making process of an individual can be divided into two transitions or sequences such that, in Transition 1, an individual chooses one of the H sub-choice sets, or A_h for some h; in Transition 2, an individual chooses alternative $j \in A_h$, i.e.

$$Pr\left(y \in A_k\right) = \frac{exp\left(\dot{X}\delta_h\right)}{\sum_{u=1}^{K} exp\left(\dot{X}\delta_u\right)} \text{ for h = 1,...H} \qquad -(1)$$

$$Pr\left(y = j \mid A_h\right) = \frac{exp\left(\dot{X}\alpha_h\right)}{\sum_{k \in A_h}^{H} exp\left(\dot{X}\alpha_k\right)} \qquad -(2)$$

where, $\delta_h \in \mathbb{R}^k$, $h=1,2, \ldots, H$ and $\alpha_j \in \mathbb{R}^k$, $j=1,2, \ldots, J$

It is possible to identify the model with normalization $\delta_h = 0$ and $\alpha_{jh} = 0$, $\forall A_h$, where j_h is the first element in A_h. This model can be derived in the context of 'utility maximizing behaviour' by specifying the utilities for each choice separately, setting A_h at the first stage and $j \in A_h$ at the second stage. It is worth noting that in the SL model, the test of the property of Independence of Irrelevant Alternatives (IIA) is not required. Estimates of adjusted odds ratios (AOR) have been used in interpretation.

Besides, Oaxaca (1973) decomposition model was used to understand the effects of JSY on institutional delivery outcomes (Oaxaca, 1973). This method considers following linear regression model

$$Y_{ig} = X_{ig}\beta_g + \varepsilon_{ig} \qquad -(3)$$

for $i=1,2,3,\ldots N_g$ and $\sum_g = N$. Blinder (1973) and Oaxaca (1973) propose the following decomposition:

$$\Delta_{OLS} = \bar{y}_A - \bar{y}_B = \bar{X}_A - \bar{X}_B\hat{\beta}_A + \bar{X}_B\hat{\beta}_A - \hat{\beta}_B \qquad -(4)$$

where $\bar{y}_g = N_g^{-1}\sum_{i=1}^{N_g} Y_{ig}$ and $\bar{X}_g = N_g^{-1}\sum_{i=1}^{N_g} X_{ig}$

The first term of the right-hand side of (4) displays the difference in outcome variable between the two groups that is due to differences in observable characteristics, whereas the second term shows the differential that is due to differences in coefficient estimates and is referred to as an estimate of discrimination by Oaxaca (1973).

Since JSY was implemented in all the districts of EAG states and every pregnant woman was eligible for it, neither difference-in-difference (DiD) or propensity score (P-score) matching methods were employed.

Results

Sample Characteristics of Bihar and All Other EAG States

The social and demographic profiles of sampled households are given in Table 12.1. The table shows that respondents to the survey predominantly lived in rural areas (91.1% in Bihar and 83.5% in total EAG states), belonging to poor (40.1% in Bihar and 42.2% in total EAG states), and Hindu upper caste communities (54.2% in Bihar and 50.8% in total EAG states), and have a low level of education. About half of the population in Bihar is illiterate while only about one out of fifteen has completed higher secondary schooling. In comparison with other EAG sates, Bihar has a slightly higher availability of doctors and other community-based healthcare providers. However, this does not hold entirely for other supply-side variables.

Status of Continuum of MCH Care Services in Bihar and Adjacent States

As shown in Figure 12.1, Bihar has lagged behind in nearly all of its important MCH parameters over the past three NFHS rounds. Only after 2005–06, percentages of women opting for institutional delivery increased noticeably in the state (from 19.9% in 2005–06 to 76.2% in 2019–21); while other essential parameter remained stumpy and found to be low in comparison with neighbouring states (IIPS, 2007; IIPS, 2017). As per NFHS 5 (2019–21), Bihar has the lowest (among the published fact sheets) percentage of institutional deliveries, where the percentage of women who received at least four prenatal check-ups is 25.2%, followed by only 57.3% of women receiving postnatal care (IIPS, 2021).

Distribution of Home Births, Institutional Delivery, and Choice of Providers by Respondents Selected Background Characteristics

According to Table 12.2, as expected, respondents belonging to rural, illiterate, non-Hindu, and economically weaker households are more likely to deliver at home. Among those who delivered at any institution, 91% were assisted through JSY. It can be seen that the uptake of institutional delivery from public sources is higher among poor, less educated, not-working women who primarily belong to rural areas. Substantial variations can also be observed among different socio-religious categories. Other than minorities, SCs are the highest in proportions (77%) to opt for public sources for

Table 12.1 Background Characteristics of Currently Married Women (Aged 15–49), AHS 2012–13, Bihar, and EAG States

Background characteristics	EAG states (Total)	Bihar
Women from rural (%)	83.48	91.08
Mean age of respondents (SD[a])	26.40 (6.87)	26.95 (5.60)
Educational attainment of women (%)		
Non literate	41.62	58.78
Up to primary	25.66	21.82
Middle	14.94	7.83
Secondary	7.20	6.02
Higher secondary and above	10.59	5.57
Working status of women at the time of survey (%)		
Working	17.42	11.68
Not working	82.58	88.32
Socio-religious category (%)		
Hindu upper caste	50.83	54.22
Hindu SC	19.26	19.10
Hindu ST	9.53	1.43
Muslims	17.13	18.07
Other minorities	3.24	7.18
Wealth quintiles (%)		
Poorest	23.47	23.63
Poorer	18.73	16.47
Middle	18.16	16.94
Richer	19.75	21.57
Richest	19.89	21.39
% of villages having self-help group (SD) [Range]	60.1(23.8) [5.5, 96.8]	53.1(4.6) [16.3, 60.7]
% of villages having PDS[b] shop (SD) [Range]	55.8 (12.8) [21.07, 82.3]	64.9 (7.8) [49.8, 82.3]
Mean number of doctors per 100,000 population (SD) [Range]	9.5 (9.1) [0, 85.32]	10.1 (6.3) [1.0, 24.1]
% of villages with ASHAs[c](SD) [Range]	78.2 (13.5) [17, 100]	80.9 (14.2) [17, 100]
% of villages with Nutritional Centres – Anganwadi Centre (SD) [Range]	77.6 (13.6) [2, 100]	79.6 (13.3) [41, 98]
% of villages with all-weather roads (SD) [Range]	61.1 (18.5) [0, 98]	59.2 (19.8) [18, 90]

[a]Standard deviation, [b]PDS: public distribution system, [c]ASHA: accredited social health activist
Source: Calculated from unit level data of AHS 2012–13

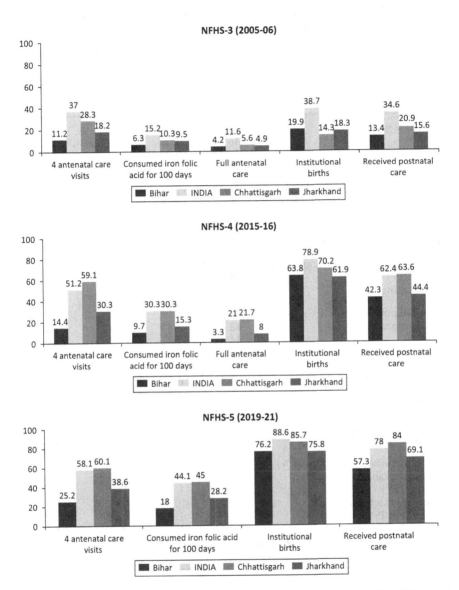

Figure 12.1 Status of Continuum of MCH Care Services (in percent) in Bihar and Adjacent States between NFHS-3 (2005–06) and NFHS-5 (2019–21)

Source: State factsheets, Bihar, and other states, NFHS-3 (2005–06) to NFHS-5 (2019–21)

Note: Mothers received postnatal care from doctor/nurse/LHV/ANM/midwife/other health personnel within 2 days of delivery (%)

Table 12.2 Distribution of Home Delivery, Institutional Delivery, and Type of Providers According to Respondent's Selected Background Characteristics, Bihar, AHS 2012–13

Background characteristics	Home delivery	Institutional delivery	Public facilities	Private facilities
Place of residence (%)				
Rural	46.92	53.08	75.25	24.35
Urban	30.77	69.23	57.10	42.90
Educational attainment of women (%)				
Not literate	48.27	51.73	77.58	22.42
Up to primary	44.32	55.68	72.41	27.59
Middle	39.53	60.47	69.77	30.23
Secondary	39.31	60.69	66.74	33.26
Higher secondary and above	35.61	64.39	55.07	44.93
Working status of women at the time of survey (%)				
Working	45.86	54.14	73.31	26.69
Not working	45.43	54.57	75.38	24.62
Socio-religious category (%)				
Hindu upper caste	43.17	56.83	71.91	28.12
Hindu SC	44.18	55.82	77.00	23.00
Hindu ST	49.09	50.91	67.91	32.09
Muslims	50.34	49.66	73.35	26.65
Other minorities	53.42	16.46	79.45	20.55
Wealth quintiles (%)				
Bottom asset quintiles	56.75	43.25	76.22	23.78
Middle asset quintiles	43.54	56.46	77.08	22.92
Higher asset quintiles	30.69	69.31	67.36	32.64
Maternity financial assistance (%)				
Janani Suraksha Yojana (JSY)	9.01	90.99	89.14	10.86
Other Govt. schemes (Other than JSY)	59.72	40.28	57.05	42.95
Not availed	77.69	22.31	17.90	82.10
Mean out-of-pocket expenditure (INR)			740	1850
% of villages with all-weather roads	66.63	65.1	52.75	64.82

Source: Calculated from unit-level data of AHS 2012–13

delivery care following Muslims (73.35 %), while STs are more likely to choose private sources (32.09%) for the same. Within institutional delivery, about 89% of respondents delivered in public institutions under the JSY scheme, this proportion is lower (57.1%) among those who availed financial assistance under any other government schemes. Mothers who have delivered in private facilities are less likely to avail any form of financial assistance. As likely, respondents in private facilities spend twice as much on OOPE (INR 1850) as those in public ones (INR 740).

Econometric Analysis

Table 12.3 estimates the AORs with 95% confidence interval obtained from sequential logit regression models after controlling for several confounding variables. The odds of choosing institutions for delivery as contrasting to delivery at home specifies the first transition, while the second transition refers to the odds of preferring private sources over public sources for delivery. The odds and transitional probabilities at the first stage indicate that women from urban residences, with higher levels of education and having any kind of work engagements are more likely to choose an institution for delivery. Respondents who are educated above the higher secondary level use institutional delivery roughly twice (AOR 1.41, $p < 0.001$) as often as not-literate respondents. The likelihood of in-facility delivery significantly increases among other general caste compositions (AOR 1.08, $p < 0.001$) compared to SCs in Bihar. Women with adequate media exposure are highly likely (by 1.92 times) to deliver in an institution. Respondents belonging to non-Hindu communities and with higher numbers of children choose to deliver at home. The availability of doctors and healthcare providers significantly increases the likelihood of using an institution for delivery by 1.03 and 1.27 times, respectively, in Bihar. Interestingly, the odds of preferring delivery at institutions decrease with the availability of all-weathered roads and villages having self-help groups. Receiving assistance under JSY found to be the best incentive for delivering in an institution (AOR 6.8, $p < 0.001$ times more) compared to those who were reluctant to receive assistance under JSY.

According to the AOR estimation of the second transition, the likelihood of giving birth in private facilities over public sources tends to proceed in the same direction as giving birth at any institution against giving birth at home, especially when individual-level stratifiers were under consideration. Results underscore that urban (1.97 times higher than rural areas), educated (2.29 times higher than its counterpart), working (1.02 times higher than its counterpart) women mainly belonging to affluent class (1.12 times more than the poor), and Hindu community are more likely to deliver in private institutions. Moreover, women belonging to scheduled tribes (which consist nearly 2% of the total population) are 1.34 times more likely to deliver in a private care than the SCs in Bihar. Notably, those who are reluctant to accept financial aid are around six times (AOR 5.71, $p < 0.001$) more likely to give birth in private facilities than their counterparts (who availed JSY or others government cash incentives). With more access to grassroot-level healthcare providers, respondents' probability to prefer private facilities increases by 1.16 times, which seems surprising. However, the availability of doctors noticeably could not able to influences mothers (AOR 0.97, $p < 0.001$) to avail safe delivery care from public facilities.

Table 12.4 demonstrates the results from the Oaxaca decomposition model executed by the year 2004 and 2014 by employing probit regression models after controlling for different socio-economic predictor variables

Table 12.3 Adjusted Odds Ratios with 95% CI of Preference for In-Facility Delivery and Choice of Specific Provider, Bihar, AHS 2012–13

Variables	Transition 1: Utilization of Institutional Delivery (Home vs. Institution)		Transition 2: Choice of provider (Public vs. Private)	
	AOR (SE^Ω)	95% CL	AOR (SE^Ω)	95% CL
Age	0.99 (0.002)	0.99–1.01	0.99 (0.003)	0.98–1.01
Place of residence				
Rural (Ref)	1.00	1.00	1.00	1.00
Urban	1.85*** (0.01)	1.83–1.87	1.97*** (0.013)	1.94–1.99
Birth order				
Single child (ref)	1.00	1.00	1.00	
Two children	3.35*** (0.045)	3.26–3.44	0.94 (0.025)	0.92–1.05
Three children	2.90*** (0.038)	2.83–2.98	0.82*** (0.020)	0.77–0.86
More than three children	2.63*** (0.036)	2.56–2.71	0.76*** (0.019)	0.72–0.80
Educational level				
Not literate (Ref)	1.00	1.00	1.00	1.00
Up to primary	1.10*** (0.004)	1.09–1.11	1.22*** (0.007)	1.20–1.23
Middle	1.29*** (0.007)	1.27–1.30	1.34*** (0.011)	1.32–1.36
Secondary	1.26*** (0.008)	1.24–1.29	1.48*** (0.013)	1.46–1.51

(Continued)

Table 12.3 Continued

Variables	Transition 1: Utilization of Institutional Delivery (Home vs. Institution)		Transition 2: Choice of provider (Public vs. Private)	
	AOR (SE$^\Omega$)	95% CL	AOR (SE$^\Omega$)	95% CL
Higher secondary and above	1.41*** (0.009)	1.39–1.42	2.29*** (0.020)	2.25–2.33
Religion				
Hindu (Ref)	1.00	1.00	1.00	1.00
Non-Hindu	0.76*** (0.008)	0.75–0.77	0.91 (0.005)	0.90–0.92
Caste				
SC (Ref)	1.00	1.00	1.00	1.00
ST	0.77*** (0.008)	0.98–0.99	1.34*** (0.218)	1.30–1.39
Others	1.08** (0.004)	0.98–0.99	1.17*** (0.007)	1.15–1.18
Occupational status				
Not working (ref)	1.00	1.00	1.00	1.00
Working	1.01*** (0.005)	1.01–1.03	1.02** (0.013)	0.95–0.96
Asset quintiles				
Bottom asset quintiles	1.00	1.00	1.00	1.00
Middle asset quintiles	1.57*** (0.01)	1.57–1.59	0.91*** (0.01)	0.89–0.92
Higher asset quintiles	2.13*** (0.03)	2.29–2.35	1.12*** (0.02)	1.17–1.20
Maternity financial assistance				
Other Govt. schemes (Other than JSY)	1.00	1.00	1.00	1.00

(Continued)

Table 12.3 Continued

Variables	Transition 1: Utilization of Institutional Delivery (Home vs. Institution)		Transition 2: Choice of provider (Public vs. Private)	
	AOR (SE$^{\Omega}$)	95% CL	AOR (SE$^{\Omega}$)	95% CL
Janani Suraksha Yojana (JSY)	6.80*** (0.13)	15.62–16.12	0.17*** (0.01)	0.16–0.17
Not availed	0.27*** (0.02)	0.25–0.26	5.71*** (0.08)	6.55–6.87
Degree of media exposure[a]	1.92*** (0.009)	1.91–1.94	1.26*** (0.005)	1.25–1.27
% of villages having self-help group	0.95*** (0.0004)	0.94–0.95	0.99*** (0.0005)	0.98–0.99
Availability of doctor [b]	1.03*** (0.0003)	1.02–1.03	0.97*** (0.0003)	0.99–1.01
Availability of community health workers[c]	1.27*** (0.007)	1.25–1.28	1.16*** (0.009)	1.14–1.18
Availability of all-weathered roads[d]	0.98*** (0.0001)	0.98–0.99	0.99*** (0.0001)	0.98–0.99
Number of cases (weighted)	1,886,958			

Source: Calculated from unit-level data of AHS 2012–13 (Women's file)
Note: ***p<0.001; **p<0.01; *p<0.05
$^{\Omega}$Standard error

[a]factor scores of household having media exposure [continuous], [b]doctors per 100,000 population [continuous],

[c]factor scores of number of in station personal at Primary Health Centres per 1,00,000 population ,number of in station para medical staff at Primary Health Centres per 10000 population, number of in station para medical staff at sub-centres per 10000 population, Percentage of villages with ASHAs, and percentage of villages with Nutritional Centres – Anganwadi Centre,

[d]percentage of villages with all-weather roads

Table 12.4 Understanding the Effects of *Janani Suraksha Yojana* on Safe Delivery in Bihar – A Decomposition Analysis

	Institutional Delivery		Delivery in Public Sector		Delivery in Private Sector	
	Absolute	Percentage	Absolute	Percentage	Absolute	Percentage
Difference between years	0.518	100	0.480	100	0.039	100
Weight = 1						
Explained by model	0.039	7.48	0.022	4.68	0.012	31.93
Unexplained (partly attributed to NHM)	0.479	92.52	0.457	95.32	0.026	68.07
Weight = 0						
Explained by model	0.022	4.24	0.016	3.30	0.015	38.90
Unexplained (partly attributed to NHM)	0.496	95.76	0.464	96.70	0.024	61.10

Note: The decompositions were carried out by year (2004 and 2014) by employing for probit regression models after controlling for the variables included in the SL models.
Source: Calculated from 60th and 71st round of NSSO data by Ghosh and Husain (2019)

incorporated in the SL model, including district fixed-effects (Ghosh and Husain, 2019). It reveals that the implementation of the JSY scheme led to an overall 94% growth in institutional delivery in Bihar, with a 96% increase in public services and a 36% decline in private facilities. While tracing the pace of institutional delivery care in Bihar, before the JSY scheme, it was restricted to 10% points in 13 years: it was at 22 % in 2005–06 and reached 12.1% in 1992–93. In comparison, the post-JSY era accounts for a 63% increase in institutional delivery, nearly tripling in the last ten years. The significant increase in the use of institutional deliveries in Bihar is mainly responsible for the success of JSY intervention in reproductive healthcare services.

Discussion

Findings indicate that the utilization of institutional delivery and the selection of public facilities are marginal among a specific socio-economic group in Bihar. For instance, women belonging to less-educated, poor, SC, non-Hindu, and rural households are less likely to deliver in any institution, while economically better-off, educated, general caste Hindus are more likely to opt for delivery services from private facilities. Supply-side aspects such as access to health professionals and availability of CHWs are not enough to meet these challenges. Regardless of their positive influence on the usage of in-facility delivery care, they have failed to encourage mothers to deliver in public facilities. At the same time, although the percentage of institutional delivery has increased manifold following the launch of the JSY programme, it would be misleading to interpret that uptake of maternal care has enhanced because of JSY. This is because increase in institutional delivery camouflages the issue of continuum of care. Essential MCH care services, including as comprehensive ANC, PNC, and other necessary care, which are critical for meeting SDG targets and establishing UHC, are severely lacking in Bihar (Figure 12.1).

Therefore, one can argue that in addition to physiographic 'access' several other dimensions of 'access' such as accessibility to knowledge, initial utilization of services (or contact with health personnel), continuity of access has critical implications for finishing the 'unfinished agenda' of MDG 4 and 5 and moving towards Universal Health Coverage (UHC) as a part of SDGs.

In the case of institutional births (in transition one), women's working status and educational attainment appeared to be as important contributing factors influencing their decisions (Ahmed et al., 2010; Mengesha et al., 2013). In addition to developing self-esteem, educated and working women are better aware of the benefits of institutional delivery for the survival of their children. The heightened awareness must be investigated in conjunction with high media exposure at the community level, for which women are better able to identify with their rights to maternal healthcare services and become more responsive to their entitlements (Sharma et al., 2014; Singh et al., 2012). Women with high media exposure in Bihar are approximately two times more likely to opt for safe delivery care than their counterparts. Respondents' place of residence and religious affiliation has a considerable effect on their decision to use in-facility services. The present study reveals that safe deliveries are more likely to occur in urban settings which can be explained by the augmented availability of infrastructure (accessibly to health facilities, better transportation) than in rural areas (Ahmed et al., 2010; Hazarika, 2011; Kumar et al., 2013).

Although education and place of residence showed significant associations, the paper tries to understand how the availability of health professionals and household economic status influence the quality of in-facility care and access to it, particularly when it comes to public facilities. According to Table 12.3, availability of doctors and community-based health practitioners increases the likelihood of obtaining institutional delivery by 1.27 and 1.03 times, respectively. The appropriate explanation is that doctors' valuable recommendations and advice contributed to a considerable behavioural shift in mothers' attitudes toward receiving in-facility birth care (Scott and Shanker, 2010). However, the decision to deliver in private healthcare facilities among affluent sections (Table 12.3) reflects a perception of better quality, whereas the choice of availing public health services among deprived sections refers to a decision based on cost rather than quality (Barua, 2005; Marar, 2019). At this juncture, where economically distressed populations are less likely to opt for institutional delivery over affluent ones and seeking out public facilities, JSY has the potential to reduce the development gaps between these sections.

However, in the second transition, the gravitation towards private services (by 1.16 times) despite the presence of government-appointed healthcare providers like ASHAs and ANMs is puzzling. The reasonable assumption would be that the increased presence of grassroot-level healthcare providers would popularize utilization of public services. One of the most important roles of CHWs, to effectively attain MDG4 and 5 (Awasthi and Nichter et al., 2015), is to act as a bridge between the doctor and members of the community to encourage the uptake of public healthcare facilities (Raj, 2015). The results from Table 12.3 indicate that this role is not being performed effectively in Bihar. Arguably, an increase in CHWs does not necessarily imply higher uptake of public healthcare and thereby quality of performance. In fact, there are a variety of factors responsible for their below average performance. It may also be reflected in the lack of continuum of care.

The matter of ensuring a steady supply of relevant and updated healthcare information has been neglected by policy initiatives. Therefore, the possibilities of continued professional development and skill-building opportunities are scarce for community health workers (Deepak et al., 2014; Kapadia-Kundu et al., 2012; Raj et al., 2015).

It is entirely plausible that experience with CHWs who provide below-average care is perpetuating a trend of preferring private healthcare facilities over public ones. If CHWs who are the first point of contact are performing ineffectively, then the likelihood of choosing private services increases. The solution here does not lie in increasing the number of CHWs but look into factors preventing the effective dispensation of services. The effects of stress caused by role stagnation among ANMs and other CHWs are also another important consideration (Purohit and Vasava, 2017).

A low desire for in-facility delivery, even in villages with self-help groups and covered by all-weather roads, cannot solely be explained by existing data (AHS, 2013; RGI, 2011); therefore, the paradox persists. Depending on the physical condition of the roads, it may seem more convenient for mothers to avoid any unpleasant obstacles by not returning to a hospital for delivery. On the other hand, a recent study stated that participation in SHGs is mainly restricted among older women where mothers-in-law ('Saas') are taking part as a proxy for daughters-in-law ('Bahu') (Dutta et al., 2021). However, the study could not construe these because of data constraints and recommends qualitative investigations for a clearer picture.

While the number of institutional deliveries has increased dramatically in Bihar, CHWs, particularly ASHAs have played an indifferent role in transferring this trend to public sources. CHWs in Bihar are not performing many responsibilities, such as checking on new mothers after delivery (Dongre and Kapur, 2013) that leads to a lower usage of postnatal care services (57.3%) among mothers. Even though private health care is an attractive option for both urban and rural populations, the latter's use is restricted due to matters of accessibility and cost (Jeffery and Jeffery, 2010; Ramani and Mavalankar, 2006). Given the concentration of private hospitals in urban areas and the economic prosperity of the Hindu general caste majority, it is not surprising that they take to mostly private hospitals (Barua, 2005; Marar, 2019). Creating demand for MCH services among marginalized sections is necessary, followed by identifying obstacles to utilize them. Needless to say, health professionals or frontline workers should offer care seekers more equitable options, such as the utilization of maternal incentives by using public institutions. The missing link which has hitherto been lacking in the evidence can be found in the effects of JSY implementation. These findings (Tables 12.3 and 12.4) suggest that the implementation of JSY has increased the proportion of institutional deliveries in Bihar (about 7 times) by bringing pregnant women to public institutions, predominantly those who are poor and marginalized (Table 12.3). It is thus contributed significantly to the ultimate goal of improving equity in MCH care outcomes. JSY has been largely successful if assessed on certain parameters, even in the most backward districts of India. One of the most important features of this scheme that has contributed to the significant increase in institutional deliveries is its incentives. The provision of free medication, as well as cash incentives to mothers and ASHAs, has increased the popularity of public health services considerably. The example of JSY illustrates how monetary incentives can elicit positive behaviour changes among the population as well as a strong extrinsic motivator for ASHAs to work more effectively (Batra, 2015).

To add, although JSY has achieved its goal of providing women with access to medically safe birthing opportunities, women's experiences with JSY are not uniform and euphoric. There are several instances where women and their families had to undergo distressing experiences and where they were exploited for money by medical or government staff (Jeffery and Jeffery, 2010; Mukherjee and Singh, 2018). Apart from problems regarding institutional deliveries, there is evidence to show lesser coverage of ASHAs in areas populated with Muslim of marginalized communities. This suggests that the socio-cultural biases of JSY workers are a hindrance to its effective implementation (Jeffery and Jeffery, 2010; Patel et al., 2018; Lim et al., 2010). Encouraging institutional deliveries without examining the underlying factors responsible for the persistence of home births is one of the shortcomings of JSY.

Alongside the limitations of JSY, the authors acknowledge the limitations that the present study has. Although the Annual Health Survey (AHS, 2013) is the largest demographic survey in the world being a point-data AHS does not appropriate for tracing the continuum of care and the cause–effect relationships among variables. Secondly, it does not provide any information on quality indicators of the functioning of the health system such as availability of drugs and other essential equipment, human resources, etc., thus could not control them in the multivariate models. Finally, none of the contextual/supply-side variables or data on quality of care is available in AHS data. However, the present study can be justified based on the proximate survey periods of two data sets, the size of the data, and the design (community-based) of the study.

Conclusions

The SDGs seek to provide universal health coverage (UHC) by identifying confounding factors for maternal and child mortality (neonatal and under five years), as well as providing financial protection from catastrophic healthcare spending (CHS). A parallel could therefore be drawn from the study. While Bihar has made considerable gains in institutional delivery, severe lack of continuum of care poses serious challenges to achieving UHC and leaves mothers vulnerable. As a result, judging equity-focused approaches in Bihar by the extent to which safe delivery is improved would be misleading. The paper also rationally argued that to ensure an equitable and universal access to MCH care, particularly safe delivery care in an underdeveloped state like Bihar, we must distil the major socio-economic loopholes from the big deck of health and awareness. Any intervention or making community health workers available, without understanding the demand-side issues, could lead to sub-optimal outcome. NHM must adequately focus on strengthening of PHCs and CHCs in delivering MCH care to achieve UHC. Improved institutional delivery care is required to prevent vulnerable populations from losing faith in public health services. Filing complaints involve time-consuming and bureaucratic procedures which are not favoured by patients, who respond instead by dropping out from public health services. The payment incentives received by women under JSY are meagre and often do not cover the cost of transportation or wages of family members lost in attending to the pregnant mother. An increase in JSY payments would compensate the mother and her family fully. With these restructuring together with spreading awareness, public services will be more appealing to mothers than they were previously. Furthermore, state policy should promote equitable access to maternal healthcare services by creating demand among marginalized groups, enhancing the efficiency of community-level healthcare providers to build trust in public health services, and providing an equal opportunity to receive JSY benefits. Adjustments and rectification in the programme would undoubtedly improve the situation.

Acknowledgements

The authors sincerely extend thanks to Noyonika Das for her assistance in the earlier version of the article.

Notes

1 Institutional delivery, in-facility births, and safe-delivery are used here interchangeably.
2 Under delivery care, institutional delivery refers to giving birth to a child in a medical institute (public or private) under the overall supervision of qualified, trained, and competent health personal where there are more amenities available and receiving of postnatal check-up within 48 hours of delivery can be assured.
3 A SHG is a locally formed financial intermediary committee usually composed of 10–20 locale women /men of a cohort group having approximately equal socio-economic conditions. They are subject to open and voluntary membership, democratic control of members, participation of members in economic activities of the group, autonomy and independence, education, training and information, and co-operation among different groups and concern for the community.

References

Ahmed, S., Creanga, A. A., Gillespie, D. G., & Tsui, A. O. (2010). Economic status, education and empowerment: Implications for maternal health service utilization in developing countries. *PloS One, 5,* e11190.
Arokiasamy, P., & Pradhan, J. (2013). Maternal health care in India: Access and demand determinants. *Primary Health Care Research & Development,* 14(4), 373–393. doi: 10.1017/S1463423612000552.
Awasthi, S., Nichter, M., Verma, T., Srivastava, N. M. et al. (2015). Revisiting community case management of childhood pneumonia: Perceptions of caregivers and grass root health providers in Uttar Pradesh and Bihar, Northern India. *PloS One,* 10(4), e0123135.
Baral, Y. R., Lyons, K., Skinner, J. V. T. E., & Van Teijlingen, E. R. (2010). Determinants of skilled birth attendants for delivery in Nepal. *Kathmandu University Medical Journal,* 8(3), 325–332.

Batra, S. (2015). Can unique incentives promote safe motherhood behaviour: An appraisal. *Indian Anthropologist*, 46(1), 31–46.

Buis, M. L. (2007). Not all transitions are equal: The relationship between inequality of educational opportunities and inequality of educational outcomes. *Available from*: https://home.fsw.vu.nl/m.buis/wp/distmare.html. Accessed 23 March 2017.

Census of India (2013). *Annual Health Survey*. AHS 2012–13 Fact Sheet, *Bihar, India*. Available *from*: http://www.censusindia.gov.in/vital_statistics/AHSBulletins /AHS_Factsheets_2012_13.html. Accessed 12 June 2017.

Census of India (2011). *District Census Handbook*. Bihar. Available from: https:// censusindia.gov.in/2011census/dchb/DCHB.html. Accessed 31 May 2018.

Das, K., & Ghosh, S. (2021). Rural–urban fertility convergence, differential stopping behavior, and contraceptive method mix in West Bengal, India: A spatiotemporal analysis. *Journal of Family History*, 46(2), 211–235. doi:10.117 7%2F0363199020959785.

Das, K., Ganguly, N., Ghosh, S. (2018). Factors affecting maternal care utilization in Empowered Action Group (EAG) States of India: Evidences from Annual Health Survey 2012–13. *Journal of Indian Anthropological Society*, 53, 161–178.

Deepak, K. K., Kumar, Y., & Adkoli, B. V. (2014). Extending professional education to health workers at grass root level: An experience from All India Institute of Medical Sciences, New Delhi. *Indian Journal of Community Medicine: Official Publication of Indian Association of Preventive & Social Medicine*, 39(1), 38–42. doi:10.4103/0970-0218.126358

Dongre, A., &Kapur, A. (2013). How is Janani Suraksha Yojana performing in backward districts of India? *Economic and Political Weekly*, 48(42), 53–59.

Dutta, M., Ghosh, S., & Hussain, Z. (2021). Saas, bahu, and ASHA Information diffusion and behavioural change in rural Bihar. International Growth Centre (IGG); IND-18013. Available from: https://www.theigc.org/wp-content/uploads /2021/07/Husain-et-al-June-2021-Policy-Brief_18013.pdf. Accessed 29 June 2021.

Ghosh, S., & Husain, Z. (2019). Has the national health mission improved utilisation of maternal healthcare services in Bihar?. *Economic & Political Weekly*, 54(31), 44–51.

Ghosh, S., Siddiqui, M., Barik, A., &Bhaumik, S. (2015). Determinants of skilled delivery assistance in a rural population: Findings from an HDSS site of rural west Bengal, India. *Maternal and Child Health Journal*, 19(11), 2470–2479. doi:10.1007/s10995-015-1768-0.

GoI (2020). *Key Indicators of Social Consumption in India, Health, NSSO Report No. 586*. New Delhi: Ministry of Statistics and Programme Implementation, Government of India, 2017–18. Available from: http://164.100.161.63/sites/ default/files/publication_reports/NSS%20Report%20no.%20586%20Health %20in%20India.pdf. Accessed 1 March 2022.

GoI (2015). *Key Indicators of Social Consumption in India, Health, NSSO Report No. 574*. New Delhi: Ministry of Statistics and Programme Implementation, Government of India. 2016. Available from: http://mospi.nic.in/download-reports ?main_cat=NzI2&cat=All&sub_category=All. Accessed 9 July 2019.

GoI (2006). *Morbidity, Health Care and the Condition of the Aged, NSSO Report No. 507*. New Delhi: Ministry of Statistics and Programme Implementation, Government of India. January-June, 2004. Available from: http://mospi.nic.in/ download-reports?main_cat=NzI2&cat=All&sub_category=All. Accessed 15 June 2019.

Gupta, S. K., Pal, D. K., Tiwari, R., Garg, R., Shrivastava, A. K., Sarawagi, R., & Lahariya, C. (2012). Impact of Janani Suraksha Yojana on institutional delivery rate and maternal morbidity and mortality: An observational study in India. *Journal of Health, Population, and Nutrition*, 30(4), 464–71. doi:10.3329/jhpn.v30i4.13416.

Hazarika, I. (2011). Factors that determine the use of skilled care during delivery in India: Implications for achievement of MDG-5 targets. *Maternal and Child Health Journal*, 15(8), 1381–1388.

International Institute for Population Sciences (IIPS) and ICF (2017). National Family Health Survey (NFHS-4), 2015–16: Bihar, India: Mumbai, IIPS. Available from: https://dhsprogram.com/methodology/survey/survey-display-355.cfm. Accessed 10 September 2018.

International Institute for Population Sciences (IIPS) and ICF (2021). National Family Health Survey (NFHS-5), 2019–20: Bihar, India: Mumbai, IIPS. Available from: http://rchiips.org/nfhs/NFHS-5_FCTS/FactSheet_BR.pdf. Accessed 10 June 2021.

Issac, A., Chatterjee, S., Srivastava, A., & Bhattacharyya, S. (2016). Out of pocket expenditure to deliver at public health facilities in India: A cross sectional analysis. *Reproductive Health*, 13(1), 1–9. doi:10.1186/s12978-016-0221-1.

Jat, T. R., Ng, N., & San Sebastian, M. (2011). Factors affecting the use of maternal health services in Madhya Pradesh state of India: A multilevel analysis. *International Journal for Equity in Health*, 10(1), 1–11. doi:10.1186/1475-9276-10-59.

Jeffery, P., & Jeffery, R. (2010). Only when the boat has started sinking: A maternal death in rural north India. *Social Science & Medicine*, 71(10), 1711–1718.

Joe, W., Perkins, J. M., Kumar, S., Rajpal, S., & Subramanian, S. V. (2018). Institutional delivery in India, 2004–14: Unravelling the equity-enhancing contributions of the public sector. *Health Policy and Planning*, 33(5), 645–653.

Joshi, C., Torvaldsen, S., Hodgson, R., & Hayen, A. (2014). Factors associated with the use and quality of antenatal care in Nepal: A population-based study using the demographic and health survey data. *BMC Pregnancy and Childbirth*, 14(1), 1–11.

Kapadia-Kundu, N., Sullivan, T. M., Safi, B., Trivedi, G., & Velu, S. (2012). Understanding health information needs and gaps in the health care system in Uttar Pradesh, India. *Journal of Health Communication*, 17(sup2), 30–45.

Kesterton, A. J., Cleland, J., Sloggett, A., & Ronsmans, C. (2010). Institutional delivery in rural India: The relative importance of accessibility and economic status. *BMC Pregnancy and Childbirth*, 10(1), 1–9.

Kumar, C., Rai, R. K., Singh, P. K., & Singh, L. (2013). Socioeconomic disparities in maternity care among Indian adolescents, 1990–2006. *PloS One*, 8(7), e69094. doi: 10.1371/journal.pone.0069094.

Lee, C., Ayers, S. L., Kronenfeld, J. J., Frimpong, J. A., Rivers, P. A., & Kim, S. S. (2010). The importance of examining movements within the US health care system: Sequential logit modeling. *BMC Health Services Research*, 10(1), 1–8.

Lim, S. S., Dandona, L., Hoisington, J. A., James, S. L., Hogan, M. C., & Gakidou, E. (2010). India's Janani Suraksha Yojana, a conditional cash transfer programme to increase births in health facilities: An impact evaluation. *The Lancet*, 375(9730), 2009–2023. doi:10.1016/s0140-6736(10)60744-1.

Marar, A. (2019). Upper caste Hindus richest in India, own 41% of total assets; STs own 3.7%, says study on wealth distribution. *The Indian Express*. February 14. Available from:https://indianexpress.com/article/india/upper-caste-hindus-richest

-in-india-own-41-total-assets-says-study-on-wealth-distribution-5582984/. Accessed 21 March 2020.

Mengesha, Z. B., Biks, G. A., Ayele, T. A., Tessema, G. A., & Koye, D. N. (2013). Determinants of skilled attendance for delivery in Northwest Ethiopia: A community based nested case control study. *BMC Public Health*, 13(1), 1–6.

Mohanty, S. K., & Kastor, A. (2017). Out-of-pocket expenditure and catastrophic health spending on maternal care in public and private health centres in India: A comparative study of pre and post national health mission period. *Health Economics Review*, 7(1), 1–15.

MoHFW (2017). National Health Policy 2017, Ministry of Health and Family Welfare, Government of India, New Delhi. Available from: https://www.nhp.gov .in/nhpfiles/national_health_policy_2017.pdf. Accessed Oct 2019.

Mukherjee, S., & Singh, A. (2018). Has the Janani Suraksha Yojana (a conditional maternity benefit transfer scheme) succeeded in reducing the economic burden of maternity in rural India? Evidence from the Varanasi district of Uttar Pradesh. *Journal of Public Health Research*, 7(1), 957. doi: 10.4081/jphr.2018.957.

Mission, N. R. H. (2005). National rural health mission (2005–2012): Mission document. *Indian Journal of Public Health*, 49(3), 175–183. PMID: 16468284.

Navaneetham, K., & Dharmalingam, A. (2002). Utilization of maternal health care services in Southern India. *Social Science & Medicine*, 55(10), 1849–1869.

Oaxaca, R. (1973). Male-female wage differentials in urban labor markets. *International Economic Review*, 693–709.

Patel, P., Das, M., & Das, U. (2018). The perceptions, health-seeking behaviours and access of scheduled caste women to maternal health services in Bihar, India. *Reproductive Health Matters*, 26(54), 114–125.

Purohit, B., &Vasava, P. (2017). Role stress among auxiliary nurses midwives in Gujarat, India. *BMC Health Services Research*, 17(1), 1–8. doi:10.1186/ s12913-017-2033-6.

Raj, S., Sharma, V. L., Singh, A., & Goel, S. (2015). The health information seeking behaviour and needs of community health workers in Chandigarh in Northern India. *Health Information & Libraries Journal*, 32(2), 143–149. doi:10.1111/ hir.12104.

Ramani, K. V., & Mavalankar, D. (2006). Health system in India: Opportunities and challenges for improvements. *Journal of Health Organization and Management*, 20(6): 560–572.

Requejo, J., Bryce, J., Victora, C. G. (2012). Building a future for women and children: The 12 report. Countdown to 2015–2012. Available from: http:// countdown2015mnch.org/documents/2012Report/2012-Complete.pdf. Accessed 16 Oct 16 *2019*.

RGI (2019). Special bulletin of maternal mortality in India 2017–19. New Delhi, India: SRS. Available from: https://censusindia.gov.in/vital_statistics/SRS_Bulletins /MMR%20Bulletin%202017-19.pdf. Accessed 30 March 2022.

Rodríguez, G. (2012). *Generalized Linear Model*. Princeton University. Available from: http://data.princeton.edu/wws509/stata/c6s4.html. Accessed 17 June 2018.

Saroha, E., Altarac, M., & Sibley, L. M. (2008). Caste and maternal health care service use among rural Hindu women in Maitha, Uttar Pradesh, India. *Journal of Midwifery & Women's Health*, 53(5), e41–e47.

Scott, K., & Shanker, S. (2010). Tying their hands? Institutional obstacles to the success of the ASHA community health worker programme in rural north India. *AIDS Care*, 22(sup2), 1606–1612. doi:10.1080/09540121.2010.507751.

Sharma, S., & Bothra, M. (2016). Maternal and child healthcare: An analysis of out-of-pocket expenditure under the Janani Shishu Suraksha Karyakaram. *Institute of Economic Growth (IEG)*, no. 366.

Sharma, S. R., Poudyal, A. K., Devkota, B. M., & Singh, S. (2014). Factors associated with place of delivery in rural Nepal. *BMC Public Health*, *14*(1), 1–7. doi: 10.1186/1471-2458-14-306.

Singh, P. K., Rai, R. K., Alagarajan, M., & Singh, L. (2012). Determinants of maternity care services utilization among married adolescents in rural India. *PloS One*, *7*(2), e31666. doi: 10.1371/journal.pone.0031666.

Sumner, A., & Melamed, C. (2010). Introduction–The MDGs and Beyond: Pro-poor Policy in a Changing World. *IDS Bulletin*, *41*(1), 1–6.

Tarekegn, S. M., Lieberman, L. S., & Giedraitis, V. (2014). Determinants of maternal health service utilization in Ethiopia: Analysis of the 2011 Ethiopian Demographic and Health Survey. *BMC Pregnancy and Childbirth*, *14*(1), 1–13. doi:10.1186/1471-2393-14-161.

UNICEF (2015). The state of world children. UNICEF Health Section, Program Division. Available from: www.unicef.org/publications/index_92018.html. Accessed 15 Oct 2020.

Uthman, O. A., Aiyedun, V., & Yahaya, I. (2012). Exploring variations in under-5 mortality in Nigeria using league table, control chart and spatial analysis. *Journal of Public Health*, *34*(1), 125–130.

Wong, K. L., Restrepo-Méndez, M. C., Barros, A. J., & Victora, C. G. (2017). Socioeconomic inequalities in skilled birth attendance and child stunting in selected low and middle income countries: Wealth quintiles or deciles? *PloS One*, *12*(5), e0174823.

World Health Organization (2019). Trends in maternal mortality: 2000 to 2017: estimates by WHO, UNICEF, UNFPA, World Bank Group and the United Nations Population Division. Geneva. ISBN 978-92-4-151648-8. Available from: https://www.unfpa.org/featured-publication/trends-maternal-mortality-2000-2017. Accessed 9 Dec 2020.

World Health Organization (2019). World health statistics 2019: Monitoring health for the SDGs, sustainable development goals. World Health Organization. Available from: https://apps.who.int/iris/handle/10665/324835. Accessed 13 September 2020.

Yamashita, T., Suplido, S. A., Ladines-Llave, C., Tanaka, Y., Senba, N., & Matsuo, H. (2014). A cross-sectional analytic study of postpartum health care service utilization in the Philippines. *PLoS One*, *9*(1), e85627. doi:10.1371/journal.pone.0085627.

Yanagisawa, S., Oum, S., & Wakai, S. (2006). Determinants of skilled birth attendance in rural Cambodia. *Tropical Medicine & International Health*, *11*(2), 238–251.

13 Men's Role in Unpaid Activities and Maternal Health Care in India

How Far Women Get Support from Men?

Aditi B Prasad and Aparajita Chattopadhyay

Introduction

Men's involvement is essential in a male-driven country like India to ensure women can access health facilities as and when needed and can practice healthy living. The need to promote positive gender norms regarding masculinity is now reflected in the global gender equality agenda. Engaging men can benefit men as well, as it relieves the strain of being the household's primary breadwinner and allows them to form healthier connections with their wives and children. Men also have a role to play in the economic empowerment of women. In a world where they still benefit from the "patriarchal dividend" (Sweetman, 2013), they can serve as true gatekeepers to greater gender equality by assisting their female family members in gaining access to resources critical to their economic empowerment and health care. Involving men is a promising starting point for overcoming unequal divisions in the field of labour and care, improving sexual and reproductive health and rights, and preventing violence against women and girls. Evidence shows that men's gender beliefs, perceptions, and practices have a profound effect on the lives of women and girls (UNFPA & Promundo, 2018).

A lot of literature tends to equate women's economic empowerment with their participation in the labour force, without considering the kind of work they do, how it impacts their unpaid responsibilities and where they stand in the skewed distribution of income and wealth (Kabeer, 2019). As gatekeepers of the household, men have a vital role in ensuring equitable division of labour in households. Further, involving men in maternal health goals is an important strategy to improve maternal health, as well as to ensure a more egalitarian world where the responsibility of childbearing and childcare is not restricted to the woman, and men are seen as playing an equal part in looking after the needs of the woman and child, removed from their perceived role as sole breadwinner and head of the family.

Why Do Unpaid Activities and Maternal Health Care Matter? A Critical Look

Gender-specific constraints, such as social norms, beliefs, and values, define social relationships of family and kinship. They contribute to the gendered

DOI: 10.4324/9781003430636-18

pattern of labour market outcomes noted in different regions of the world (Kabeer, 2021). Men's higher labour force participation in most regions of the world, relative to women, reflects the breadwinning responsibilities ascribed to them in most cultures. Women's labour force participation, on the other hand, varies considerably across the world. Although the economy is growing, education levels are rising, fertility rates are declining, and women are not participating in the formal economy.

Women tend to be over represented in occupations perceived as unskilled and "low-valued", particularly in care jobs (Elson, 2017). Their contribution to the family and society remains invisible and unrecognized and, in conventional terms, yields no economic benefits. This devaluation of "women's work" is reflected in the house. In countries with a high proportion of multi-generational households, men spend less than an hour on average, while women take care of children, the elderly, the sick or the disabled for an average of 4.5 hours a day (NSSO, 2020). The devaluation of women's workforce has increased the gender classification of paid and unpaid work, leaving women unpaid, having little household bargaining power, and prospering men, businesses, and the economy (Kamdar, 2020).

The global debate on the domestic roles of men and women dates back to the International Conference on Population and Development (ICPD) in Cairo (1994) and the World Conference on Women in Beijing (1995). The paradigm shift from women being seen as solely responsible for their health to their spouse's involvement to ensure that the woman can gain access to quality healthcare was also brought about by ICPD 1994. It was a pathbreaking initiative that led to a dialogue on women's health rights being initiated. This Conference acted as a catalyst to advance the cause of ensuring a more equitable and egalitarian view of women's work and health without the pressure of demographic targets as the central theme of policies.

Since the 1960s, a substantial amount of research findings pointed out that enhancing gender disparities in paid and unpaid work is a contributing factor to promoting women's economic empowerment and overall human development. As a result, policy attention and resources have been devoted to addressing gaps in health, education, labour markets, labour rights, and access to credit and markets. Despite these initiatives, gender disparities in the division of labour between paid and unpaid work continue to persist, with men spending more of their work time in remunerative employment and women performing most of the unpaid work (Antonopoulos, 2008; Himmelweit, 1995; Kabeer, 2021).

It is a standard assumption that to improve the levels of female labour force participation, investment in female education and employability and decreasing fertility rates is the only solution. Yet, the burden of unpaid work and the time spent on unpaid care activities is often missed out of the equation. It is also common for studies to associate women's economic empowerment with their labour force participation, without taking into account the kind of work they do, where they stand in the skewed distribution of income and wealth, and how it impacts their unpaid responsibilities (Kabeer, 2019).

Long hours at home spent cooking, cleaning, and caring for family limits the amount of time individuals can spend in paid work. Women spend far more hours on unpaid household and caregiving activities than men do (OECD, 2017). While unpaid care and domestic work is a global phenomenon, it is especially prevalent in India. Globally, Indian women's unpaid care and domestic work hours are second only to women in Kazakhstan, according to the latest report by Oxfam India (2019).

Economic policies are fundamentally biased against women and the types of work they do. Although women make up the majority of the world's low-paid workers, they are often undervalued in economic policymaking (Kidder et al., 2017). These policies overlook the unpaid work of women and discredit women's informal paid work. For effective economic empowerment for women to occur, women must enjoy their rights to control and benefit from resources, assets, income as well as their own time. In addition, women face several social barriers which restrict them from engaging in the paid labour force, threatening their autonomy.

One of the most universal and persistent barriers for women and girls to achieve economic equality is the exclusion in economic policymaking of unpaid activities, including unpaid care and domestic activities. The unpaid care workers, primarily women, are denied official recognition as workers and remain invisible and excluded from the Indian development policy (Neetha & Palriwala, 2019).

Gender Differentials in Paid and Unpaid Activities

In this study, "work" that is remunerated in cash or kind (in the shape of wages, salaries, and profit) is defined as a paid activity, while tasks performed without any direct remuneration are termed as unpaid activities.

Unpaid activities have the following components – (i) household maintenance including, cooking, cleaning and shopping; (ii) care of persons of own household such as looking after children, the elderly, sick, disabled or simply other adults requiring care; (iii) voluntary services or services rendered free to other households or the community.

The discourse on women's unpaid activities is particularly relevant in the Indian context because women's labour force participation rate (LFPR) is very low and has seen a declining trend over the last decade probably because the majority of them are moving into the domain of domestic duties. In India, merely 22 per cent of women are engaged in the labour force, and 70 per cent of them are associated with farm activities that are informal in nature with little or no economic remuneration or social recognition (Mehrotra & Sinha, 2017). Furthermore, the burden of unpaid work is worsened by the lack of adequate public provisioning in critical sectors, such as energy, health, water and sanitation, food security, and livelihoods (Hirway, 2015). Moreover, the failure of the State to provide alternatives for care and domestic assistance increases the burden of unpaid activities, which leads to restraining women's choices for paid work (Das et al., 2015; Singh & Pattanaik, 2020). Macro-level gender inequality, as measured by wage discrimination and barriers to entry into preferred jobs, is a disincentive to women entering the labour force (Das, 2006).

Men's Involvement in Maternal Health Care

Men's involvement in women's health has been a less understood and little-researched issue as compared to other areas of sexual and reproductive health (Ntabona, 2002). Nonetheless, there is literature that has looked at the issue from a theoretical standpoint and through ethnographic work in various parts of the developing world.

A lot of men only involve themselves in maternal health issues when complications arise (Ganle & Dery, 2015). Education of women and strong conjugal bonds enable higher participation of men in maternal health activities (Nagawa, 1994). Areas of participation of men in maternal care can include accompanying woman for antenatal care (ANC) visits, being present in the delivery room, supporting her during childbirth and helping her access postnatal care, taking care of expenses related to childbirth and her healthcare needs and joint participation in decision-making regarding maternal health (Varkey et al., 2004).

Stigma, lack of knowledge regarding reproductive health, hesitance due to social roles, and work-related responsibilities deter men from participating in maternal health. These can be mitigated through encouraging joint decision-making regarding reproductive health (Mullany, 2010), and enabling better communication between couples. In certain settings, women also act as barriers when they resist participation of men in maternal care due to ingrained idea of child caring and maternity as primarily a woman's job, and to avoid negative stereotyping, while also fearing that hitherto safe social spaces for women could turn into insecure ones (Ganle et al., 2016).

Men themselves show better physical and psychological health when recognized in their new roles as fathers and caregivers (Plantin et al., 2011). Making programmes couple-friendly instead of simply women-centric can help men play a more involved role in maternity and childcare. Improvements in formal education can also play an important role in making men more involved in maternal health (Craymah et al., 2017). Knowledge of maternal health and involvement of husband in maternal health issues have shown a clear correlation (Rahman et al., 2018; Turan et al., 2011).

Multiple qualitative studies show that designing activities to engage men in maternal nutrition programs are important to maximize impact. A study by Singh & Ram (2009) in rural Ahmednagar, Maharashtra, found that interventions to encourage male involvement in low socioeconomic group help in improving maternal health. Other studies have also shown that involvement of men in ANC translates into good maternal health of wife (Rahman et al., 2018). Husbands accompanying women when receiving health services are positively correlated with the use of skilled maternal and neonatal healthcare services. Chattopadhyay (2012) and Chattopadhyay & Govil (2020) used NFHS data to find role of men's involvement in maternal health for certain Indian states. They invoke the irony that as "gatekeepers of care" men may take decision regarding women's health needs, but are ultimately not involved in her healthcare. A woman's disadvantage as a homemaker is evident when in most cases; she does not have the decision-making power over most resources including finances, transport, faces restrictions over movement, and cannot leave children alone even if she wishes to access health care.

According to the Fourth World Conference on Women held in Beijing in 1995, men's knowledge, attitudes, and behaviours influence not just their health but also that of their partners and spouses. Male involvement definitely leads to better health outcomes for women in developing countries (Yargawa & Leonardi-Bee, 2015), as evident through the various studies. Even UNFPA, in 1998, observed that men have a prominent role to play in wife's health and morbidity during reproductive phase. This critical role must be taken account of while drafting policies and programmes so that the mutual responsibility of spouses in the reproduction process is highlighted.

The responsibility of caregiving can be shared by both the spouses, and while prevailing cultural and societal barriers in the form of gender roles, norms and practices regarding accepting this view exist, involvement in maternal health can be seen as an opportunity for a safe motherhood, better communication between spouses, and overall empowerment of women.

Therefore, this study explores evidences on the gendered patterns and role of men in unpaid activities and maternal healthcare utilization. Additionally, it also looks into the current scenario of unpaid activities and maternal healthcare utilization in India.

Conceptual Model

The study is based on an extension of the conceptual model given by Agénor & Canuto (2012). Figure 13.1 shows a gender-based overlapping generation's model to address interactions between the gendered division of labour, women's time allocation, women's health and economic growth. Due to ascribed social norms and the gendered division of labour, women allocate their time between four alternatives: market work, raising children, human capital accumulation, and home production.

The time spent on health, education, and parenting affect women's health and education and children's health and education. In the family, fathers prefer current consumption relatively, while mothers prefer their children's health. For example, family-wide preference parameters for consumption and child health depend on women's bargaining power. Women's bargaining power is dependent on and restricted by men in a position of power, such as

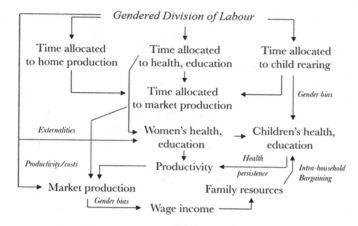

Figure 13.1 Conceptual Model for Gendered Division of Labour

the household head at an individual level. Power can also be exercised collectively, such as the authority of men in the labour market and the public sphere. Gender bias in the workplace is captured by assuming that women earn only a fraction of their marginal income. The difference in economic outcomes in the market between men and women is related to the gender bias experienced at home as a child.

Interestingly, men have a role to play in almost all interactions. Inter- and intra-generational health persistence in the sense of women's health affect their children's health, and health in childhood affects health in adulthood. In the Indian setting, men control the access of all household members to resources, which makes the need for men's involvement inseparable from any real progress. By engaging in unpaid activities and maternal healthcare, men will play an active role in women's lives and, by extension, their children's lives.

Data and Methods

The chapter is based on the reports of varying rounds of NSS, including India's first Time Use Survey (2019). Time Use Survey is an important source of information about the activities performed by the population and the time duration for which such activities are performed. One distinguishing feature of the survey from other household surveys is that it can capture the time distribution of different aspects of human activities, be it paid, unpaid or other activities, with accuracy, which is otherwise not possible in labour surveys.

Recently, the National Statistical Office (NSO) conducted the Time Use Survey for the period of January 2019–December 2019 in all states and UTs of India. The survey collected information on time use, covering a period of 24 hours starting from 4:00 AM on the day before the date of the interview to 4:00 AM on the day of the interview, for each member of the selected household aged six years and above.

On the other hand, to understand men's role in maternal care, the chapter looks into the basic statistics of the recently published NFHS-5 (2019–21) report. The fifth round of the survey was conducted in 28 states and 8 union territories, with a sample of 6,36,699 households, 7,24,115 women aged 15–49 years, and 1,01,839 men aged 15–54 years. The survey was conducted under the aegis of the Ministry of Health and Family Welfare, Government of India, with International Institute for Population Sciences, Mumbai, as the nodal agency. Simple bivariate analysis is applied to understand the pattern and trends.

Results

The 68th round of NSS gives an insight into the unpaid domestic duties of women in some major states of India. The survey classified the women who attended domestic duties only and those who were also engaged in free collection of goods, sewing, tailoring, weaving, etc., for household use, in addition to domestic duties. These women were involved in unpaid labour or subsistence production and were not a part of the formal economy or the labour force (NSSO, 2014).

Among women aged 15 years and above, about 60 per cent in rural areas and 64 per cent in urban areas were engaged in domestic duties and were not a part of the labour force. The proportion of women engaged in domestic duties has continued to increase over time in both rural and urban areas. This increase has been supplemented with continuously declining female labour force participation rates.

In rural areas, the proportion increased from 35.3 per cent in 61st (2004–05) round to 40.1 per cent in 66th (2009–10) round which further increased to 42.2 per cent during 68th (2011–12) round. At the same time, the proportion of women engaged in domestic duties in urban areas increased by about 3 percentage points between 61st (2004–05) and 68th (2011–12) rounds. Between NSS 50th round (1993–94) and 68th round (2011–12), the LFPR (Labour Force Participation Rate) for rural females decreased by 8 percentage points and 1 percentage point for rural females and urban females respectively (NSSO, 2014).

In both rural and urban areas, about 92 per cent spent most of their time on domestic duties. The main reason cited by women to be engaged in domestic duties and not the formal workforce was the "unavailability of another member to carry out the domestic duties", followed by "unable to afford hired help" and "social and/or religious constraints". For most women, outsourcing unpaid care activities, such as cooking, cleaning or fetching water is not an affordable or realistic option. Their household's daily wellbeing depends on them to carry out these activities (Ferrant et al., 2014). The women who can afford to do so outsource their domestic services to other women and assume the role of supervisors, while the social norm related to the care work remains the same – that it is the primary responsibility of a woman to undertake care work (Dutta & Nandy, 2020).

Table 13.1 gives the percentage of persons aged 15–59 who participated (i.e., participation rate) in different activities during the reference period of 24 hours. Although the participation rates of men and women are similar for socialization and community participation, leisure, and self-care and maintenance, there are some stark differences in other aspects.

The participation rate of men in employment and related activities is more than thrice of that of women. This has direct implications on women's autonomy and productivity and the economy and society as a whole. Although the production of goods and services for own final use is included in economic activities, it is often unpaid (subsistence production). Women are more likely to get involved in unpaid economic activities than men. Furthermore, the extended SNA (or non-economic) unpaid activities, such as domestic and caregiving services for household members, are predominantly done by women.

Table 13.2 shows the gaps in average time (in minutes) spent by men and women aged 15–59 on different activities. In India, women spend 315 minutes per day only on unpaid domestic activities for household members, while men spend a mere 95 minutes on the same activity.

As shown in Table 13.2, women do most of the unpaid activities, while men tend to devote most of their time to paid work. While these general patterns have been changing slowly, they are still the prevalent patterns in much of the world (Antonopoulos, 2008). It is interesting to note that when combined with unpaid work, women work longer hours than men in general.

Figure 13.2 illustrates that women's entry into paid work has not been accompanied by a comparable change in the gender division of unpaid labour in the domestic economy. At large, women remain responsible for a great deal of the unpaid domestic (and caregiving) activities. The available evidence overwhelmingly suggests that women tend to retain responsibility

Table 13.1 Percentage Aged 15–59 Participating in Different Activities in a Day

Description of the activity	Male	Female
Employment and related activities	70.9	21.8
Production of goods for own final use	15.6	22.7
Unpaid domestic services for household members	28.9	92.3
Unpaid caregiving services for household members	16.2	32.8
Unpaid volunteer, trainee, and other unpaid work	2.9	2.2
Learning	14.3	10.9
Socializing and communication, community participation, and religious practice	93.4	92.6
Culture, leisure, mass-media, and sports practices	86.9	83.8
Self-care and maintenance	100.0	100.0

Data Source: Based on Time Use Survey 2019

Table 13.2 Average Time (in Minutes) Spent in a Day Per Participant Aged 15–59

Description of the activity	Male	Female
Employment and related activities	470	343
Production of goods for own final use	198	115
Unpaid domestic services for household members	95	315
Unpaid caregiving services for household members	73	137
Unpaid volunteer, trainee, and other unpaid work	103	100
Learning	421	414
Socializing and communication, community participation, and religious practice	146	136
Culture, leisure, mass-media, and sports practices	144	151
Self-care and maintenance	711	704

Data Source: Based on Time Use Survey 2019

for these activities even if they take up paid employment. As a result, working women tend to work longer hours each day than working men.

The unequal gender distribution of the unpaid activity burden is recognized by the United Nations as an infringement of women's rights and a serious obstacle to empowerment and hence economic development.

According to Dewan et al. (2017), the unpaid caregiving activities of women in India contributes to about 35% of India's GDP and is equivalent to about 182% of the total government tax revenue. Currently, Indian women's paid contribution to the GDP is 17%, which is not only far below the average 37% but is also lower than that of China (41%) and sub-Saharan Africa (39%). Globally, women spend three times more time on unpaid care work than men. However, in India, it is 9.8 times more (NITI Aayog, 2017).

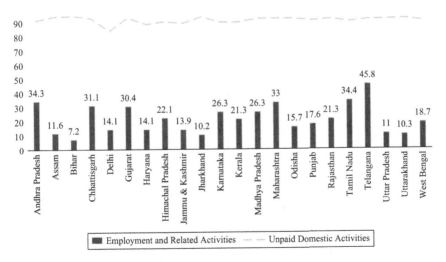

Figure 13.2 Double Burden of Work on Women

Data Source: Based on Time Use Survey, 2019

Unpaid tasks are not counted as part of economic activity because they are difficult to measure based on values in the marketplace. Yet, their economic value is substantial, with estimates ranging from 10 to 60 per cent of GDP (Georgieva et al., 2019). If women were to spend less time on unpaid caregiving activities in India, they would add around USD 300 billion to the GDP (Agrawal, 2019).

Figure 13.3 shows the percentage of females aged six years and above participating in different activities in a day for different levels of education. It is evident that women's participation in unpaid domestic and caregiving activities is notably high where there is low involvement in learning. Here, the graph shows that only 1.7% of illiterate women spend time on learning while 88.9% of illiterate women participate in unpaid domestic activities. A probable reason for such high participation of illiterate women in unpaid activities could be few work opportunities for them in the labour market due to no technical skills. On the other hand, 44.5% of the women who have studied till below primary participate in learning, while 52.6% participate in unpaid domestic activities. There are no significant changes in the participation of women in unpaid caregiving activities, which reiterates that women participate in unpaid caregiving activities irrespective of their educational attainment.

It is also interesting to note that with an increasing level of education, the participation of women in learning declines and that in unpaid domestic

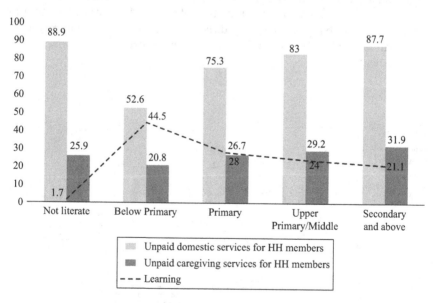

Figure 13.3 Females Aged 6 Years and Above Participating in Different Activities in a Day at Different Levels of Education (%)

Data Source: Based on Time Use Survey, 2019

and caregiving activities increases. Adolescent girls do more housework than boys, which can make it difficult for them to finish secondary school (UNESCO, 2016). Thus, as women advance to higher levels of education, it becomes difficult for them to give time to learning due to their burden of unpaid work.

Men's Involvement in Maternal Healthcare Utilization: Empirical Patterns

Significant improvements in maternal care indicators and men's participation in maternal care have been observed in India between NFHS-4 in 2015–16 and NFHS-5 in 2019–21 (IIPS & ICF, 2017; IIPS, 2022). Women having four or more ANC visits increased from 51.2% in 2015–16 to 58.5% in 2019–21. About 93% of women had at least one antenatal check-up in 2019–21, compared with 83% in 2015–16. In 2015–16, among women who received ANC, about 67% were accompanied by their husbands, while in 2019–21, this number increased to more than 77% (an increase by ten percentage points).

Antenatal Care

ANC is essential for protecting women's health and their unborn children. Figure 13.4a shows the presence of men during ANC in a set of heterogeneous states. Here, Rajasthan from West India, Maharashtra from Central India, Bihar, from East India, Arunachal Pradesh from Northeast India and Karnataka from South India were chosen to investigate the regional variation in men's presence during ANC. Almost 77% of men in India were present during any antenatal check-up of their child. This proportion rises to 90.6% in Karnataka and 84.1% in Rajasthan, while it is merely 55.7% in Bihar.

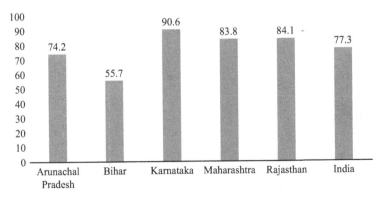

Figure 13.4a Men Who Were Present at Any Antenatal Check-Up (%), 2019–21

Furthermore, almost 82% of men were present during ANC if they had only one child, compared to only 62% of men with four or more children (Table 13.3). Interestingly, men are more actively involved during the birth of their first or second child. However, this enthusiasm seems to fade with more children. 81.4% of urban fathers were present during any ANC, compared to 75.7% of rural fathers. Interestingly, fathers with ten or more years of schooling showed more involvement with their presence during ANC (85.3%), while only 60.6% of men with no schooling were present for any ANC. Similarly, the richest fathers were more engaged (87.5%) than the poorest fathers (62.5%).

When husbands were asked for likely reasons for their partners' not receiving, the most common reason was the cost of ANC, as shown in Table 13.4: 27.5% of husbands reported that ANC cost too much, followed by 21.2% of husbands who felt that ANC was not necessary. Family not allowing ANC was also a common reason (15.5%).

Table 13.3 Male Involvement in Maternal Care by Background Characteristics, India (NFHS 5, 2019–21)

Background characteristic	Percentage of men who were present at any antenatal check-up	Percentage ever told what to do if child's mother had any pregnancy complication
Father's age		
<20	79.0	60.0
20–34	77.0	63.7
35–49	78.6	65.2
Number of children ever born		
1	81.7	67.8
2–3	77.7	63.2
4 or more	62.1	54.9
Residence		
Urban	81.4	66.1
Rural	75.7	63.0
Father's schooling		
No schooling	60.6	49.8
<5 years complete	69.2	60.2
5–7 years complete	72.1	61.9
8–9 years complete	77.2	64.6
10–11 years complete	85.3	69.3
12 or more years complete	84.9	68.5
Wealth status		
Poorest	62.5	57.3
Poorer	74.3	60.5
Middle	80.1	66.1
Richer	85.1	67.4
Richest	87.5	69.9

Table 13.4 Main Reason for not Receiving ANC Reported by Husbands (NFHS-5, 2019–21)

N	756
Family-related reasons	
Husband did not think it was necessary/did not allow	21.2
Family did not think it was necessary/did not allow	15.5
Child's mother did not want check-up	7.8
Has had children before	2.7
Programme-related reasons	
Costs too much	27.5
Too far/no transportation	8.6
No female health worker available	2.9
Other/don't know	13.9

Pregnancy Complications

Table 13.3 shows that older men aged 35–49 were more informed about what to do if the child's mother has any pregnancy complications (65.2%) than younger men aged less than 20 years (60%). Only 55% of men with four or more children were told how to manage pregnancy complications, compared to 68% of men with only one child. A plausible reason could be that men with more children were informed about it during their hospital visits for their previous children. Uneducated and poor fathers were the least informed about what to do if their partner has some pregnancy complications (49.8% – no schooling; 57.3% – poorest), compared to men with ten or more years of schooling (69.3%) and belonging to the richest wealth quintile (69.9%). Over 75% of men in Maharashtra were informed about what to do if their child's mother has any pregnancy complications, followed by 72.2% of men in Rajasthan (Figure 13.4b). However, this proportion drops sharply to 40.4% of men in Bihar, which presents a rather concerning picture.

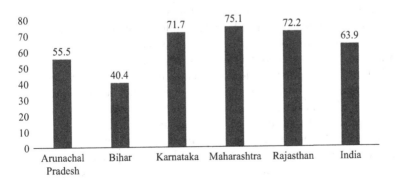

Figure 13.4b Men Ever Told What to Do If Child's Mother had Any Pregnancy Complication (%), 2019–21

Discussion

Helmed as the heads of the household and gatekeepers of care, men play a critical role in addressing the gendered division of labour in household as well as improving the maternal health outcomes and utilization of women. In a traditional Indian household, men have control over access of all household members to resources, which makes them the key link to achieving the sustainable development goals (SDGs) at the household level. SDGs reiterate the importance of ensuring universal access to sexual and reproductive healthcare services. SDGs also recognize the importance of unpaid care and domestic work through public services, infrastructure, and social protection policies as well as shared responsibility within the household. To understand how far women, get support from men, this paper explored men's role in unpaid work and maternal health care of women in India.

Women in India are overwhelmingly burdened by unpaid work accompanied by a declining female labour force participation, which is famously referred to as the defeminization of missing labour force (Abraham, 2013; Rangarajan et al., 2011). In India, despite the laws on equality in property ownership and in wages, the bitter truth of deprivation of women and the widespread prevalence of unequal wages is several times justified in society. In contrast to other "re-emerging" economies, the already poor participation of women in the workforce has been declining. In the last decade, 21 million women have exited the workforce in India (Dewan et al., 2017).

Several social factors are at play here. For instance, the male breadwinner norm can potentially harm female labour force participation. The idea behind a male breadwinner model is centred on men being the primary provider and women naturally assuming the roles of primary caretakers. This phenomenon has given birth to the complex power dynamics in the labour market. Women are typically encouraged to work within the four walls of their house, while men go out to earn. Naturally, it also gives the impression that women do not really "work" and tend to simple house chores. Yet, it couldn't be further from the truth.

Unpaid work is a never-ending drudgery for women, which is often bolstered by inadequate infrastructure, lack of employment opportunities and acceptance of unpaid work as a duty by women. When women have to walk long distances to fetch water and firewood or spend a long time lighting the stove, it limits their participation in social and political activities and leisure. Furthermore, the burden of managing these duties forces women to undertake low-paid and low-quality jobs in the informal market. The lack of basic physical infrastructures such as water, sanitation, roads, and transportation has significantly increased women's time spent on household chores. This gender divide in unpaid work is further linked to unequal employment opportunities and persistent wage gaps. While the lack of basic physical infrastructure and gender stereotypes have a critical role in the gendered division of labour, the upbringing of women also has a role to play. When engaging the subject of unpaid work, we rarely acknowledge the contribution women make in endorsing it, even in the absence of men. In the traditional Indian household setting, women take on the burden of household duties and child-rearing while men earn for the family. Even within a modern context, this deep-rooted construct keeps creating obstacles for women to achieve an equitable distribution of household labour. Evidence shows that even highly educated couples with egalitarian beliefs about the division of labour tend to adopt traditional roles, i.e., men prioritize breadwinning and their careers (Bianchi et al., 2012; Donnelly et al., 2016; Sayer, 2005). At the same time, women shoulder most of the childcare and household chores.

There are strong links between women's economic empowerment and their unpaid activities. Since women are primarily responsible for unpaid activities in their household, it limits their choice of employment. When they do find paid work, the "double burden" of paid activities on top of managing their unpaid activities, adversely impacts the physical and mental wellbeing of women (Sengupta & Sachdeva, 2017). This double work shift means less time for studying, resting, leisure, engaging in social relations, and so on. Women's dominance in unpaid work tends to reduce their status in the labour market. Empirical studies in developing countries have shown that the skewed participation of women in unpaid work, including the care of household members, often prevents women from entering the labour market. Even if they do manage to enter the labour market, they bear the burden of unpaid work and are denied equal competition with men (Esquivel et al., 2008; Hirway, 2008). Since women struggle with traditional norms of caregiving and taking care of households, they lag behind in education and skills, further limiting their paid work opportunities. Women tend to pick up stereotypical jobs such as teaching, nursing and clerical jobs, which are often low-paying or are self-employed as unpaid family helpers with menial job conditions.

Due to the increasing nuclearization of households, there are fewer adult women to lend support to unpaid care and domestic work, putting greater pressure on single/fewer women to perform these tasks (Oxfam India, 2019). Such time deprivation, or commonly known as "time poverty", is indeed a problem. Many women still have their autonomy restricted because much of their time is committed to caring for their households, reducing the time that could be used for paid work. In addition, domestic work also restricts time available for socialization, which is a way to receive information about the labour market (Antonopoulos & Hirway, 2009). In cases where women do take up paid jobs, they are overburdened with domestic labour in addition to their work commitments. Consequently, many women face "time poverty"; i.e., they experience such acute time pressure and anxiety that they often do not get to choose how to allocate their time or indulge in leisure (Kamdar, 2020; Sanghera, 2019).

In shrinking families, such unequal distribution of caring responsibilities between women and men within the household further turns into unequal opportunities in terms of time to participate equally in paid activities. Gender inequality in unpaid care work is the missing link in the analysis related to gender gaps in labour outcomes such as participation rates, quality of employment, and wages (Ferrant et al., 2014). In recent decades, women in many countries have experienced increased freedom in choosing what to do with their own lives, including participation in the labour market. However, this has not been accompanied by a reduction of their responsibilities in the domestic sphere (Antonopoulos & Hirway, 2009).

Another interesting takeaway is the relationship between educational attainment and unpaid domestic and care giving activities of women. Education has a big role in changing a society's gendered norms, which further impacts women's work status (Marphatia & Moussié, 2013). Intriguingly, the participation rate of women in unpaid domestic and caregiving activities between primary school and higher secondary level of education has increased significantly. The higher burden of unpaid work is prominent for urban females aged six years or more than rural females. Increasing educational attainment improves women's skill set and makes it challenging to find suitable employment. The low opportunity cost of unpaid work in a market economy, mostly in urban areas, restricts the choice of women to go for paid work, and they tend to take up all the unpaid domestic and caregiving work. On the other hand, women with no education are unable to find proper jobs due to lack of education and end up taking on the drudgery of unpaid work. Here, the role of men becomes rather critical. With men taking on their share of unpaid duties of the household, women have better opportunities to enter the labour market. An adult literacy programme in rural Nepal boosted the acknowledgement of women's unpaid work by family and community by involving marginalized women and men in gathering data on women's use of time (Marphatia & Moussié, 2013). In some areas, this helped to establish a more equitable division of women's unpaid care duties. Unpaid care and domestic work fall within the ambit of gender inequality leading to unequal opportunities for women in the labour market (Mehrotra & Sinha, 2017). It is a retrogressive development, both for women's autonomy and for an economy undergoing structural transformation. This is because most paid jobs went to men, and the unpaid jobs were left for women to take up.

In short, unless labour policies are designed with women's unpaid work and social barriers in mind, gender disparities in labour market outcomes cannot be eliminated. Another important area of gender inequality is the time burden of women's unpaid work and overall work. The first step in ensuring gender equality and women's empowerment is to make unpaid services visible in data and policymaking. This means governments need to conduct regular time-use surveys to understand the amount and characteristics of unpaid work. Unpaid work is excluded from traditional GDP data, so it is important to cash this work so that its contribution to human wellbeing can be compared to paid work. Another approach is to reduce the pain of unpaid work by improving technology and infrastructure and access to basic services. Unpaid work is usually neglected in macroeconomic policies. There is a strong need to address this oversight. The lack of public sector facilities such as basic infrastructure, nursing homes, daycare facilities, and affordable private sector services is driving women out of the workforce, increasingly burdened with care and household chores. The states where the participation of women in paid work is higher have a better childcare provision system. For instance, states like Andhra Pradesh, Tamil Nadu, and Maharashtra have a high proportion of functional creches under the Rajiv Gandhi National Creche Scheme (RGNCS) for children of working mothers. These are also the states which see a high proportion of women involved in paid employment and related activities. The policy on paid leave for parenthood (maternal and paternal) has implications for new parents. There is a need for more studies to explore the impact of shorter paternity leaves and longer maternity leaves on women. There have been speculations that extension of maternity leaves further makes it difficult for women/new mothers to rejoin the workforce and get stuck in the drudgery of unpaid work. However, such findings cannot be justified with available evidence as of now. Therefore, the current need of the hour to address the burden of unpaid work on women is flexible working arrangements, parental leave, affordable child care, social security, pension credits, tax allowances, and care services for the elderly.

Healthy reproduction and childcare are possible only if the individual and their partner are both concerned with the illness and the benefits of care (Bloom et al., 2000). Therefore, without the participation of men, it is difficult to improve women's access to health care and the labour market (Bhalerao et al., 1984). Studies show that the husband's knowledge of pregnancy and childbirth was a significant determinant of the wife's maternal healthcare utilization, regardless of the stage of development the husband is in.

India has shown tremendous improvement in maternal healthcare utilization with the active participation of husbands/partners. The present study shows that more than nine in every ten pregnant women received at least ANC, with more than three-fourths of them (77%) accompanied by their partners. National Rural Health Mission, a Government of India health initiative that expanded MCH services to disadvantaged rural areas, played a crucial role in this progress (Taneja et al., 2019). However, there are stark differences at the state level, with Bihar severely lagging.

Regional variances in ANC use could be attributed to differences in the economy, education, access, and distance to health facilities, and the quality of the services provided (Ogbo et al., 2019; Pathak et al., 2010; Rani et al., 2008). One of the pressing issues in the poor utilization of maternal healthcare services in Bihar is inadequate infrastructure, which is failing the mothers. It is often amplified by poor communication between the mother and healthcare providers, especially in the absence of husbands. Lack of separate, well-equipped rooms, shortage of qualified staff, and overwhelmed healthcare workers lower pregnant women's effective and efficient healthcare utilization. A low patient–healthcare worker ratio may cause healthcare providers to multitask, which increases their workload and thus fail to provide services to the patients while maintaining a satisfactory level. Men often act as catalysts and facilitators for maternal healthcare utilization, but the biggest problem remains involving men in discussions. Due to rigid social norms, states like Bihar often tend to alienate men from maternal healthcare despite men controlling access to sexual and reproductive health information and services, finances, transportation, and other resources. For a better understanding, studies that evaluate region-specific determinants of ANC uptake and men's involvement in ANC utilization may be required to inform an equal distribution of MCH resources and policy at the subnational level in India.

Consistent with previous studies (Chattopadhyay, 2012; Chattopadhyay & Govil, 2020), the present study found a strong need to address the involvement of rural, poor, and illiterate men in maternal health. The low participation of men in these strata further translates into poor maternal healthcare utilization for women. Past studies (Ganle & Dery, 2015) have identified four main barriers to men's involvement in maternal healthcare utilization, including: a) masculinity and male role conflicts; 2) cultural beliefs and practices; 3) health services factors such as unfavourable opening hours of services, poor attitudes of healthcare providers, and lack of space to accommodate male partners in health facilities; and 4) the high cost associated with accompanying women to seek maternity care. Along similar lines, this study shows that family-related reasons were the main reasons for women's non-utilization of maternal health care, i.e., the partner and/or family did not think that ANC was necessary. This concerning finding could be a result of limited exposure to safe motherhood initiative programs. The reproductive health of a woman in India is a matter of family concern. There is a need for awareness programmes with men at the centre, as disinterest and insufficient knowledge of men are catastrophic to maternal health in the long run. Following family apathy, the cost of ANC, transportation issues and lack of female healthcare workers threaten complete ANC utilization of women. Transportation poses a huge challenge as health centres are spread far across rural areas. In such cases, the family does not prefer to allow women to go to the health centre without the husband. Therefore, women's ANC checkups depend on the availability of their husbands. Furthermore, if no female health workers are available, patients do not feel comfortable enough to consent to a check-up. Considering the cultural dynamics, it is important to have female health workers present during the check-up of pregnant women. Also, there is a need to train the staff of the sub-centres and primary healthcare centres (PHCs) in maternal healthcare services, to ensure having auxiliary nurse midwives (ANM workers) in each clinic and to strengthen the motherhood awareness initiatives, especially for men.

Therefore, there is no doubt about the appropriateness of husband inclusion in the MCH policy. Even the landmark study by Raju & Leonard (2000) shows that women need and want the support of their partners to access reproductive health services. Men are interested in participating in reproductive health issues, especially when it concerns their children and families. Therefore, healthcare providers, including outreach workers, need specialized training to support male participation further. There is ample evidence that male ignorance, apathy, and lack of interest act as barriers to achieving the goals of MCH. The dynamics of power relations within households are key factors in this regard. There is a need to empower women, value men equally, and disseminate good knowledge among men. Therefore, the support of men in all aspects is a necessary prerequisite for quality maternal health care and childcare.

Conclusion

Addressing the disproportionate burden of unpaid care and family work by women is not only the responsibility of households and communities but also the responsibility of the state. Public policies that allocate resources to recognize, reduce, and reallocate unpaid care services in terms of money, services, and time are called care policies. These include the direct provision of child and aged care services, the transfer of social protection and care-related benefits to workers with family responsibilities, unpaid caregivers, or people in need of care. They also include strengthening infrastructure to reduce women's hardship, such as water access, sanitation, and energy supply. At the household level, the valuation of unpaid work and redistribution of the division of labour is possible only when men are consciously engaged.

Public investment in basic infrastructure and family-friendly policies expand women's opportunities for productive employment, overcoming their socioeconomic disadvantage. Promoting a more equitable share of unpaid care and family activities between women and men would also help challenge stereotypes and change social norms, potentially transforming the household.

References

Abraham, V. (2013). Missing labour or consistent "de-feminisation"? *Economic and Political Weekly*, 99–108.

Dewan, R., Sehgal, R., Kanchi, A., & Raju, S. (2017). *Invisible work, invisible workers: The sub-economies of unpaid work and paid work*. UN Women and ActionAid.

Agénor, P.-R., & Canuto, O. (2012). Access to infrastructure and women's time allocation: Evidence and a framework for policy analysis. *Policy Paper*, 45.

Agrawal, M. (2019). It is not your job: Unpaid care work in India. https://www.oxfamindia.org/blog/unpaid-care-work-in-india

Antonopoulos, R. (2008). *The unpaid care work-paid work connection*. Levy Economics Institute, Working Papers Series.

Antonopoulos, R., & Hirway, I. (Eds.). (2009). *Unpaid work and the economy: Gender, time-use and poverty in developing countries*. Palgrave Macmillan.

Bhalerao, V. R., Galwankar, M. M., Kowli, S. S., Kumar, R. R., & Chaturvedi, R. M. (1984). Contribution of the education of the prospective fathers to the success of maternal health care programme. *Journal of Postgraduate Medicine*, 30(1), 10.

Bianchi, S. M., Sayer, L. C., Milkie, M. A., & Robinson, J. P. (2012). Housework: Who did, does or will do it, and how much does it matter? *Social Forces*, 91(1), 55–63.

Bloom, S. S., Tsui, A. O., Plotkin, M., & Bassett, S. (2000). What husbands in northern India know about reproductive health: Correlates of knowledge about pregnancy and maternal and sexual health. *Journal of Biosocial Science*, 32(2), 237–251.

Chattopadhyay, A. (2012). Men in maternal care: Evidence from India. *Journal of Biosocial Science*, 44(2), 129–153. https://doi.org/10.1017/S0021932011000502

Chattopadhyay, A., & Govil, D. (2020). Men and maternal health care utilization in India and in selected less-developed states: Evidence from a large-scale survey 2015–16. *Journal of Biosocial Science*, 53(5), 724–744.

Craymah, J. P., Oppong, R. K., & Tuoyire, D. A. (2017). Male involvement in maternal health care at Anomabo, central region, Ghana. *International Journal of Reproductive Medicine*, 1–8.

Das, M. B. (2006). Do traditional axes of exclusion affect labor market outcomes in India? Available at SSRN 1919070.

Das, M. S., Jain-Chandra, M. S., Kochhar, M. K., & Kumar, N. (2015). *Women workers in India: Why so few among so many?* International Monetary Fund.

Donnelly, K., Twenge, J. M., Clark, M. A., Shaikh, S. K., Beiler-May, A., & Carter, N. T. (2016). Attitudes toward women's work and family roles in the United States, 1976–2013. *Psychology of Women Quarterly*, 40(1), 41–54.

Dutta, D., & Nandy, A. (2020). *On women's backs: India inequality report 2020*. Oxfam India.

Elson, D. (2017). Recognize, reduce, and redistribute unpaid care work: How to close the gender gap. *New Labor Forum*, 26(2), 52–61.

Esquivel, V., Budlender, D., Folbre, N., &Hirway, I. (2008). Explorations: Time-use surveys in the south. *Feminist Economics*, 14(3), 107–152.

Ferrant, G., Pesando, L. M., & Nowacka, K. (2014). *Unpaid care work: The missing link in the analysis of gender gaps in labour outcomes*. OECD Development Center.

Ganle, J. K., &Dery, I. (2015). 'What men don't know can hurt women's health': A qualitative study of the barriers to and opportunities for men's involvement in maternal healthcare in Ghana. *Reproductive Health*, 12(1), 1–13.

Ganle, J. K., Dery, I., Manu, A. A., & Obeng, B. (2016). 'If I go with him, I can't talk with other women': Understanding women's resistance to, and acceptance of, men's involvement in maternal and child healthcare in northern Ghana. *Social Science & Medicine*, 166, 195–204.

Georgieva, K., Alonso, C., Dabla-Norris, E., & Kochhar, K. (2019). *The economic cost of devaluing "womens work."* https://blogs.imf.org/2019/10/15/the-economic-cost-of-devaluing-womens-work/

Ghosh, J. (2009). Informalization and Women's Workforce Participation. In *The Gendered Impacts of Liberalization: Towards" Embedded Liberalism"?*, ed. S. Razavi (pp. 163–190). New York: Routledge.

Himmelweit, S. (1995). The discovery of "unpaid work": The social consequences of the expansion of "work." *Feminist Economics*, 1(2), 1–19.

Hirway, I. (2008). Equal sharing of responsibilities between men and women: Some issues with reference to labour and employment. Paper Prepared and Presented at the Expert Group Meeting on 'Equal Sharing of Responsibilities between Men and Women, Including Care-Giving in the Context of HIV/AIDS', United Nations Division for the Advancement of Women, Geneva, 6–9.

Hirway, I. (2015). Unpaid work and the economy: Linkages and their implications. *Indian Journal of Labour Economics*, 58(1), 1–21.

Kabeer, N. (2008). *Paid work, women's empowerment and gender justice: Critical pathways of social change.* Pathways of Empowerment working papers (3). Institute of Development Studies, Brighton.

Kabeer, N. (2019). Women's empowerment and the question of choice. *Journal of International Affairs*, 72(2), 209–214.

Kabeer, N. (2021). Gender equality, inclusive growth, and labour markets. In *Women's economic empowerment: Insights from Africa and South Asia* (pp. 13–48). Routledge.

Kamdar, B. (2020). *India's women bear the burden of unpaid work: With costs to themselves and the economy: The diplomat.* https://thediplomat.com/2020/11/indias-women-bear-the-burden-of-unpaid-work-with-costs-to-themselves-and-the-economy/

Kidder, T., Romana, S., Canepa, C., Chettleborough, J., & Molina, C. (2017). *Oxfam's conceptual framework on women's economic empowerment.* Oxfam. https://doi.org/10.21201/2017.9682.

Marphatia, A. A., &Moussié, R. (2013). A question of gender justice: Exploring the linkages between women's unpaid care work, education, and gender equality. *International Journal of Educational Development*, 33(6), 585–594.

Mehrotra, S., & Sinha, S. (2017). Explaining falling female employment during a high growth period. *Economic & Political Weekly*, 52(39), 54–62.

Mullany, B. C. (2010). Spousal agreement on maternal health practices in Kathmandu, Nepal. *Journal of Biosocial Science*, 42(5), 689–693.

Nagawa, E. S. (1994). Absent husbands, unsupportive in-laws and rural African mothers. *Reproductive Health Matters*, 2(4), 46–54.

National Sample Survey Organization. (2014). *Participation of women in specified activities along with domestic duties (68th round, July 2011–June 2012).*

National Sample Survey Organization. (2020). *Time use survey.*

Neetha, N., & Palriwala, R. (2019). Unpaid care work: Analysis of the Indian time use data. In *Time use studies and unpaid care work* (pp. 114–139). Routledge.

NITI Aayog. (2017). *Towards building a more inclusive society. Three year action agenda 2017–18 to 2019–20; Chapter 22.*

Ntabona, A. B. (2002). *Involving men in safe motherhood: The issues.* World Health Organization.

OECD. (2017). *The pursuit of gender equality: An uphill battle.* OECD Publishing. https://doi.org/10.1787/9789264281318-en

Ogbo, F. A., Dhami, M. V., Ude, E. M., Senanayake, P., Osuagwu, U. L., Awosemo, A. O., Ogeleka, P., Akombi, B. J., Ezeh, O. K., & Agho, K. E. (2019). Enablers and barriers to the utilization of antenatal care services in India. *International Journal of Environmental Research and Public Health*, 16(17), 3152.

Oxfam India. (2019). *Mind the Gap: The State of Employment in India.* Oxfam.

Pathak, P. K., Singh, A., & Subramanian, S. V. (2010). Economic inequalities in maternal health care: Prenatal care and skilled birth attendance in India, 1992–2006. *PloS One*, 5(10), e13593.

Plantin, L., Olykoya, A., & Ny, P. (2011). Positive health outcomes of fathers' involvement in pregnancy and childbirth paternal support: A scope study literature review. *Fathering: A Journal of Theory, Research, and Practice about Men as Fathers*, 9(1), 87–102.

Rahman, A. E., Perkins, J., Islam, S., Siddique, A. B., Moinuddin, M., Anwar, M. R., Mazumder, T., Ansar, A., Rahman, M. M., & Raihana, S. (2018). Knowledge and involvement of husbands in maternal and newborn health in rural Bangladesh. *BMC Pregnancy and Childbirth, 18*(1), 1–12.

Raju, S., & Leonard, A. (2000). *Men as supportive partners in reproductive health: Moving from rhetoric to reality.* Population Council.

Rangarajan, C., Kaul, P. I., & Seema. (2011). Where is the missing labour force? *Economic and Political Weekly,* 68–72.

Rani, M., Bonu, S., & Harvey, S. (2008). Differentials in the quality of antenatal care in India. *International Journal for Quality in Health Care, 20*(1), 62–71.

Sanghera, T. (2019). *Time poverty: Unpaid work keeps Indian women out of jobs, disempowered.* https://www.business-standard.com/article/current-affairs/time-poverty-indian-women-spend-a-huge-portion-of-their-day-on-unpaid-work-119032500121_1.html

Sayer, L. C. (2005). Gender, time and inequality: Trends in women's and men's paid work, unpaid work and free time. *Social Forces, 84*(1), 285–303.

Sengupta, S., & Sachdeva, S. (2017). *From double burden of women to a "double boon": Balancing unpaid care work and paid work.* (GrOW Research Series Policy Brief). New Delhi, India: Institute of Social Studies Trust.

Singh, A., & Ram, F. (2009). Men's involvement during pregnancy and childbirth: Evidence from rural Ahmednagar, India. *Population Review, 48*(1), 83–102.

Singh, P., & Pattanaik, F. (2020). Unfolding unpaid domestic work in India: Women's constraints, choices, and career. *Palgrave Communications, 6*(1), 1–13.

Sweetman, C. (2013). Introduction: Working with men on gender equality. *Gender & Development, 21*(1), 1–13.

Taneja, G., Sridhar, V. S.-R., Mohanty, J. S., Joshi, A., Bhushan, P., Jain, M., Gupta, S., Khera, A., Kumar, R., & Gera, R. (2019). India's RMNCH+ A Strategy: Approach, learnings and limitations. *BMJ Global Health, 4*(3), e001162.

Turan, J. M., Tesfagiorghis, M., &Polan, M. L. (2011). Evaluation of a community intervention for promotion of safe motherhood in Eritrea. *Journal of Midwifery & Women's Health, 56*(1), 8–17.

UNESCO. (2016). *Global education monitoring report summary 2016: Education for people and planet: Creating sustainable futures for all.* United Nations Educational, Scientific and Cultural Organization.

UNFPA, & Promundo. (2018). *Engaging men in unpaid care work: An advocacy brief for Eastern Europe and Central Asia|Promundo.* https://promundoglobal.org/resources/engaging-men-unpaid-care-work-advocacy-brief-eastern-europe-central-asia/

Varkey, L. C., Mishra, A., Das, A., Ottolenghi, E., Huntington, D., Adamchak, S., Khan, M. E., & Homan, F. (2004). *Involving men in maternity care in India* (p. 62). Population Council.

Yargawa, J., & Leonardi-Bee, J. (2015). Male involvement and maternal health outcomes: Systematic review and meta-analysis. *Journal of Epidemiology and Community Health, 69*(6), 604 LP–612. https://doi.org/10.1136/jech-2014-204784

14 Quality of Maternal Health Care in Public Hospitals of Uttar Pradesh

A Case Study of Lucknow District

Sonia Verma and C S Verma

Introduction

Mothers and children were first recognized as vulnerable groups in the primary healthcare movement by the Alma Ata statement in 1978 (World Health Report, 2005). This was a significant change in the healthcare system because it highlighted the importance of health as a human right, highlighted justice in the distribution of resources, and increased access through decentralized services geared at promoting community involvement, addressing local health issues, and providing preventative and promotional healthcare (Cooper et al., 2004). Further, the Cairo conference (1994) defined women's health by giving women's rights top priority and encouraging safer childbirth. The historic Programme of Action (POA) was a turning point in human history, from worries about population control and fertility regulation to the promotion of women's human and reproductive health and rights within a development context. Maternal and child health services are a subset of reproductive health services, and by the Year 2015, governments were to offer universal access to these services as part of primary health care.

At the United Nations Millennium Summit in 2000, a declaration was made with the goal of halving the number of people living in severe poverty by 2015. It is a well-acknowledged fact that all of the Millenium Development Goals were interconnected and supportive of one another to varying degrees. It was realized that in order to enhance maternal health, goal five must reduce the maternal mortality ratio by 75 per cent between 1990 and 2015 (Freedman et al., 2005; World Health Report, 2005). Maternal health is a result of the interaction between our biology and the physical, socioeconomic, cultural, and political environments in which we live, or in other words, it is a socially determined act. As a result, socioeconomic class inequalities as well as biological variances contribute to differences in people's health status. Many aspects of health may be influenced by social class, colour, ethnicity, gender, and other social determinants, including risk and vulnerability, health-seeking behaviour, and access to health care (Ravindran, 2012).

India is responsible for at least 25 per cent of all maternal deaths reported internationally since the Safe Motherhood Initiative started. As per the latest data from Sample Registration System (2018–20), MMR in India is reduced

DOI: 10.4324/9781003430636-19

to 97 per 100,000 live births, but achieving the targets of sustainable development, the country is still far off. Furthermore, MMR is varying among the states and it is significantly high in Empowered Action Group (EAG) states. The recent data on MMR show 137 per 1000 live birth in the EAG states, in southern states MMR is 49, and for others, it is 76 per 1000 live birth. Though there has been several periodic initiative taken for the improvement of the MMR in the state but nothing much could be achieved. Along with the health system issues, economy, geography and socio-cultural challenges made it difficult to implement health sector reform uniformaly across the state/s. The situation worsen in the EAG states as they lag behind some of the better performing states.

As an SDG mandate, the MMR is not only an important indicator of maternal health of a population but also the development index for any nation. Maternal health is a major public health concern in India, and monitoring MMR is necessary due to large inter and intra-state differences. Results from a sizable study demonstrated that the MMR did not decline over time point to a critical public health issue. It has been discovered that pregnancy-related illnesses and birth complications are the main causes of death and disability among women of reproductive age. The health of mothers and newborns is negatively impacted by malnutrition, poverty, illiteracy, filthy living conditions, diseases, and unrestrained fertility. Ineffective public health services and poor infrastructure are other factors contributing to subpar obstetric care. The accurate evaluation of the issue could be followed thanks to the availability of MMR estimates and causes of maternal mortality (Chhabra, 2014).

Maternal mortality is a complex phenomenon that are influenced by a number of factors, including economic position, educational attainment, age, caste, religion, and lack of information, in varied contexts (Kuswaha et al., 2008). The importance of maternal health care to the overall healthcare system is well established. To achieve faster and more equitable improvements in maternal and child health outcomes across the country, the government of India launched the National Rural Health Mission (NRHM) in 2005, which expanded into the National Health Mission (NHM) in 2013 (Department of Health and Family Welfare 2013–14). The programme focused on infrastructural and human resources strengthening across public health facilities to expand coverage of maternal and child healthcare services. Interventions included a nationwide conditional cash transfer programme, which was launched to promote institutional delivery with an emphasis on free provision of drugs, diagnostics, and drop-back facilities for pregnant women and mothers. In addition, a large network of community health workers was established to improve healthcare knowledge and awareness and as well as linkages between communities and the public health system (Department of Health and Family Welfare 2013–14).

However, there has not been much empirical research done in specific nations to determine how different aspects of the health system can affect maternal health outcomes (Banerjee, 2003). Quality of healthcare facilities is one of the important aspects to understand the improved health outcomes. It has been well established globally that unless there is sufficient quality facility available at institutions it is unlikely to improve maternal and neonatal birth outcomes at facilities. The idea of quality of care is intricate and multifaceted. The term "quality of care" has a wide range of meanings, from "degree to which health services for individuals and populations increase the chance of desired health outcomes and are compatible with current professional knowledge" to "degree to which expectations or goals have been reached" (Samuel et al., 1994). Ability to access effective care on an efficient and equitable basis for the optimization of health benefit/well-being for the entire population is a definition of quality of care at the population level (Cambell et al., 200). There are only two questions that capture all aspects of care quality. First, is the care accessible so that a person may access it when they need it. Second, is the care they receive effective in terms of both clinical and interpersonal relationships? When used at the individual level, this concept of quality of care is suitable.

India's most populous state, Uttar Pradesh (UP) one of the EAG states, consists of about 200 million residents, or about one-sixth of the country's total population. The MMR in Uttar Pradesh for the years 2012–13 was 258 per 100,000 live births, according to the Annual Health Survey (AHS). In 2013, there were 50 infant deaths for every 1000 live births. In UP, the rates of maternal and newborn mortality are both decreasing. From 517 maternal deaths per 100,000 live births in 2001–02 to 258 in 2012–13, the maternal mortality rate has decreased by almost half. Similar to this, since 2006, the infant mortality rate has decreased by 23 points, from 73 per 1,000 live births to 50 in 2013. The utilization of key maternal and child health services has also been improving in the state. The proportion of institutional deliveries has almost tripled from 21% in 2002–04 to 57% in 2012–13.

In addition to the commencement of the *"Hausla"* campaign to rescue mothers and children across the state, the Government of Uttar Pradesh (GoUP) has relaunched its effort to enhance reproductive, maternity, neonatal, child, and adolescent health (RMNCH+A) in its 25 high-focus districts throughout the state. Investment in health and development with a focus on RMNCH+A through the National Health Mission has been a significant priority of the Government of Uttar Pradesh (GoUP). In order to improve RMNCH+A in UP, the NHM has brought attention, resources, and technical initiatives. The NHM has brought focus, resources, and technical strategies for improving RMNCH+A in UP, as it has elsewhere in India. While government investment in health and development has increased significantly over the past ten years and outcomes have improved significantly as well, more work needs to be done to increase the quality and coverage of essential health services in order to meet the state's lofty health and development goals.

In this study, an attempt is made to understand the quality of care in health facilities that influences maternal health outcomes in Uttar Pradesh.

In this study, the term "quality of care" is an attempt to draw a connection between the institution where the child was born and the health facilities that are critical to making birthing a good experience. As there are a number of events that go around a number of factors that may seem irrelevant but play an important role in the overall birthing experience. The gravity of the phenomenon varies based on other external factors like location of the hospital, skilled/unskilled manpower, availability of emergency services, and the behavior of the treating health personnel and so on.

From the literature, we have learnt that the range for the quality of care in maternal health is huge; however, the present study has discussed the factors that should be present in the health facility for quality maternal health. The idea behind such an approach is to understand how the quality of maternal health is governed by the facilities present in the health centres which guide success of institutional delivery and hence better birthing experience for the mothers. It is important to understand that it is never that the numbers (MMR) are important and but to explore the story behind those numbers to know the mechanisms contributing to poor outcomes.

Methods

The data for the present study were collected in 2018 in the month of November and December by using a cross-sectional study design on a pre-tested questionnaire by interviewing women who had delivered children during the past 15 days in the government health facilities of Lucknow district of Uttar Pradesh. A different set of questionnaire was administered for the service provider as well. It was not surprising that most of the service providers did not participate in the study on the pretext of busy schedules.

The district is the capital city of the most populous state of India. Since the health facilities in the district carry most of the patients hailing from the neighbouring district, almost all the health facilities were found to be overburdened with the caseload.

To make the research more feasible, it was deemed to select not more than four facilities in different geographical locations considering the proximity and convenience of inflow of the patients from the neighbouring district. From the four health facilities, a total of 36 women were selected as a study sample, nine from each facility. The two service providers who agreed to participate in the study were one staff nurse of a CHC and one pharmacist of the CHC.

It was very challenging to have a conversation with women who gave birth in the health facility as most of the women with normal (vaginal) delivery leave the hospital even before the completion 24 hours of the delivery. Most of the caesarean cases stay back in the health facility for two–three days post-delivery. Pseudo-names have been used while presenting the results in order to maintain confidentiality.

Results

The background details of the respondents (patients) show that most of the women were of the age group of 15–24 years and belonged to the rural area. These women were primary educated, which means they were able to write their names and simple sentences in their mother tongue, i.e. Hindi. The last row of table 14.1 shows the respondent's experience with the quality of care received at the particular facility.

Though the indicators *"access to quality care"* entails other components that are important to consider while deliberating on it, they are discussed further in detail in the coming section. The major issues emerged during the interview related to quality of care are explained below

Shortage of Specialist Professionals

It is not a hidden fact that the country or to be more precise, the state of Uttar Pradesh is having severe dearth of the medical specialist, but the condition become serious when it comes to the public health facility. The health facilities selected for the study though were present in the urban fringes of the city, but these facilities were mostly catering the rural patients. While data collection it was found that the specialist required during the child birth especially in caesarean section were on-call. This implies that whenever there was requirement of the specialist they were informed about the requirement and based on their availability they attended the patients. It was also found that when there were no specialist present in the facility, the cases were either referred to nearest district

Table 14.1 Responses of the Care Seekers

Age Group (Years)	No.	%
15–24	19	52.77
25–34	13	36.11
35–45	4	11.11
Place of residence		
Urban	5	13.889
Rural	31	86.11
Education level		
Illiterate	5	13.88
Primary	16	44.44
Secondary	15	41.667
Access to quality care		
Good	14	38.88
Poor	22	61.11
Total number of women	**36**	**100**

hospital or were denied from admitting/attending. The two instances were recorder from the field-

> "*Yesterday a pregnant woman came to the hospital in the midnight for delivery, she was lying next to me the staff in the hospital (Staff-nurse) tried very hard for normal delivery but the case was complicated and C section was required, but the Madam who does the C-section was herself on maternity leave. So, she was sent to Big (District) Hospital.*"
> (Meera/23 years old/Primi mother)

> "*No body wants to come here, as there are not good staff, if I could have afford, I too would have gone to the Private hospital like other.*"
> (Somu/27 years old/mother of three)

Although most of the public health facilities where deliveries (child birth) happen operate 24/7, this was not the case in the study sample hospital.

> "*Mostly staffs Nurse are available in the night shift; Maam (Doctor) leaves the hospital by afternoon as soon as OPD gets over.*"
> (Julia/31 years/staff nurse)

Insufficient Necessary Infrastructure

During the data collection, it became evident that the present infrastructure is not sufficient to cater for the patients. It was observed the mother in labour-pain was lying on the floor, waiting for "4cm cervix dilation" as beds were not allotted to them. The toilets in some of the hospitals were so dirty that anyone can easily catch urinary tract infection if used.

> "*We stay here for emergency services but there is no room for us to stay, and the washrooms are so bad that we don't use it.*"
> (Anita/32 years/staff nurse)

Lack of Emergency Services

Blood banks are one of the most important and critical emergency facility that was found to be missing from almost all the health facilities visited. The lack of emergency services leads to most of the denial of the patients. The respondents' knowledge about the emergency services was poor and it seems they did not find it an important component of safe delivery.

> "*Though my blood (haemoglobin) was very less, was 8gm, ANM madam (who does ANC) told me blood transfusion will be (might be) required during my delivery, but see doctor managed my delivery with-out it (blood). We just expect decent behaviour from the hospital staff rest we can manage on our own.*"
> (Durga/25 years/mother of three)

Absence of Ambulance Transportation Services

It was recorded that most of the people visited the hospital and went back to their homes by their own conveyance. Most of the respondents who agreed to respond informed that the ambulance service was not readily available and also they charged the patient for ferrying them to the hospital and dropping them back to their houses. This was the reason they preferred using their own vehicle.

It was also noted that there was an ambulance parked on one of the hospital premises and probing further it was found that the appointment of the driver and ambulance technician is in process, that's why the ambulance is yet to start its fleet.

Though efforts were made to take the in-depth interview with the service providers in these facilities, most of them turned down the request on the pretext of work workload and those who agreed to respond were not very comfortable with recording their interview.

Quality Care

While interviewing the hospital staff with regard to utilization of services by patients and role of service provider, it was stated that provision of quality service delivery has a direct relation with service utilization.

> *"The women who received good quality of care from the health personnel are more likely to use antenatal care, compared to the women who received poor quality of care. The use of antenatal care was also significantly associated with quality of care received by the women."*
> (Dev/37 years/pharmacist)

> *"there are no basic facilities available in the hospital and the hospital premises, hence no doctor wants to stay here during the night time."*
> (Suraj/26 years/hospital staff)

Discussion

Interviews with the respondents who came for delivering their babies showed their dissatisfaction with the quality-of-service delivery and facilities provided at the hospital. The respondents were mainly young women who travelled from rural areas. More than three-fourths of respondents stated the quality of service provided in facilities is not good. Lack of staff, unavailability of doctors during the need, and lack of ambulance facilities are stated as the major challenges of accessing health services from institutions. The provider's behaviour with the client also is observed to be an important aspect of quality of care that affects the use of services.

The study found very low quality of delivery care across the study facilities. The analysis indicates crucial deficiencies in staffing, infrastructure, referral systems, and routine and emergency care practices. The facilities lacked skilled healthcare providers and those present in the facilities were not available for 24 h per day which hampered even the referral facility for the pregnant women to higher-level facilities if needed. These are concerning given facts for quality of maternal health in any population.

The quality of care has an independent and significant effect on the use of antenatal care indicating emphasis should be laid on providing good quality care in order to improve the health of pregnant women. The government should continue the communication programme highlighting the importance of antenatal care on print and electronic channels of mass media.

Overall, the study shows quality of maternal care in the public hospitals of Lucknow district is compromised due to a shortage of specialist doctors and necessary infrastructure. The situation is further aggravated by inappropriate geographical locations of the health centres.

Pre- and post-delivery care of mothers is as important as the delivery itself. However, hospital care in PHCs and CHCs needs substantial improvement. The absence of blood banks even at the combined hospitals restricts doctors from taking risks in tackling complicated cases. Due to these bottlenecks, patients who utilize the maternal services in these institutions do not get the sense of accomplishment of staying in the hospitals. A focused approach towards maternal health would require adequate human resources, equipment, and commitment to improving maternal health.

Maternal mortality has generally been accepted as an indicator of how well a health system functions (Srivastva et al., 2014), but at the same time those who have experienced the services provided by the health system also narrates a lot about it. The quality of maternal health these women have experienced tells a lot about the important things that are missing. The reflections obtained from them have clearly shown that the present health system needs further preparation in order to provide quality maternal healthcare services for the pregnant women.

Conclusion

Maternal mortality is widely accepted as a key indicator of health and socioeconomic development. It is a reflection of the whole national health system and represents the outcome of its cons and pros along with its other characteristics such as intersectoral collaboration, transparency, and disparities. Decreasing maternal mortality requires dealing with various factors other than individual determinants including political will, reallocation of national resources (especially health resources) in the governmental sector, education, and attention to the expansion of the private sector trade and improving spectrums of governance. These findings are believed to be beneficial for sustainable development in the Post-2015 Development Agenda.

Social determinants of health play a large role in women's ability to achieve maternal and reproductive health. It is therefore important to consider the role of social, cultural, health system, and economic factors that impact maternal health, and ultimately maternal mortality. At least 20% of the burden of disease among children under five is attributable to conditions directly associated with poor maternal and reproductive health, nutrition, and quality of obstetric and newborn care (Lule et al., 2005). Strengthening maternal and reproductive health services can also benefit the health system as a whole, enhancing access and use of a broader number of reproductive healthcare services (Lule et al., 2005).

Research on maternal mortality suffered from robust methodological design to produce knowledge about macrostructural causes of maternal mortality. Although health care plays a critical role in maternal mortalities, the effects of other factors, e.g. female education and accessibility to health facilities, should not be neglected. However, the reasons for higher declines in MMR in some countries and the absence of progress in others have not been fully discovered.

References

Banerjee, B. (2003). A qualitative analysis of maternal and child health services of an urban health centre, by assessing client perception in terms of awareness, satisfaction and service utilization. *Indian Journal of Community Medicine, 28*(4), 153–156.

Campbell, S. M., Roland, M. O., & Buetow, S. A. (2000). Defining quality of care. *Social Science & Medicine, 51*(11), 1611–1625.

Census of India. (2011). *Provisional Population Totals; Rural Urban Distribution.*

Chhabra, P. (2014 Jul). Maternal near miss: An indicator for maternal health and maternal care. *Indian Journal of Community Medicine, 39*(3), 132–7. doi: 10.4103/0970-0218.137145. PMID: 25136152; PMCID: PMC4134527.

Cooper, D., Morroni, C., Orner, P., Moodley, J., Harries, J., Cullingworth, L., & Hoffman, M. (2004). Ten years of democracy in South Africa: Documenting transformation in reproductive health policy and status. *Reproductive Health Matters, 12*(24), 70–85.

Estimates by WHO, UNICEF, UNFPA, The World Bank and the United Nations Population Division; Trends in maternal mortality: 1990 to 2013.

Freedman, L. P. (2005). Achieving the MDGs: Health systems as core social institutions. *Development, 48*(1), 19–24.

Gabrysch, S., & Campbell, O. M. (2009). Still too far to walk: Literature review of the determinants of delivery service use. *BMC Pregnancy and Childbirth, 9*(1), 1–18.

Govt. of India, & National Population Policy. (2000). *Department of Family Welfare, Ministry of Health and Family Welfare.* New Delhi: GOI. https://upnrhm.gov.in/Home/RCH

Kushwaha, P., Mehnaz, S., Ansari, M. A., & Khalil, S. (2016). Utilization of antenatal care services in periurban area of Aligarh. *International Journal of Medical Science and Public Health, 5*(10), 2004–2008.

Lule, E., Ramana, G. N. V., Ooman, N., Epp, J., Huntington, D., & Rosen, J. E. (2005). Achieving the millennium development goal of improving maternal health: Determinants, interventions and challenges. In *National Family Health Survey-3* (pp. 2005–2006). Uttar Pradesh: International Institute of Population Sciences.

Ravindran, T. K. (2012, June). Universal access: Making health systems work for women. In *BMC Public Health*, *12*(1), 1–7. BioMed Central.

Samuel, O., Irvine, D., & Grant, J. (Eds.). (1994). *Quality and Audit in General Practice: Meanings and Definitions.* Royal College of General Practitioners.

Srivastava, A., Bhattacharyya, S., Clar, C., & Avan, B. I. (2014). Evolution of quality in maternal health in India: Lessons and priorities. *International Journal of Medicine and Public Health*, *4*(1). https://upnrhm.gov.in/assets/site-files/Annual _Health_Report_2012-13_New.pdf

Vora, K.S., Mavalankar, D.V., Ramani, K.V., Upadhyaya, M., Sharma, B., Iyengar, S., Gupta, V., & Iyengar, K. (2009 Apr). Maternal health situation in India: A case study. Journal of health, population, and nutrition., 27(2):184–201. doi: 10.3329/ jhpn.v27i2.3363. PMID: 19489415; PMCID: PMC2761784.

World Health Organization. (2005). *The World Health Report: 2005: Make Every Mother and Child Count.* World Health Organization.

15 Assessment of Health System Governance in Empowered Action Group States in India

Pravin Kumar

Introduction

Health is a critical measure of development and plays a crucial role in shaping the human capital of a nation (Becker, 2007). Health is enshrined as a fundamental human right in the constitution of many countries, and most are a signatory to at least one human rights treaty that includes the right to health and several rights related to conditions necessary for health (Siddiqi et al., 2009, p.15). Therefore, it is the right of the citizens of a country to get efficient healthcare services from the state. The World Health Organization (1946) defines *health* as "A state of complete physical, mental and social well-being and not merely the absence of disease or infirmity" (WHO, 2020, p.1). According to this definition, it is the responsibility of the state to manage the HSG to improve health indicators for population well-being. After almost seventy years of acceptance of the World Health Constitution, the health scenario of developing countries including India has yet to be satisfactory. The Lancet Commission report (2016) on the Global Healthcare Access and Quality Index(GHAQI) between 1990 and 2016 shows that overall, in 2016, the score for India's healthcare access and quality was 41.2 (up from 24.7 in 1990), placing it 145th out of 195 countries. However, India's gap between the highest and lowest healthcare access and quality scores increased from 1990 to 2016 (from a 23.4-point difference to a 30.8-point difference) (Lancet, 2018).

The World Bank and the WHO published a joint research report in 2017. The research report shows, "Almost 100 million people are pushed into extreme poverty each year because of debts accrued through healthcare expenses". The research also found that more than 122 million people worldwide are forced to live on $3.10 a day, the benchmark for "moderate poverty", due to healthcare expenditure. Since 2000, this number has increased by 1.5% a year (The Guardian, 14 Dec 2017). About 800 million people spend at least 10 per cent of their household budget on health expenses for themselves, a sick child or another family member (New Indian Express, 14 Dec 2017). The report mentions that around 49 million people in India are pushed into extreme poverty yearly due to healthcare expenses (*New Indian Express*, 14 Dec 2017). The study by the

DOI: 10.4324/9781003430636-20

Public Health Foundation of India (PHFI) shows that "about 55 million Indians were pushed into poverty in a single year because of having to fund their healthcare, and 38 million of them fell below the poverty line due to spending on medicines alone" (*The Economics Times*, 13 Jun 2018). United Nations has identified the eight Millennium Development Goals (MDGs) for its member countries to be achieved by 2015, and India is a signatory of it. Among the eight MDG goals, three were based on health indicators, i.e. Goal 4: Reduce child mortality; Goal 5: Improve maternal health; Goal 6: Combat HIV/AIDS, malaria and other diseases. At the end of the duration of the MDGs, the United Nations has given a new agenda to its member countries. The new agenda is called SDGs; in this agenda, seventeen goals will be achieved by its member countries by 2030 and the third goal of SDGs is on health.

The present chapter assesses the health sector performance of the EAG states of India from the MDGs to the SDGs era and the challenges ahead. More specifically, the paper assesses the HSG among EAG states in India.

Conceptual Framework and Working Definition

India is a country with huge cultural, political, and environmental diversity observed across the states. In 2001, the Ministry of Health and Family Welfare Government of India certified in a press conference that the EAG sets up to facilitate the preparation of area-specific programs in eight states. These included Bihar, Jharkhand, Madhya Pradesh, Chhattisgarh, Orissa, Rajasthan, Uttar Pradesh, and Uttaranchal (later Uttarakhand). These states needed to catch up in controlling population growth to manageable levels. The EAG states become crucial in influencing India's socioeconomic transformation because they account for almost half (46%) of the Indian population (Singh & Keshari, 2016, p.44) and 61% of the poor (living below the poverty line).

The most conspicuous feature of the demographic characteristics of the EAG states is their high fertility, infant mortality rate, maternal mortality ratio, population growth rate, low literacy rate, and high literacy gender differential (Som & Mishra, 2014, p.34). Among the EAG states, Uttar Pradesh and Bihar are the worst-performing states in terms of access to public sources of health care, as around 83% of inpatients (in both rural and urban areas) in these states are dependent on private sources of health care. Though the situation is similar in Jharkhand, the inpatients of mainly rural areas of Odisha and Uttarakhand have better access to public sources of health care. The dependency on private sources of health care is also higher in Madhya Pradesh, Rajasthan and Chhattisgarh (Kumar & Singh, 2016, p.271). As per the *Lancet* report on the GHAQI (2016), Goa and Kerala had the highest scores in 2016, each exceeding 60 points. In contrast, Assam and Uttar Pradesh had the lowest, each below 40 (Lancet, 2018). It signifies that analyses of health governance are critical, especially in the low-performing states, EAG states of India.

Health systems contain three categories of actors: government, providers, and beneficiaries/clients. Health governance involves the rules that determine the roles and responsibilities of each of these categories of actors and the relationships, structures, and procedures that connect those (Mutale et al., 2013, p.2). WHO defines Health Governance (2007) as governance which is "ensuring strategic policy frameworks exist and are combined with effective oversight, coalition building, the provision of appropriate regulations and incentives, attention to system design, and accountability" (Lopez et al., 2011, p.2). Health governance is "the actions and means a society adopts to organise itself to promote and protect the population's health, involves numerous actors, and is subject to multiple constraints (Fehr et al., 2017, p.1).

There are generally three accepted health system goals: improved health status through more equitable access to quality health services and preventive and promotion programs, responsiveness to the legitimate patient and public expectations, adequate financing that protects against financial risks for those needing health care (WHO, 2000; Roberts et al., 2004; Brinkerhoff et al., 2014, p.2). World Health Report (2000) points out that health system has a responsibility not just to improve people's health but also to protect them against the financial cost of illness and treat them with dignity. Health systems thus have three fundamental objectives. These are improving the health of the population they serve, responding to people's expectations, and providing financial protection against the costs of ill health (WHR, 2000, p.8). Health systems' governance concerns the actions and means adopted by society to organise itself to promote and protect the health of its population (Siddiqi, 2009, p.14). The HSG thus can be defined as "the initiative taken by central and state governments like regulatory, structural, institutional, systematic, financial, partnerships with various stakeholders and that initiative impacted, improvement in health indicators".

In this chapter, the HSG of the EAG states is assessed. It discusses the availability and gap in healthcare policy, regulation, finance, healthcare resources, and improvement in health indicators. Also, it attempts to identify the issues and challenges and find the possible ways to achieve SDGs and UHC among the EAG states in India. The secondary data were used for this paper between 2000 and 2022, and data were collected from research papers and documents including National Health Profile, National Family Health Survey, National Health Account, Sample Registration Survey Bulletin, and Household Healthcare Utilization and Expenditure in India: State Fact Sheets and research papers.

Health System Governance Among the EAG States

Many research studies have applied the World Health Organization and USAID framework for HSG. The WHO in World Health Report 2000 focused on features of the health system, i.e. (1) stewardship (often referred to as *governance* or *oversight*), (2) financing, (3) human and physical resources, and (4) organisation and management of service delivery (World Health Report, 2000; Islam, 2007, p.1). USAID identifies three areas for HSG: (1) setting strategic direction and objectives; (2) making policies, laws, rules, regulations, or decisions, and raising and deploying resources to accomplish the strategic goals and objectives; and (3) overseeing and making sure that the strategic goals and objectives are accomplished (WHO, 2014, p.9). The scholar has chosen to assess the HSG in the EAG state on four initiatives taken by the government. These include Healthcare Policy, Finance, Human Resources, Healthcare Infrastructure, and Health indicators (Output).

This section discusses the HSG in the EAG states. The discussion of this section is on Healthcare Policy and Healthcare Protection Schemes, Healthcare Infrastructure, Healthcare Human Resources, and Health Indicators among the EAG states.

Healthcare Policy and Healthcare Protection Schemes

Table 15.1 depicts the healthcare regulations and protection schemes by the state governments among the EAG states. It considers the healthcare policies of the EAG states regarding investment from both public and private agencies.

This table suggests most EAG states have yet to have a clear state health policy, though Rajasthan has Health Vision 2025, and Madhya Pradesh, Uttar Pradesh, and Uttarakhand have drafted a state health policy. The state healthcare private investment policy is available in Rajasthan, Madhya Pradesh, and Odisha, but Bihar, Chhattisgarh, Jharkhand, Uttar Pradesh, and Uttarakhand lack any such provision. The state health-specific public–private partnership policy is available in Jharkhand and Uttar Pradesh, but Bihar, Chhattisgarh, Madhya Pradesh, Rajasthan, and Uttarakhand do not have such provisions. The state government-sponsored healthcare protection schemes available are "Dr. Khoobchand Baghel Swastyha Sahayata Yojana (DKBSSY)" in Chhattisgarh, "Bhamashah Swasthya Bima Yojana/ Mukhyamantri Chiranjeevi Swasthya Bima Yojana" in Rajasthan, "Biju Swasthya Kalyan Yojana" in Odisha, and "Atal Ayushman Yojna and Golden Card Yojana" in Uttarakhand. No government health protection scheme is implemented for the poor in Bihar, Jharkhand, Madhya Pradesh, and Uttar Pradesh. However, the central government healthcare protection scheme "Ayushman Bharat Pradhan Mantri Jan Arogya Yojana" is available in the six EAG states (Bihar, Chhattisgarh, Jharkhand, Madhya Pradesh, Uttar Pradesh, and Uttarakhand) except two states Odisha and Rajasthan.

Public Health Expenditure Among the EAG States

Table 15.2A and 15.2B present the status and variations in public health expenditures for 2014–15 and 2018–19 within empowered action group states. Table 15.2A shows that the percentage of health expenditure in total health expenditure is highest in Uttarakhand, and it is lowest in Bihar (16.5%).

Table 15.1 Healthcare Regulations and Healthcare Protections Schemes

National State	State Health Policy	State Healthcare Private Investment Policy	State Health-Specific Public-Private Partnerships	State Government Health Protection Schemes
Bihar	Bihar: Road Map For Development of Health Sector A Report of the Special Task Force on Bihar 2007	NA	NA	NA
Chhattisgarh	NA	NA	NA	Dr. Khoobchand Baghel Swastyha Sahayata Yojana (DKBSSY)
Jharkhand	NA	NA	Policy Guidelines on Public Private Partnerships for Establishing Medical Colleges, Super Specialty Hospital, Nursing Schools/ Colleges/ Paramedical Institutes	NA
Madhya Pradesh	State Health Policy (Draft)	Madhya Pradesh Health Sector Investment Promotion Scheme, 2020/ Healthcare Investment Policy 2019	NA	NA
Odisha	NA	Odisha Healthcare Investment Promotion Policy 2016	NA	Biju Swasthya Kalyan Yojana

(Continued)

Table 15.1 (Continued)

National State	State Health Policy	State Healthcare Private Investment Policy	State Health-Specific Public-Private Partnerships	State Government Health Protection Schemes
Rajasthan	Health Vision 2025	Policy to Promote Private Investment In Health Care Facilities-2006	NA	Bhama Shah Swasthya Bima Yojana/Mukhyamantri Chiranjeevi Swasthya Bima Yojana
Uttar Pradesh	The Uttar Pradesh Health Policy, 2018 Delivering on Health - Towards building a Robust, Resilient and Responsive health system	NA	Uttar Pradesh Public-Private Partnership Policy	NA
Uttarakhand	Draft, Uttarakhand State Public Health Policy, 2020	NA	NA	Atal Ayushman Yojna and Golden Card Yojana

Source: State Health Department and allied Websites

Table 15.2A Public Health Expenditure 2014–2015

EAG States	% of THE	% of GSDP	% of GGE	Per Capita in Rs.	In crores
Bihar	16.5	1.0	4.1	338	3689
Chhattisgarh	27.9	1.0	5.2	880	2376
Jharkhand	23.9	0.8	4.4	480	1631
Madhya Pradesh	25.5	1.0	5.1	640	4799
Odisha	21.5	1.0	5.2	735	3233
Rajasthan	30.7	1.1	5.9	904	6511
Uttar Pradesh	19.0	1.2	5.4	581	12209
Uttarakhand	36.2	0.9	5.9	1534	1534

The percentage of health expenditure to Gross State Domestic Product (GSDP) is highest in Uttar Pradesh (1.2%) while lowest in Jharkhand (0.8%). The percentage of government general expenditure is equal in Rajasthan and Uttarakhand (5.9%), while the lowest is in Bihar (4.1%). Among all the EAG states, per capita expenditure is lowest in Bihar (Rs 338), and it is highest and almost three times higher in Uttarakhand than in Bihar (Rs 1534).

It has been observed from Table 15.2B that there was a sharp increase in public health expenditure in Bihar between 2014–15 and 2018–19.

Bihar ranks lowest in 2014–15 in terms of percentage of total health expenditure; it is third highest in 2018–19 (44.5%). While Uttarakhand recorded the highest (61.0%), Uttar Pradesh ranks lowest (24%). There is an increase in the percentage of health expenditure to GSDP. Bihar ranks highest among all the EAG states with 1.5%. However, the EAG states spent less than the national average. In terms of per capita, Uttarakhand spent more than other EAG states (Rs. 2093), and it is lowest in Bihar (Rs. 674). However, for other EAG states like Rajasthan, Odisha, Madhya Pradesh, and Jharkhand, the per capita health expenditure is more than Rs. 1000.

Table 15.2C displays the increase/decrease in public health expenditure in the empowered action group states between 2014–15 and 2018–19. The

Table 15.2B Public Health Expenditure 2018–2019

EAG States	% of THE	% of GSDP	% of GGE	Per Capita in Rs.	In crores
Bihar	44.5	1.5	5.5	674	8,090
Chhattisgarh	46.7	1.3	5.7	1,433	4,155
Jharkhand	33.5	1.2	6.1	1005	3,717
Madhya Pradesh	40.8	1.0	4.9	1,031	8,458
Odisha	40.9	1.2	5.6	1,343	6,043
Rajasthan	43.7	1.4	7.0	1,696	13,061
Uttar Pradesh	24.8	1.2	5.3	863	19,418
Uttarakhand	61.0	1.0	6.0	2,093	2,302

Table 15.2C Increase/Decrease in Public Health Expenditure

EAG States	% of THE	% of GSDP	% of GGE	Per Capita in Rs.	In crores
Bihar	28.0	0.5	1.4	336	4401
Chhattisgarh	18.8	0.3	0.5	553	1779
Jharkhand	9.6	0.4	1.7	525	2081
Madhya Pradesh	15.3	0.0	-0.2	391	3659
Odisha	19.4	0.2	0.4	608	2810
Rajasthan	13.0	0.2	1.1	792	6550
Uttar Pradesh	5.8	0.0	-0.1	282	7209
Uttarakhand	24.8	0.1	0.1	559	768

percentage of total health expenditure increased by 28% since 2014–15 in Bihar, and the lowest increase was in Uttar Pradesh (5.0%). Hence, the highest gross state domestic product percentage increased in Bihar (0.5%) and was stable in Uttar Pradesh (0%). It has been seen the health expenditure as a percentage of general government expenditure increased in Jharkhand (+1.4) and decreased in Uttar Pradesh (-0.1). On the contrary, the per capita health expenditure increased in all the EAG states. The table indicates the highest increase in per capita expenditure in Rajasthan (792) and the lowest in Uttar Pradesh (282). The table also shows the expenditure on health in crore, with the highest increase in Uttar Pradesh (7209) and the lowest in Uttarakhand (768).

State-Wise Households Expenditure Among EAG States

Table 15.3 shows the household expenditure on health (inpatients and outpatients) during the last 30 days. The Out-of-Pocket Expenditure (OOPE) was highest in Rajasthan in 2004, while it was lowest in Jharkhand, and in 2018, Uttar Pradesh spent the highest (2371) and lowest expenditure was in Bihar (1212). It has been found from the table that medical expenditure on inpatient and outpatient care in 30 days had the highest increase in Jharkhand (+577) among the EAG states and the decrease was more in Rajasthan (-358). Furthermore, the table shows the household expenditure on inpatient care in 365 days was highest in Rajasthan (18426) and lowest in Jharkhand (5798) in 2004. On the other hand, in 2018, it was highest in Uttar Pradesh (22064) and lowest in Bihar (9907). Between 2004 and 2018, the highest increase was in Uttar Pradesh (+9146) and the decline was more in Rajasthan (−399). This signifies Rajasthan made a significant improvement in reducing the financial burden occurred due to out-of-pocket expenditure. The household expenditure on health (outpatients) during the last 15 days was highest in Rajasthan (1094) in 2004, while Jharkhand

Table 15.3 Trend of Medical Expenditure on Inpatient and Outpatient Care (₹) of Households at 2018 Prices in the EAG States of India, 2004–18

National and States	Medical Expenditure on inpatient and outpatient care in 30 days		Increase/Decrease Between 2004–18	Medical Expenditure on Inpatient care in 365 days		Increase/Decrease Between 2004–18	Medical Expenditure on Outpatient care in 15 days		Increase/Decrease Between 2004–18
	2004	2018		2004	2018		2004	2018	
India	1950	2063	+113	15969	21157	+5188	793	888	+95
Bihar	1333	1212	-121	6956	9907	+2951	571	649	+78
Chhattisgarh	1637	1448	-189	12565	20225	+7660	702	495	-207
Jharkhand	1222	1799	+577	5798	14558	+8760	539	883	+344
Madhya Pradesh	1629	1780	+151	12136	13174	+1038	689	999	+310
Odisha	1345	1493	+148	10508	15380	+4872	601	688	+87
Rajasthan	2577	2219	-358	18426	18027	-399	1094	1164	+70
Uttar Pradesh	2025	2371	+346	12918	22064	+9146	883	1068	+185
Uttarakhand	2029	1698	-331	12983	20563	+7580	850	661	-189

Source: Trend in Out-of-Pocket Expenditure and Catastrophic Health Spending in India 2004–2018 (Mohanthy, 2018, pp.42–43).

(539) recorded the lowest. In 2018, the highest was spent by Rajasthan (2371) and the lowest by Chhattisgarh (495). It has been found from the table that medical expenditure on an outpatient in the last 15 days had the highest increase among EAG states in Jharkhand (+344) and a decrease in Chhattisgarh (–207).

Health Human Resources Among the EAG States

Table 15.4 shows the human resources in the health, distribution of doctors, nurses and auxiliary nurse midwifery (ANM), and the number of people handled by one doctor, one nurse, and one ANM.

The table highlights the highest load of the population per doctor in Jharkhand (1/5830.70) and the lowest was in Uttarakhand (1/1271.07). Furthermore, the highest load of the population per nurse and midwife was in Bihar (1/11113.58) and the lowest in Rajasthan (1/396.06). The highest population load on one ANM in Bihar (1/10389.38) and the lowest in Odisha (1/650.85).

Table 15.5 and Figure 15.1 show the Availability of and Gap in Health Infrastructure among the EAG States.

Table 15.5 shows Madhya Pradesh has large number of functional divisional hospitals (92), whereas it was acutely short in Uttar Pradesh. On the other hand, Uttar Pradesh has the highest number of functional district hospitals (168) among all the EAG states, whereas the number was lowest in Uttarakhand (13). In terms of the number of medical colleges, Rajasthan performs better with highest number (39) among the EAG states.

Figure 15.1 shows the shortage percentage of the primary health centres, community health centres, and sub-health centres among all EAG states

Among all EAG states, primary health centres, community health centres, and sub-health centres in Rajasthan were found to be more than the required position, which can be called a surplus. The number of community health centres in Odisha, and sub-health centres in Uttarakhand were more than the required position that is surplus. The highest percentage of shortage of primary health centres was found in Jharkhand (74.0%). In contrast, the highest shortage of community health centres was found in Bihar (66.0%). Similarly, the highest shortage of sub-health centres was found only in Bihar (53.0%). Among the EAG states, if the surplus states are left out, then the lowest percentage of shortage of primary health centres was found in Uttarakhand (3.0%), the lowest percentage of shortage of community health centres was also found in Uttarakhand (16.0%), and the lowest percentage of shortage of sub-health centres was found in Chhattisgarh (6.0%).

Table 15.4 Healthcare Human Resources among EAG States

National State	Projected Population of the Country	Registered Doctors	Doctors/1000 Population	Registered Nurses and Midwives	Nurses and Midwives/1000 Population	Registered ANM	ANM /1000 Population
India	1,36,06,81,968	1234205	1/1102.47	2,272,208	1/598.83	934,583	1/1455.92
Bihar	12,30,83,000	45795	1/2687.69	11075	1/11113.58	11847	1/10389.38
Chhattisgarh	2,94,93,000	9555	1/3086.65	21984	1/1341.56	14782	1/1995.19
Jharkhand	3,84,71,000	6598	1/5830.70	4977	1/7729.75	7896	1/4872.21
Madhya Pradesh	8,45,16,000	40171	1/2103.90	118793	1/711.45	39563	1/2136.23
Odisha	4,40,33,000	24780	1/1776.95	82189	1/535.75	67654	1/650.85
Rajasthan	7,92,81,000	46253	1/1714.07	200171	1/396.06	108688	1/729.43
Uttar Pradesh	23,09,07,000	82299	1/2805.70	111860	1/2064.24	75671	1/3051.45
Uttarakhand	1,13,99,000	8968	1/1271.07	15519	1/734.51	9410	1/1211.37

Source: National Health Profile 2021; State/UT wise Aadhaar Saturation (Overall) - All Age Groups 31 January, 2022.

Table 15.5 Status of Health *Infrastructures (Hospitals)*

National State	Functional Divisional Hospitals	Functional District Hospitals	Functional Medical College and Hospitals
India	1224	764	307
Bihar	45	36	10
Chhattisgarh	12	27	8
Jharkhand	13	23	6
Madhya Pradesh	92	51	10
Odisha	33	32	7
Rajasthan	25	28	39
Uttarakhand	19	13	3
Uttar Pradesh	0	168	20

Source: RHS 2020–21, p.121

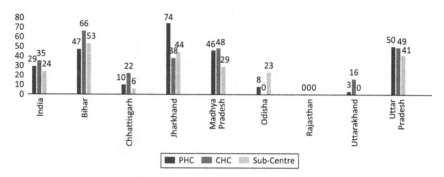

Figure 15.1 Percentage Shortage in Health Infrastructure
Source: RHS 2020-21, 0 indicates surplus

Status of Health Indicators Among Empowered Action Group States

Table 15.6A shows the health indicators among the EAG states from 1999 to 2022. This table has been taken from the NFHS, SRS and statistics on the Indian states. The improvement/reduction in health indicators among the EAG states based on the data given in Table 6.

Changes in Performance of Health Indicators between 2003 and 2022

Table 15.6B shows the difference in health indicators between 2000–04 and 2020–22. The comparison between the health indicators for the marked duration highlights the improvement in health indicators in the current table.

It has been found out the reduction/improvement in health indicators; in the crude birth rate, the highest reduction in Utter Pradesh (7.7) and the

Table 15.6A Health Indicators 1999–2022 in India

National State	Crude Birth Rate (1999)	Crude Death Rate (1999)	Life Expectancy Rate (2001–2005)	Total Fertility Rate NFHS2	Maternal Mortality Rate (2001–2003)	Infant Mortality Rate (NFHS2)	Under-five mortality rate (U5MR) (NFHS)	Institutional Delivery Rate (NFHS3) 2005–06
India	26.0	8.6	64.3	2.85	301	67.6	94.9	38.7
Bihar	31.5	8.9	64.2	3.49	371	72.9	105.1	19.9
Chhattisgarh	26.9	9.6	59.7	NA	379	80.9	122.7	14.3
Jharkhand	26.3	8.9	64.2	NA	371	54.3	78.3	18.3
Madhya Pradesh	31.1	10.4	59.7	3.31	379	86.1	137.6	26.2
Odisha	24.1	10.7	60.8	2.46	358	81.0	104.4	35.6
Rajasthan	31.1	8.4	64.5	3.78	445	80.4	114.9	29.6
Uttar Pradesh	32.8	10.5	60.8	3.99	517	86.7	122.5	20.6
Uttarakhand	19.6	6.5	60.8	NA	517	37.6	56.1	32.6
Health Indicators 2020–22	SRS Bulletin	SRS Bulletin	RBI	NFHS5	SRS 2022	NFHS5	NFHS5	NFHS5
India	19.5	6.0	69.4	2.0	103	35.2	41.9	88.6
Bihar	25.5	5.4	69.1	3.0	130	46.8	56.4	76.2
Chhattisgarh	22.0	7.9	65.2	1.8	160	44.3	50.4	85.7
Jharkhand	22.0	5.2	69.1	2.3	61	37.9	45.4	75.8
Madhya Pradesh	24.1	6.5	66.5	2.0	163	41.3	49.2	90.7
Odisha	17.7	7.3	69.3	1.8	136	36.3	41.1	92.2
Rajasthan	23.5	5.6	68.7	2.0	141	30.3	37.6	94.9
Uttar Pradesh	25.1	6.5	70.9	1.9	167	50.4	59.8	83.4
Uttarakhand	16.6	6.3	65.3	2.4	101	39.1	45.6	83.2

Source: National Family Health Survey 2; Sample Registration Survey and Handbook of Statistics on the Indian States 2020–2021

Table 15.6B Health Indicators between 1999–2022 in India as well as the EAG States

National State	CBR (2022)	CDR (2022)	LER	TFR	MMR (SRS 2017–2019)	IMR (NFHS5)	USMMR (NFHS5)	IDR (NFHS5)
India	6.5	2.6	+5.1	0.85	198	32.4	53.0	+49.2
Bihar	6.0	3.5	4.9	0.15	241	37.7	48.7	56.3
Chhattisgarh	4.9	1.7	5.5	N A	219	36.6	72.3	71.4
Jharkhand	4.3	3.7	4.9	N A	310	16.4	32.9	57.5
Madhya Pradesh	7.0	3.9	6.8	1.31	216	44.8	88.4	64.4
Odisha	6.4	3.4	8.5	0.66	222	44.7	63.3	56.6
Rajasthan	7.6	2.8	4.2	1.78	304	50.1	77.3	65.3
Uttar Pradesh	7.7	4.0	10.1	2.09	350	36.3	62.7	62.6
Uttarakhand	3.0	0.2	5.5	N A	416	+1.5	10.5	50.8

Source: Analysis result of table 06: 2022

lowest in Uttarakhand (3.0). The similarly highest reduction in crude death rate is in Uttar Pradesh (4.0), and the lowest was in Uttarakhand (0.2). Furthermore, the highest increase in life expectancy rate was recorded in Uttar Pradesh (10.1) and the lowest in Rajasthan (4.2). The highest reduction in total fertility rate has been observed in Uttar Pradesh (2.09), and it was the lowest in Bihar (0.15). The maximum reduction in maternal mortality rate was in Uttarakhand (416) and the minimum in Odisha (216). The infant mortality rate decreased maximum in Rajasthan (50.1) but increased in Uttarakhand (+1.5). The highest reduction in the under-five mortality rate (U5MR) is noticed in Madhya Pradesh (88.4) and the lowest in Uttarakhand (10.5). The highest reduction in the institutional delivery rate is found in Chhattisgarh (71.4) and is the lowest in Uttarakhand (50.8).

Discussion and Conclusion

In this section, the state's ranking according to their policy, investment, OOPE on health, health infrastructure, health human resources, and the result in health indicators are discussed and analysed.

Ranking of the EAG States According to their Performance

Following are the rankings of states based on the increase and decrease in public health expenditure between 2014 to 2015 and 2018 to 2019 in eight EAG states.

Columns 2–4 of Table 15.7A represent the ranking of the EAG states in increasing order according to the level of health expenditure by the state for the period 2014–2019. The rankings are done for total health expenditure, percentage share in general health expenditure, and per capita health expenditure. The table shows Bihar ranks highest position in total health expenditure, while the health expenditure was lowest in Uttar Pradesh. The public spending as per capita health expenditure is increasing in Rajasthan among all the EAG states, and it was lowest in Uttar Pradesh. Columns 6–8 represent the ranking of states in decreasing order according to household health expenditure. The household OOPE for health decreasing substantially in Rajasthan as it ranks 1, and among all the EAG states, OOPE in last 30 days was highest in Jharkhand. Likewise in the case of inpatient care, Rajasthan performs better and the expenditure was lowest in Uttar Pradesh. On the other hand, in the case of outpatient visit, the household expenditure was lowest in Chhattisgarh during this period and it was highest in Jharkhand.

In terms of shortfall in health infrastructure, Jharkhand ranks highest in the shortfall in PHC, whereas Bihar ranks highest in shortage of CHC and sub-centres. On the contrary, Rajasthan performs better among all the EAG states in terms of number of PHCs as there is surplus. Likewise, there is surplus CHC and sub-centres found in Odisha and Uttarakhand, respectively.

Table 15.7A A Ranking of State Based on Public and Household Expenditure

State	Percentage of total health expenditure	The percentage of general government expenditure	Per capita expenditure in rupees	Household medical expenditure on inpatient and outpatient care in 30 days	Household medical expenditure on inpatient care in 365 days	Household medical expenditure on outpatient care in 15 days
	Increasing Order			Decreasing Order		
Bihar	01	02	07	4	3	4
Chhattisgarh	04	04	04	3	6	1
Jharkhand	07	01	05	8	7	8
Madhya Pradesh	05	08	06	6	2	7
Odisha	03	05	02	5	4	5
Rajasthan	06	03	01	1	1	3
Uttarakhand	02	06	03	2	5	2
Uttar Pradesh	08	07	08	7	8	6

Source: Author's estimation

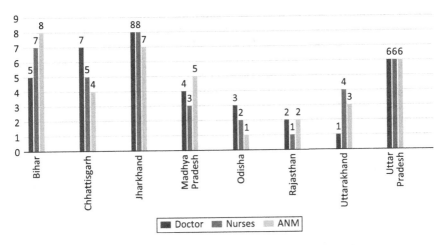

Figure 15.2 Ranking of State Based on Patients and Health Human Resources Ratios

Source: Author's estimation

The functional medical colleges and the health centres better equipped in the state Rajasthan.

Figure 15.2 depicts the ranking of states according to the number of patients per human resources such as doctors, nurses, and ANM. The figure shows Rajasthan and Odisha rank lowest, indicating there was less shortfall in these states. On the contrary, Bihar, Jharkhand, and Uttar Pradesh score higher such as 5, 6, 7, and 8 and in all three categories. Among the states, the doctor–patient ratio, nurse–patient ratio, and ANM–patient ratio were lowest in Uttarakhand, Rajasthan, and Odisha, respectively. Table 15.7B

Table 15.7C shows the highest reduction in crude birth rate and death rate found in Uttar Pradesh, and the decline was lowest in Uttarakhand. Improvement in life expectancy and decline in TFR was much higher in Uttar Pradesh. The maternal mortality rate decreased maximum in Uttarakhand; however, the decline was much slower in IMR, U5MR, and IDR in the state as it ranks lowest.

The analysis shows that the improvement in health indicators of the state is the result of not only the impact of government initiatives but also the individual's OOPE on health. This suggests the pattern of health spending in these states has not changed significantly and the household remains the main source of healthcare financing. The increase in OOPE affects the financial condition of poor households, and hence, pushes people to fall below poverty line (BPL). According to the Census of 2011, about 46 per cent of the population lives in the EAG states and more than half population of EAG states are forced to live below the poverty line every financial year.

Table 15.7B Ranking of State Based on Health Infrastructure

State	Medical College	District Hospital	PHC	CHC	Sub Health Centre
Bihar	05	06	03	01	01
Chhattisgarh	04	03	05	05	06
Jharkhand	02	02	01	04	02
Madhya Pradesh	06	07	04	03	04
Odisha	03	05	06	08	05
Rajasthan	08	04	08	07	07
Uttarakhand	01	01	07	06	08
Uttar Pradesh	07	08	02	02	03

Source: Author's estimation

Table 15.7C Ranking of States Based on the Reduction in Mortality Rates

State	CBR	CDR	LER	TFR	MMR	IMR	U5MR	IDR
Bihar	05	03	06	05	05	04	06	07
Chhattisgarh	06	06	04	NA	07	05	03	01
Jharkhand	07	03	07	NA	03	07	07	05
Madhya Pradesh	03	02	03	03	08	02	01	03
Odisha	04	02	02	04	06	03	04	06
Rajasthan	02	05	08	02	04	01	02	02
Uttarakhand	08	08	05	NA	01	08	08	08
Uttar Pradesh	01	01	01	01	02	06	05	04

Source: Author's estimation

Millennium Development Goal and Success Rate Among the EAG States

Table 15.8 shows the target to be achieved under the SDGs goal. The state-wise difference between target and achievement in EAG states suggests the states are very far from achieving the targets as compared to India. Even after a lapse of more than two decades, the health index of these eight states has yet to be able to achieve the national average. The United Nations announced the MDGs, in which eight goals were to be achieved by the United Nations member country by 2015. Out of these eight goals, three goals were related to health. The United Nations then set a new target of achieving the SDGs by 2030. Of the 17 goals, the third target was related to health. In this study, it was found that even after seven years more than the target of the MDGs, these eight states of the EAG states could not achieve the target of the MDGs. There are only seven years left to meet the SDG targets, and hence, the question arises will these EAG sates be able to achieve the SDGs in next few years?

Table 15.8 Difference between SDGs Target and Achievement

National State	MDGs MMR Target	SDGs MMR Target	Achieved MMR	To be Achieved MMR	MDGs U5MMR Target	SDGs U5MMR Target	Achieved U5MMR	To be Achieved U5MMR	MDGs IMR Target	SDGs NNMR Target	Achieved IMR	Achieved NMR	To be Achieved NMR
India	90	70	103	33	42	25	41.9	16.9	27	12	35.2	24.9	12.9
Bihar	90	70	130	60	42	25	56.4	31.4	27	12	46.8	34.5	22.5
Chhattisgarh	90	70	160	90	42	25	50.4	25.4	27	12	44.3	32.4	20.4
Jharkhand	90	70	61	09	42	25	45.4	20.4	27	12	37.9	28.2	16.2
Madhya Pradesh	90	70	163	93	42	25	49.2	24.2	27	12	41.3	29.0	17.0
Odisha	90	70	136	66	42	25	41.1	16.1	27	12	36.3	27.0	15.0
Rajasthan	90	70	141	71	42	25	37.6	12.6	27	12	30.3	20.2	7.8
Uttar Pradesh	90	70	101	97	42	25	59.8	20.6	27	12	50.4	35.7	23.7
Uttarakhand	90	70	167	31	42	25	45.6	34.8	27	12	39.1	32.4	20.4

Source: Findings of the study 2022

Suggestions

Despite various interventions and reforms, the EAG states are far from achieving the SDG targets. To achieve the targets the government should adopt technical, institutional, organisational, and financial innovations in health sectors. Firstly, there is a need to increase the budget share on health to reduce the OOPE. Secondly, the state government should formulate state health policy, state health-specific private investment policy, and state health-specific public–private partnership policy, where there is a gap in these provisions. Thirdly, there is a need to fill the shortage of health infrastructure in rural areas. Fourthly, the state government needs to evaluate their initiatives regularly by the third party like educational institutions or research professionals. Central and state governments need to identify the poor indicators of each state and try to work accordingly to fill the gap. Lastly, awareness can change society because knowledge and information empower and secure individual rights. Therefore, the state government can start an awareness campaign and encourage people to utilise services from public hospitals. In a way, the EAG states will progress towards achieving universal health coverage and SDGs of leaving no one behind.

References

Becker, G. S. (2007). Health as Human Capital: Synthesis and Extensions. *Oxford Economic Papers*, 59(3), 379–410. Retrieved from http://www.jstor.org/stable /4500116.

Government of Chhattisgarh. (2018). Dr. Khoobch and Baghel Swasthya Sahayata Yojana. Raipur. Retrieved from https://dkbssy.cg.nic.in/dkbssydoc/DKBSSY_Final _Guidelines_Signed_rotated.pdf.

Government of India. (2001, 4). Sample Registration System. *Bulletin*. New Delhi. Retrieved from https://censusindia.gov.in/nada/index.php/catalog/42702.

Government of India. (2004). National Health Accounts India. New Delhi. Retrieved from https://www.niti.gov.in/planningcommission.gov.in/docs/reports/genrep/ health/National_Health_Account_04_05.pdf.

Government of India. (2007). Bihar: Road Map for Development of Health Sector A Report of the Special Task Force on Bihar. New Delhi. Retrieved from https://niti .gov.in/planningcommission.gov.in/docs/aboutus/taskforce/tsk_bhs.pdf.

Government of India. (2011, 6). Special Bulletin on Maternal Mortality in India 2007–09. New Delhi. Retrieved from http://www.censusindia.gov.in

Government of India. (2015a). Health in India Government of India NSS 71st Round January–June 2014. New Delhi. Retrieved from https://ruralindiaonline.org/en/ library/resource/health-in-india-nss-71st-round-january-june-2014.

Government of India. (2015b). Key Indicators of Social Consumption in India Health NSS 71″ Round (January–June 2014). New Delhi. Retrieved from http://microdata .gov.in/nada43/index.php/catalog/135.

Government of India. (2017a). Achieving Millennium Development Goals Target Year Fact Sheet -India. New Delhi. Retrieved from www.mospi.gov.in

Government of India. (2017b). National Health Accounts Estimates for India 2014–15. New Delhi. Retrieved from https://nhsrcindia.org/sites/default/files/2021-06/ NHA Estimates Report -14-15.pdf.

Government of India. (2017c). National Health Policy 2017. New Delhi. Retrieved from https://www.nhp.gov.in/nhpfiles/national_health_policy_2017.pdf

Government of India. (2017d). Voluntary National Review Report on Implementation of Sustainable Development Goals. Retrieved from https://sustainabledevelopment .un.org/content/documents/26352VNR_2020_Uganda_Report.pdf

Government of India. (2018a). Ayushman Bharat Pradhan Mantri Jan Arogya Yojana. Retrieved from https://www.pmjay.gov.in/

Government of India. (2018b). Sustainable Development Goals Index Baseline Report 2018. New Delhi. Retrieved from https://sdgindiaindex.niti.gov.in/assets /Files/SDG_India_Index_Report_2018.pdf

Government of India. (2019). Key Indicators of Social Consumption in India: Health NSS 75th Round (July 2017–June 2018). New Delhi. Retrieved from http://164.100.161.63/sites/default/files/publication_reports/KI_Health_75th _Final.pdf

Government of India. (2020a). COVID-19 and its Spatial Dimensions in India III. Retrieved from https://rbidocs.rbi.org.in/rdocs/Publications/PDFs/03CH_271020 206C458AE369944258A62779FF5A2F5362.PDF.

Government of India. (2020b). Health in India NSS 75th Round July 2017–June 2018. New Delhi. Retrieved from https://www.mospi.gov.in/documents/213904 /301563//NSS Report Number 586 Health in India1606229312083.pdf/d3724e8 b-5970-0559-9ed9-12378a6cc7b3

Government of India. (2020c). National Family Health Survey (NFHS-5) 2019–20 Fact Sheets Key Indicators 22 States/UTs from Phase-I. New Delhi.

Government of India. (2020d). National Family Health Survey(NFHS-5) 2019–20 Fact Sheets Key Indicators 22 States/UTs From Phase-I. New Delhi. Retrieved from https://main.mohfw.gov.in/sites/default/files/NFHS-5_Phase-I.pdf

Government of India. (2021a). Handbook of Statistics on Indian States 2020–21. Retrieved from https://rbidocs.rbi.org.in/rdocs/Publications/PDFs/0HSIS241121 FL7A6B5C0ECBC64B0ABF0A097B1AD40C83.PDF

Government of India. (2021b). National Family Health Survey (NFHS-5) 2019–21 Compendium of Fact Sheets Key Indicators India and 14 States/UTs (Phase-II). New Delhi. Retrieved from https://main.mohfw.gov.in/sites/default/files/NFHS-5 _Phase-II_0.pdf

Government of India. (2021c). *National Family Health Survey-5 2019–21 India Fact Sheet*. New Delhi.

Government of India. (2021d). *National Family Health Survey-5 2019–21 State Fact Sheet*. New Delhi.

Government of India. (2021e). *National Health Accounts Estimates for India 2017– 18*. New Delhi. Retrieved from https://nhsrcindia.org/sites/default/files/2021-11/ National Health Accounts- 2017–18.pdf

Government of India. (2021f). National Health Profile 2021. New Delhi. Retrieved from https://www.cbhidghs.nic.in/showfile.php?lid=1160

Government of India. (2021g). Rural Health Statistics 2020–21. New Delhi. Retrieved from https://hmis.nhp.gov.in/downloadfile?filepath=publications/Rural-Health -Statistics/RHS%202020-21.pdf

Government of India. (2021h). SDG India Index & Dashboard 2020–21 Partnerships in the Decade of Action. New Delhi. Retrieved from https://sdgindiaindex.niti.gov .in/assets/Files/SDG3.0_Final_04.03.2021_Web_Spreads.pdf

Government of India. (2022a). National Family Health Survey (NFHS-5) 2019–21 India Volume I. New Delhi. Retrieved from http://rchiips.org/nfhs/NFHS-5Reports /NFHS-5_INDIA_REPORT.pdf

Government of India. (2022b, 9). National Health Accounts Estimates for India 2018–19. New Delhi. Retrieved from https://nhsrcindia.org/sites/default/files/2022 -09/NHA 2018-19_07-09-2022_revised_0.pdf

Government of India. (2022c, 5). Sample Registration Bulletin. May 2022. New Delhi. Retrieved from https://censusindia.gov.in/nada/index.php/catalog/42687

Government of India. (2022d). Special Bulletin on Maternal Mortality in India 2017– 19. Retrieved from https://censusindia.gov.in/nada/index.php/catalog/40525

Government of India. (2022e, 1). State/UT Wise Aadhaar Saturation 31 January 2022. New Delhi. Retrieved from https://uidai.gov.in/images/StateWiseAge_AadhaarSat _Rep_31012022_Projected-2021-Final.pdf

Government of Madhya Pradesh. (2019). Madhya Pradesh Health Sector Investment Promotion Policy-2019. Bhopal. Retrieved from https://health.mp.gov.in/sites/ default/files/2020-07/Nivesh_Niti_2019.pdf

Government of Madhya Pradesh. (2020). Madhya Pradesh Health Sector Investment Promotion Scheme - 2020. Bhopal. Retrieved from https://health.mp.gov.in/sites/ default/files/2020-07/Nivesh_Scheme_2020.pdf

Government of Madhya Pradesh. (2022). State Health Policy for Madhya Pradesh (Draft). Bhopal. Retrieved from http://www.dif.mp.gov.in/zoldweb/ InvestOpportunity/HealthPolicyMP_Draft.pdf

Government of Odisha. (2016). Health Care Investment Promotion Policy 2016. Bhubaneshwar. Retrieved from https://investodisha.gov.in/download/Health-Care -Investment-Promotion-Policy.pdf

Government of Odisha. (2018). Biju Swasthya Kalyan Yojana Odisha. Bhubaneshwar. Retrieved from http://www.bsky.odisha.gov.in/bsky_schemes/english/

Government of Rajasthan. (2006). Policy to Promote Private Investment in Health Care Facilities-2006. Jaipur. Retrieved from https://education.rajasthan.gov.in/ content/dam/doitassets/education/medicaleducation/medicaleducation/myfolder/ Hindi/ActandPolicies/2006 -Policy to Promote Investment in Health Care Facility 2006_com.pdf.pdf

Government of Rajasthan. (2021). Mukhyamantri Chiranjeevi Swasthya Bima Yojana. Retrieved from https://chiranjeevi.rajasthan.gov.in/#/home

Government of Rajasthan. (2022). Health Vision 2025. Jaipur. Retrieved from https:// education.rajasthan.gov.in/content/raj/education/medical-education-department/ en/Vision2025.html

Government of Uttar Pradesh. (2018). The Uttar Pradesh Health Policy, 2018 Delivering on Health -Towards Building a Robust, Resilient and Responsive Health System. Lucknow. Retrieved from http://ayushmanbharat.mp.gov.in/ uploads/media/UP_Health_Policy_Draft_Final_18_Jan_01_00am_CET.pdf

Government of Uttarakhand. (2020). Draft, Uttarakhand State Public Health Policy, 2020. Dehradun. Retrieved from https://www.ukhsdp.org/assets/pdf/State _ Public_Health_Policy _Draft-converted.pdf

Islam, M. (2007). Health Systems Assessment Approach: A How-To Manual. Management Sciences for Health. Retrieved from http://healthsystems2020.org

.Formoreinformation,pleasecontactinfo@healthsystems2020.org.Web:www.msh .org/rpmplusiiiCONTENTS

Kumar, V., & Singh, P. (2016). Access to Healthcare among the Empowered Action Group (EAG) states of India: Current status and impeding factors. *The National Medical Journal of India*, 29(05), 267–273. Retrieved August 06, 2017, from http://www.nmji.in/article.asp?issn=0970258X;year=2016;volume=29;issue=5 ;spage=267;epage=273;aulast=Kumar;type=0

Lopez, I. M., Wyss, K., & Savigny, D. D. (2011). An approach to addressing governance from a health system framework perspective. *BMC International Health and Human Rights*. Retrieved March 2019, from https://bmcinthealthhum rights.biomedcentral.com/track/pdf/10.1186/1472-698X-11-13

Mathew, S., & Moore, M. (2011, 05). State Incapacity by Design: Understanding the Bihar Story. *IDS Working Paper*, 2011(366). Institute of Development Studies. Retrieved 04 20, 2016, from http://www.ids.ac.uk/files/dmfile/Wp366.pdf

Fullman, N., Yearwood, J., Abay, S. M., Abbafati, C., Abd-Allah, F., Abdela, J., ... & Chang, H. Y. (2018). Measuring performance on the Healthcare Access and Quality Index for 195 countries and territories and selected subnational locations: a systematic analysis from the Global Burden of Disease Study 2016. *The Lancet*, 391(10136), 2236-2271. Retrieve from https://www.thelancet.com/action/ showPdf?pii=S0140-6736%2818%2930994-2

Mishra, S., Pandey, C. M., Chaubey, Y. P., & Singh, U. (2013). Determinants of Child Malnutrition in Empowered Action Group (EAG) States of India. *Statistics and Applications*, 1–9. Retrieved February 2019, from http://ssca.org.in/media/1. _Determinants_of_Child_Malnutrition_tQ0smd0.pdf

Mohanthy, S. K. (2021). Trend in Out-of-Pocket Expenditure and Catastrophic Health Spending in India, 2004–18. Mumbai. Retrieved from https://www.iipsindia.ac.in /sites/default/files/Report_Trend_in_OOP.pdf

Mukharji, A., & Mukharji, A. (2012). Bihar: What Went Wrong? And What Changed? Working Paper, National Institute of Public Finance and Policy, New Delhi. Retrieved June 29, 2015, from http://www.nipfp.org.in/media/medialibrary /2013/04/WP_2012_107.pdf

Press Information Bureau. (2001). Empowered Action Group on Population Stabilization to Focus on Bihar and Uttar Pradesh Special Session to be Held at Patna. Retrieved from https://archive.pib.gov.in/archive/releases98/lyr2001/ rjun2001/20062001/r200620011.html

Sameen, S., Masud, T. I., Nishtar, S., Peters, D. H., Sabri, B., Mohamud, K. B., . . . & Jama, A. M. (2009). Framework for assessing governance of the health system in developing countries: Gateway to good governance. *Health Policy*, 90(01). Retrieved March 2019 https://academic.oup.com/heapol/article/32/5/710/3061529

Som, K. S., & Mishra, R. P. (2014). BIMARU States: Need a Rethinking. *IOSR Journal of Humanities and Social Science*, 19(7), 34–41. Retrieved April 01, 2016, from http://iosrjournals.org/iosr-jhss/papers/Vol19-issue7/Version-1/F019713441 .pdf

The Lancet. (2018). Healthcare Access and Quality Profile India. *The Lancet*. Retrieved January 2019, from http://www.healthdata.org/sites/default/files/files/ county_profiles/HAQ/2018/India_HAQ_GBD2016.pdf

UNICEF, & World Health Organization. (1978). *Alma Ata Conference 1978 Primary Health Care*. Retrieved from https://www.unicef.org/media/85611/file/Alma-Ata -conference-1978-report.pdf

United Nations. (2015). India and the MDGs Towards a Sustainable Future for All. Retrieved from https://www.unescap.org/sites/default/files/India_and_the_MDGs _0.pdf

USAID. (2012). *The Health System Assessment Approach: A How to Manual Version 2.0*. Retrieved from https://www.hfgproject.org/wp-content/uploads/2015/02/ HSAA_Manual_Version_2_Sept_20121.pdf

World Health Organization. (2000). *The World Health Report 2000 Health Systems: Improving Performance*. Geneva. Retrieved from https://apps.who.int/iris/ bitstream/handle/10665/42281/WHR_2000-eng.pdf?sequence=1&isAllowed=y

World Health Organization. (2003). Millennium Development Goals the Health Indicators: Scope, Definition and Measurement Methods. Geneva. Retrieved from http://www3.who.int/whosis/menu.cfmMeasles

World Health Organization. (2014). Health Systems Governance for Universal Health Coverage Action Plan. Geneva. Retrieved from https://apps.who.int/iris/ bitstream/handle/10665/341159/WHO-HSS-HSF-2014.01-eng.pdf?sequence=1 &isAllowed=y

World Health Organization. (2020). *Constitution of World Health Organization 1946*. Geneva. Retrieved from https://apps.who.int/gb/bd/pdf_files/BD_49th-en.pdf

World Health Organization, & World Bank. (2017). *Tracking Universal Health Coverage: 2017 Global Monitoring Report*. Retrieved from https://apps.who.int/ iris/bitstream/handle/10665/259817/9789241513555-eng.pdf

News paper

Economics Times. (13th June, 2018). Health Spending Pushed 55 Million into Poverty in a Year: Study. Retrieved January 2019, from https://economictimes.indiatimes .com/news/politics-and-nation/health-spending-pushed-55-million-into-poverty-in -a-year-study/articleshow/64568199.cms?from=mdr

Porecha, M. (2016, December 05). Bihar Spends Lowest, HP Highest on Healthcare. Retrieved August 21, 2018, from http://www.dnaindia.com/health/report-bihar -spends-lowest-hp-highest-on-healthcare-2279699

The Guardian. (14th December, 2017). Almost 100 Million People a Year 'Forced to Choose Between Food and Healthcare'. Retrieved January 2019, from https:// www.theguardian.com/global-development/2017/dec/14/almost-100-million -people-a-year-choose-food-healthcare-extreme-poverty

The New Indian Express. (14th December, 2017). Over Half the People Pushed into Poverty Worldwide Due to Healthcare Expenses Are from India: WHO Report. Retrieved January 2019, from http://www.newindianexpress.com/nation/2017 /dec/14/over-half-the-people-pushed-into-poverty-worldwide-due-to-healthcare -expenses-are-from-india-who-re-1727419.html

Times of India. (13th June, 2018). Health Spending Pushed 55 Million Indians into Poverty in a Year: Study. Retrieved January 2019, from https://timesofindia .indiatimes.com/india/health-spending-pushed-55-million-indians-into-poverty-in -a-year-study/articleshow/64564548.cms

Websites

http://nrhmrajasthan.nic.in/
http://rchiips.org/nfhs/

http://rchiips.org/nfhs/factsheet_NFHS-5.shtml
http://rchiips.org/nfhs/pub_nfhs-2.shtml
http://statehealthsocietybihar.org/
http://up-health.in/en/
http://www.cghealth.nic.in/cghealth17/
http://www.nrhmorissa.gov.in/
http://www.udyogmitrabihar.in/priority-sectors/healthcare/
http://www.udyogmitrabihar.in/priority-sectors/healthcare/
https://health.mp.gov.in/en
https://health.odisha.gov.in/
https://health.uk.gov.in/
https://health.uk.gov.in/pages/display/114-nrhm---national-rural-health-mission -
https://jrhms.jharkhand.gov.in/
https://nhm.gov.in/
https://pmjay.gov.in/resources/publication
https://rajswasthya.nic.in/Index-2.htm
https://state.bihar.gov.in/health/CitizenHome.html
https://upnrhm.gov.in
https://www.jharkhand.gov.in/health
https://www.mohfw.gov.in
https://www.nhmmp.gov.in
https://www.niti.gov.in/verticals/health-and-family-welfare

Emerging Concerns and a Way Forward

Sandhya R. Mahapatro

Health and nutrition well-being of the population plays an important role in shaping the demography and human capital of a nation. Ending preventable maternal and child death thus is one of the global agenda. Over the past decade socioeconomic development and introduction of health care interventions leading to progress in maternal and child health and nutrition. India has made significant strides in maternal and child health after implementation of National Health Mission in 2005. The extent to which the country has succeeded in meeting health care challenges are reflected in health indicators. Although the countries' progress in maternal and child health, is considerable, regional variations have been observed. The issue of maternal and child health and nutrition is of special interest to focus on empowered action group (EAG) states as these states achieved little from an MDG perspective, lag behind many other states and are far from SDG targets. with the concerted efforts of government progress in MCH indicators is occurring, however, is certainly not adequate and leaves much to be desired. Despite numerous interventions and plans, the burden of maternal and child mortality is disproportionately higher in these states. For instance, the recent Sample Registration System (SRS) data (2081–20) shows that maternal mortality ratio (MMR) has been declining in India and is below 100 (97). However, MMR in EAG states and Assam is 137; while the southern states recorded 49, it is 76 for the rest of the states. Why there is still discussion on the health and nutrition of women and children in the EAG states, why are these states lagging behind other states? What attributes for these does the cultural values behaviour and attitude of Individual intersecting with structural conditions in the environment resulted in poor health outcomes? or is it due to the fragmented attention of government with a lack of appropriate initiatives to scale up services? This calls for a critical understanding of maternal and child health and nutrition from a regional perspective.

This edited volume delves into the areas that cause poor health and nutrition of women and children, analyses the performance of health systems and discusses the way-outs for progress to continue the existing ones or the innovative strategies to be adopted to improve maternal and child health (MCH) indicators in India, especially in EAG states. The chapters in this volume cover a range of perspectives on maternal and child health such as

DOI: 10.4324/9781003430636-21

the regional pattern and their progress over time, the social determinants, the inhibitors or enablers to access to health and nutritional services and policy gaps. The importance of the sociodemographic, economic determinants and characteristics of communities – in determining health and nutrition status and the role of public policies, flagship programmes that can help reduce the burden of poor health in these low-performing states have been discussed. This concluding section discusses the major observations and suggestive measures drawn from the preceding chapters.

Except for Uttar Pradesh, Bihar and Jharkhand, all other EAG states have reached replacement-level fertility. Increasing utilization of maternal and child health services and family planning measures would help in reaching SDG targets on maternal and child health. With the programmatic interventions, nutritional indicators such as stunting, wasting and underweight gradually are declining; however, anaemia rate is still a challenge in these states. The utilization of services among the poor and marginalized provided under Integrated Child Development Services (ICDS) is better in states like Odisha, whereas Bihar's performance is worst among EAG states. Improvement in the functioning of the scheme and its proper monitoring is thus required for its better utilization. The increasing facility delivery though tremendous across the EAG states, may not alone result in improved health outcomes. The emphasis on postnatal care is important as the use of post natal care (PNC) services is one of the most neglected components of maternal health that results in maternal health deprivation. Labour migration is one of the common features in most of the EAG states. It has been observed that migrants' children in left-behind families had a higher risk of stunting and being underweight. The mechanisms that are attributing to poor nutrition among migrant children needs more exploration. Moreover, substantial effort is needed to improve continuum of care which is severely lacking in these states.

To overcome the barriers to service utilization, the government has rolled out various interventions under National Health Mission with an aim to provide health and nutritional services in the continuum. Despite various redistributive policies, the evidences drawn from the chapters suggest healthcare services are pro-rich, and though the health needs are high, the lower socioeconomic group may not access healthcare in the same way as the better-off group. Although government schemes were launched to provide egalitarian access to health care overcoming the economic constraints, financial hardship is still found to be the major access barrier. Increasing healthcare costs accompanied by the rise of the private sector and systemic inefficiencies of health programmes made healthcare services unaffordable for the poor. The inequities in healthcare services also arise due to reasons beyond the economic one. Discrimination in the provision of service delivery in a way increases the unmet need for healthcare services. The interventions that aim to provide food and nutritional security to vulnerable households should be more specific, focused and more inclusive. An intersectional approach to understanding the dynamics of health inequalities is desirable to identify the more vulnerable group and design interventions accordingly.

It is well established that the health sector development is critical for the socioeconomic development of a region. Although there is an extensive system of health delivery, it is dysfunctional in many ways, mostly lacking infrastructure in these states. Undoubtedly, significant improvements have been made to build infrastructure after the launch of NRHM in 2005, but there is still a lot of scope for its progress. One of the chapter findings highlights that, during the transitional period of MDG to SDG, inadequacy in infrastructure was found more in Bihar, Uttar Pradesh, and Jharkhand as compared to other EAG states. Although the percentage of health expenditure is increasing, these states rank lower in per capita health expenditure. Along with imbalances in the allocation of resources, inadequate public expenditure restricts the capacity of the state to provide quality health services. These pose a major challenge in the effective implementation of strategies. Such institutional loopholes led to poor performance of health indicators in some of the EAG states. The National Health Policy 2017 envisaged health budget of the country should be 2.5% to 3% of Gross Domestic Product (GDP), and Indian Economic Survey 2020–21 also recommended for this target. Of course, in the COVID situation, at least the allocation should increase up to 5% of GDP. The Indian government, however, had spent 2.1% of GDP in the financial year 2021–22[1] which is estimated to increase to 2.5% by 2025. This is much lower than the minimum expenditure required specifically in the COVID era and far from the target. Although out-of-pocket expenditure is declining, to make health system more resilient and cater to the needy, government must ensure enhancing the allocation of healthcare resources both physical and financial. It is thus pertinent to address the systemic inefficiencies of health system that encourage the privatization of healthcare services, make health expenditure catastrophic, and accentuate poverty and health inequality.

The continuous increased attention and interventions by government, international bodies and civil societies have resulted in a decline in mortality rates and undernutrition. This underscores the potential contribution of government and development agencies in addressing the barriers to maternal and child health services. With a view to bringing about a breakthrough in poor healthcare, community-based interventions were introduced for behavioural change and upscaling utilization of services, and financing schemes were launched to reduce the cost of services. The conditional cash transfer schemes to a fair extent improve the health and nutrition of the poor; however, they should be reached to the unreached to reduce inequalities and impoverishment. A study finding from Bihar shows the poorest belonging to the marginalized class were the least advantaged in accessing the benefits of Janani Evam Baal Suraksha Yojana (BSY), and there is thus a need to revisit the distribution mechanisms of cash incentives that could not reach the marginalized and the lower class (Mahapatro, 2022).

In India, Maternal and Child healthcare was prioritised in seventh five year plan, however was not given sufficient attention. The agenda of MCH was reiterated in the International Conference on Population and Development (ICPD) held in Cairo (1994) where India was also a signatory. Since then, major initiatives have been taken for strengthening the health system and upscaling the MCH services across the states. Despite these attempts, policy gaps still persist and MCH issue is unacceptably emerging as a challenge. Currently, we are in the mid-period of Millennium Development Goals (MDGs) and Sustainable Development Goals (SDGs) and only a few years are left to achieve the targets of SDGs. The renewed commitment to reduce mortality rates under SDG era underscore exploring the complex intersections of sociocultural, behavioural attributes and institutional bottlenecks that poses challenges for universal access to maternal and child health services specifically in the EAG states in India.

In this book, it is suggested that the programmes and strategies such as male involvement in maternal care, women empowerment, and care policies to reduce unpaid work of women were the important aspects that need to be researched more for improvement in health and nutrition status. There is a need to strengthen the Information, Communication and Technology (ICT) platform and grievance redressal mechanisms to overcome the implementation challenges of the interventions. The reduction in inequalities in MCH care utilization requires more deliberate effort by the government such as policy measures to address the demand side barriers alongside political will and good governance. Unless the political economy of the healthcare system of these states is addressed systematically, it may be difficult to develop the appropriate roadmap. The suggestions as presented in the book provide a roadmap for action that can be pursued to improve the health, nutrition and well-being of women and children in such states. Moreover, more micro-level inquiries and location-specific actions are required to develop strategies that help in achieving the SDGs targets in maternal and child health and nutrition in these states.

Note

1 https://swachhindia.ndtv.com/budget-2022-a-macro-view-of-the-money-allo-cated-to-healthcare-sector-66568/

Reference

Mahapatro, S.R. (2022). *Towards Newborn Survival: Challenges and Priorities.* Palgrave Macmillian (Imprint), -Springer Publication.

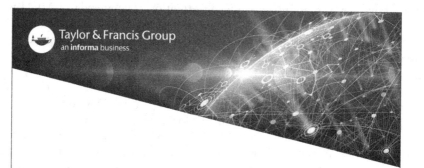

.

Printed in the United States
by Baker & Taylor Publisher Services